defying age

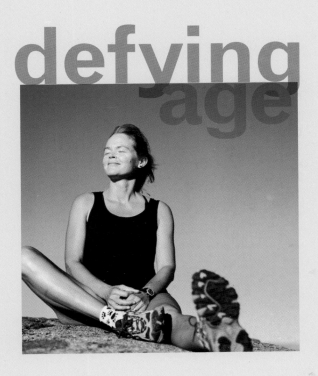

Dr. miriam stoppard

defying age

how to think, act, & stay young

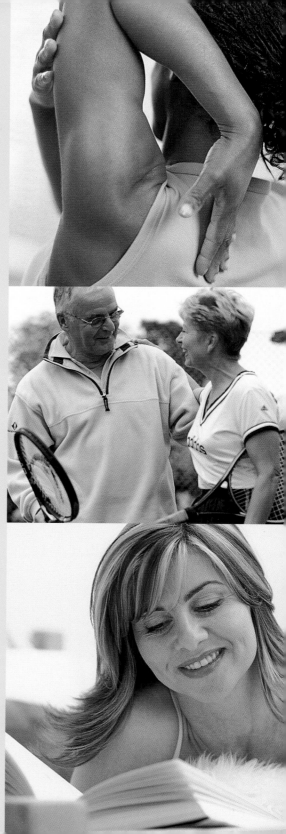

LONDON, NEW YORK, MUNICH,
MELBOURNE, DELHI

Designer **Kathryn Gammon**
Editor **Jinny Johnson**

Brand Manager for Dr. Miriam Stoppard
Lynne Brown
Senior Designer and Art Direction on
Photography **Rosamund Saunders**
Senior Editors
Peter Jones, Jennifer Williams
US Medical Consultant
Michael L. Malone, M.D.
Americanizers
Jane Perlmutter, John Searcy
DTP Designer **Karen Constanti**
Production Controller **Mandy Inness**
Production Manager **Lauren Britton**
Jacket Editor **Caroline Reed**
Jacket Designer **Nicola Powling**

First American Edition, 2004
00 01 02 03 04 05 10 9 8 7 6 5 4 3 2 1

Published in the United States by
DK Publishing, Inc., 375 Hudson Street,
New York, New York 10014

First published in Great Britain in 2003
by Dorling Kindersley Limited,
80 Strand, London WC2R 0RL

A Cataloging-in-Publication record of this book is
available from the Library of Congress
ISBN 0 7894 9691 7
ISBN 0 7566 1784 7 (Paperback)

Reproduced by GRB, Italy
Printed and bound by Tien Wah Press, Singapore

Discover more at

www.dk.com

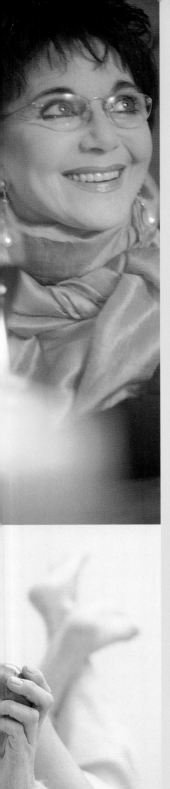

CONTENTS

FOREWORD
by Robert N. Butler, M.D.

It could be argued that life is a game of chance: We can't choose our
parents, which means we don't get to choose our genes. We don't
control our early environment, so we can't avoid exposure to infections
and toxins. On the other hand, life still gives us enormous
opportunities for choice. For example, we now live longer without
falling prey to acute diseases than at any other time in recorded history,
giving us the opportunity to maximize our potential as healthy, vital
individuals and to minimize or even eliminate factors that might keep
us from reaching our full potential as we grown older.

There are many ways to address the challenges of our later years and
still be attentive to both health and attractiveness. But in order for us to
meet the challenges and take advantage of opportunities available to us
in our later years we need information.

Within these user-friendly and beautifully illustrated pages, *Defying Age*
informs us of the directions that our lives can take and the choices
we can make. Dr. Miriam Stoppard's voice is knowledgeable, empathic,
and empowering.

From health promotion and disease prevention to personal learning
styles, Dr. Stoppard is an informative guide to everything one needs to
know to remain healthy and energetic into old age. She encourages us
to embark on a lifestyle that promotes growth and life-enhancing
experiences, which in the long run may be the best legacy we have to
give our children and the generations that follow.

Robert N. Butler, M.D.,
International Longevity Cente – USA
Professor of Geriatrics, Mount Sinai Medical Center, New York,
Founding Director, National Institute on Aging

miriam's INTRODUCTION

The other day I was thinking about that classic Frank Sinatra song **It Was a Very Good Year**. The singer is an old man looking back on his youthful years, his best years, the very good years.

Spine-tingling though it is, it's an old-fashioned view of our middle years and the last quarter of our lives. This isn't a time for pining about lost vigor or reverberating about old conquests – professional, personal, and romantic. EVERY year can be a **very good year** – this book tells you how.

Nowadays we're still full of spirit and promise. There are new vistas open to us, fresh fields to conquer and many more years of life to be lived to the fullest. We have spending power, wisdom, experience and we know who we are. The scene is set to enjoy life as never before. And we can, with a little planning, a little effort, a little knowledge, and a little common sense. I've tried in this book to give you some suggestions about planning and some pointers as to where you should

"the scene is set to enjoy life as never before"

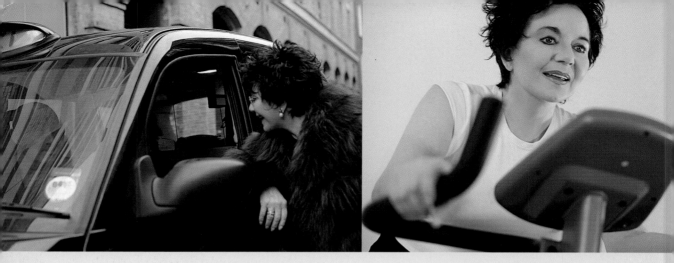

apply effort to stretch your life beyond your given quotient. And that is in your power, believe me.

years of life and fitness

Granted, some aspects of health require long-range planning to be free of illnesses that make us old. I'm thinking here specifically of warding off osteoporosis, or brittle bones, which, without a modicum of planning, will affect almost all women after menopause and men too in their seventies and eighties. If you're reading this book in your fifties, it's too late for the long-range planning: to preempt osteoporosis you have to maximize peak bone mass with weight bearing exercise *before* you reach 35.

But it's not too late to keep your bones healthy and strong. All you need to do is spend an hour a day on your feet - walking, gardening, dancing, doing t'ai chi or housework. Women who do this once a week have less osteoporosis than women who don't exercise at all, women who exercise twice a week have less than women who exercise only once a week, and so on. It's the same for most diseases we associate with age — very small changes in lifestyle can protect against high blood pressure, heart disease, strokes, Alzheimer's, diabetes, and cancers.

For we're not programmed to die. There's no "death" gene. We age and fade away by default. We're killed softly and slowly by the erosion of our genetic blueprint, DNA, which suffers thousands of assaults from internal and external forces daily. We can protect our DNA from some of those "hits," internally with power foods and a diet rich in unrefined carbohydrates and externally by avoiding smoking, sun, and pollution.

aging isn't inevitable

We know that aging isn't inevitable. We all have friends with more optimism and zest for life than people half their age. What are their secrets? Well, they're all explained in the pages that follow. And I have to add that they wouldn't be as well explained without the generous help I've had from my colleague, Professor Tom Kirkwood.

For me, the style of this book is as important as the content. I've worked hard with my editorial and design teams at DK to achieve exactly the same feel I'd want to give a book for 20- and 30-year-olds. Because that's how we can all feel — youthful, optimistic, and energized — not just in our twenties and thirties, but in our sixties, seventies, eighties, and beyond.

Enjoy your extra years of life!

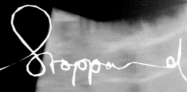

"we can all feel youthful, optimistic, and energized"

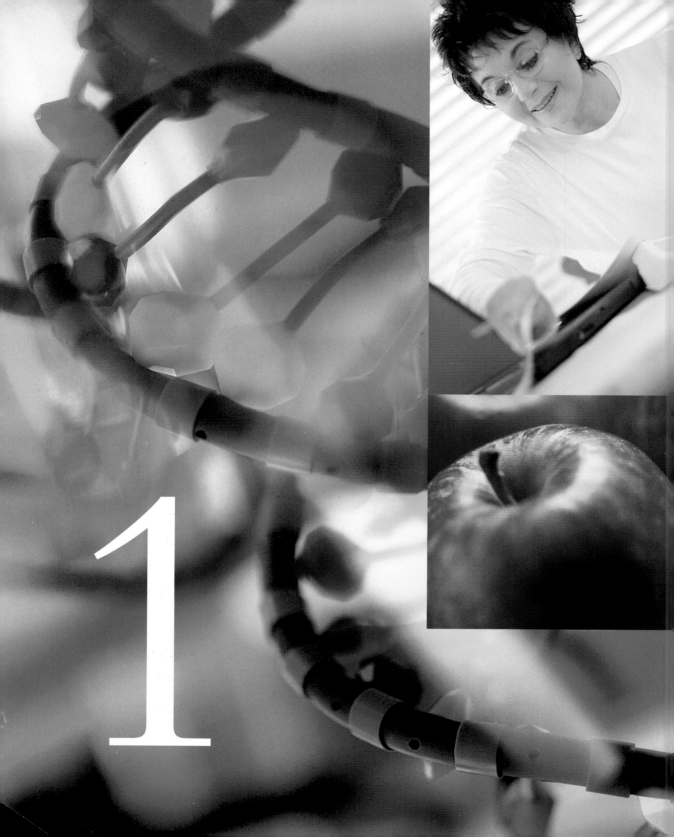

1

HOW WE NEED
NOT AGE

While we know of no pill or injection that can slow down aging, **there's no need to be downhearted.** And although the prospects may be not too bright for extending human life span much beyond 100, we can all *increase our odds* of living to that age. We have so many tools and tricks at our disposal to defy age that I hardly know where to begin. *Most are simple and require little effort: gentle daily exercise –* gardening will do – **an optimistic attitude to life,** eating delicious *antioxidant-rich foods*, leading an active social life, protecting yourself from sunlight and cigarette smoke. These small adjustments make extra years a bargain for the price. **It's within your power to live longer.**

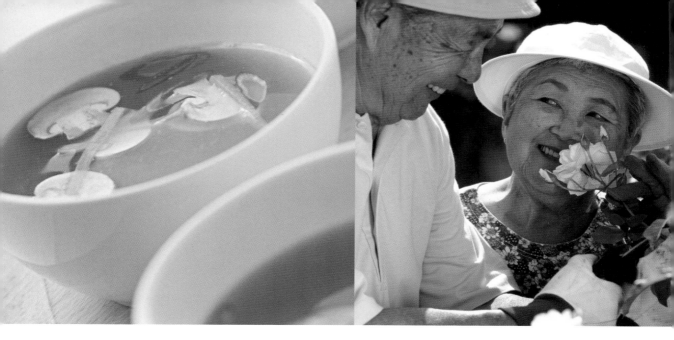

CAN WE *defy* AGE?

THERE'S PROBABLY NO SINGLE MECHANISM TO AGING. IN FACT, ONE SCIENTIST LISTED NEARLY 300 DIFFERENT THEORIES. IT FOLLOWS THAT THERE CAN BE NO SINGLE GENE RESPONSIBLE FOR AGING.

In fact we have NO death genes. **Aging is NOT inevitable**. We are NOT programmed to die. The conclusion is that we can do a lot to determine the time we die. We can lengthen or shorten our lives by how we live.

That's because longevity lies more in your hands than it does your genes. **You're in the driver's seat** when it comes to setting the limit on your own mortality.

Yes, a particular anti-aging feature on chromosome 4 is more common in people who live to 100, or more, years. It turns out, however, that it's hardly crucial, because half the people who live to 100 don't carry it. Genes account for no more than a quarter of any

difference in life span between two people. This means that someone who dies at 100 rather than 80 can thank their lifestyle for 15 of the extra years and their genes for just five.

the Okinawan lifestyle

But if lifestyle is so important, what's the best lifestyle? We can learn much from looking at the **Okinawan** people, who live on a chain of islands stretching from Japan to Taiwan. The 1.3 million inhabitants have the **longest life expectancy** on the planet, with four times as many centenarians as Western countries, and their lifestyle holds many clues to long life. People in Okinawa still show signs of age of

MAGIC INGREDIENTS IN THE OKINAWAN LIFESTYLE

Reference: *The Okinawa Way*, Bradley Willcox, D. Craig Willcox, Makato Suzuki

- ◆ **Okinawans don't drink alcohol or smoke.**
- ◆ **Okinawans eat little meat.** Three-quarters of their food comes from plants, with a lot of fruit, vegetables, and fiber. We're encouraged to eat five portions of fruit and vegetables a day – with rice and bean sprouts they eat well over ten. **They eat very little fat and refined sugars**.
- ◆ **They practice a cultural habit called** *hara hachi bu* – they stop eating at the very first hint of fullness. This means they eat 20 percent less food than we do or 400–500 fewer calories per day.
- ◆ **Most Okinawans aren't sedentary.** They dance, walk, do gardening, or engage in gentle martial arts.
- ◆ **Okinawans don't turn to alcohol** or antidepressants. To combat stress and anxiety they meditate and lean on the strong family and community support they've evolved.
- ◆ **It's difficult to prove,** but studies suggest that optimists tend to outlive pessimists and religious types outlive atheists. The spiritual life promotes long life, but then so does a willful, cantankerous frame of mind.

course, but they're better at curtailing the classic life-threatening symptoms of old age. So, for instance, **heart problems and strokes are virtually unknown** and hormone-linked cancers are much rarer than in the West.

The reason we know that genes aren't so crucial is that Okinawans who migrate to the West and take up the Western lifestyle lose their knack for living a long time.

youth's arch enemy

One explanation for aging is the free radical theory first outlined by Dr. Denham Harman in the 1950s. **Free radicals** are simply molecules of oxygen which have lost an electron in a chemical reaction. Free radicals form in all cells of the body. They're extremely unstable and are aggressively searching for an electron to make them whole again. When they raid other molecules for electrons they create more free radicals. And they'll steal electrons from anything – fats, proteins, and especially from DNA, our

genetic blueprint. The interest to us is that the theory says **that free radical damage ages cells.**

free radical damage = aging

Free radicals are the toxic waste of normal body functions like breathing or digesting food and they're deadly. Every time a free radical satiates itself by stealing an electron it damages healthy cells. Free radicals are also **generated by the external environment**: sunlight and cigarette smoke speed up the generation of free radicals inside our cells and they're capable of damaging every single component of a cell including DNA. Whenever a free radical steals an electron from a DNA molecule, the DNA takes a "hit." In any one day DNA may take 10,000 hits and it's the **resultant accumulated damage** that's thought to cause aging.

Free radicals also attack fats in cell membranes and some scientists believe that **age-related diseases** such as Alzheimer's and arthritis are due to this particular kind of free radical damage.

the role of oxygen in our cells

Without oxygen we wouldn't live very long so it's hard to think of it as a poison, but it is. Oxygen poisons by oxidizing, which is what makes a fire burn, a knife get rusty, butter go rancid, and an apple turn brown. **The energy we depend on for life** is released when oxygen "burns" inside our cells – think of the heat that comes off a fire.

Out of every 100 oxygen molecules that we breathe in, two or three are siphoned off to become **free radicals.** Free radicals aren't all bad – they're part of the weapons our **immune system** uses to kill invaders – but they inflict wholesale damage and it's indiscriminate. You could say that free radicals are like wild animals rampaging around our bodies.

So, we have the theory that **aging is the result of free radical damage** inside our cells, most importantly to DNA. This made scientists think that accumulated damage then led to faulty DNA which, if not repaired, could lead to disease and cancer.

our amazing DNA repair system

Happily, DNA is reproducing itself all the time with incredible accuracy. A mistake is made in only about one in a billion sequences. Imagine copying out all 20 volumes of the Encyclopedia Britannica with no more than a few wrong letters and you'll get some idea of how meticulously our DNA copying enzymes check for errors. DNA copying enzymes constantly scan the new DNA and when they spot an error

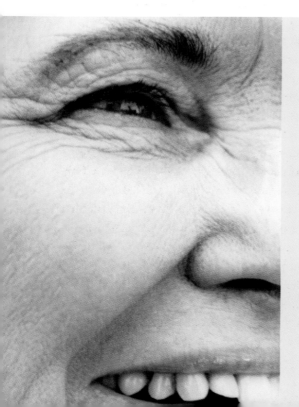

A WINDOW on your body

One effect of free radicals is on collagen in the skin. A stretchy protein, **collagen** gives your skin its **youthful suppleness, elasticity, and tautness,** but chemically speaking it's an easy target for free radicals. Over the years, free radical attack on collagen changes its structure. Normally, collagen molecules are arranged in parallel bundles, which slide over one another, and this gives the skin its plumpness and recoil. But free radicals stiffen the chemical cross-linkages between bundles, making the collagen stiff and inelastic. The skin begins to look "old."

In addition to our own homegrown free radicals, sunlight liberates more free radicals and increases the onslaught on collagen from outside. Whenever the sun is shining, your skin is absorbing sunlight and free radicals are being activated. Sunlight also triggers an enzyme that destroys the fat in skin cells, liberating a chemical called arachidonic acid involved in inflammation. This further accelerates skin aging.

they fall on the incorrect sequence, slice it out, and splice in the correct one. In spite of this formidable **DNA repair kit** our DNA gets more and more tattered as we go through life. Scars accumulate and gene malfunctions form. As a result, genes that should be turned on are turned off and vice versa. **This, in a nutshell, is what causes aging and age-related diseases.**

how the body defends itself against free radicals

With all this free radical bombardment from inside and out you might ask how our cells survive at all. The reason most of us enjoy long healthy lives is that the body has developed its **own unique defense system for fighting free radicals.** This defense system is powered by antioxidants. Our own bodies manufacture far more potent antioxidants than anything you can find in a health food store – vitamin pill or food. Simply put, they prevent damage by donating to free radicals the electron they're searching for. So **our own antioxidants work by rendering free radicals harmless.**

Once a free radical joins an antioxidant, it's stable. It no longer scavenges electrons from cellular components and damages them. With as many as 10,000 hits per day by free radicals to its DNA, every cell would be decimated if it weren't for our DNA repair systems and **our homegrown army of antioxidant defenses.** The big guns are **antioxidant enzymes** made in the cells themselves, the chief being superoxide dismutase, catalase, and glutathione peroxidase, which are helped by vitamins, especially vitamins C and E.

How do **WRINKLES** form?

Inside your skin cells the damage from free radicals activates messenger chemicals that tell DNA to turn on inflammation. Each time this happens, the inflammation leaves behind a tiny scar and when these scars join together you have a wrinkle. This is one of the reasons why sunshine, particularly tanning, leads to wrinkled skin.

antioxidant burn out

If we can produce these super antioxidants that neutralize free radicals, **why do we still age?** Well, normally we can keep pace with the production of free radicals as long as the system isn't overwhelmed, but under certain circumstances our own antioxidants get overpowered. The onslaught from internal free radicals caused by infections, illness, accidents, surgery, plus external free radicals like heavy smoking, exposing our skin to bright sunlight, and so on means the body can't keep pace. This blitz on our antioxidant reserves is called **oxidative stress.** If we could minimize oxidative stress, or at least slow it down, we might have a way to prevent age-related damage to our cells and organs.

But BEWARE! Loading up on antioxidants by popping vitamin pills and supplements is far from the complete answer to halting aging, and has failed to work in animal studies.

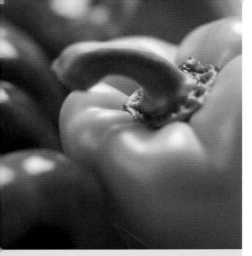

CELL *aging*

IN THE LATE 1970S, ANOTHER THEORY OF AGING EMERGED: THE MEMBRANE HYPOTHESIS OF AGING. IT PROPOSED THAT FREE RADICAL DAMAGE TO THE OUTER LAYER OF THE CELL – THE CELL MEMBRANE – WAS THE MAIN FACTOR IN CELL AGING, NOT FREE RADICAL DAMAGE TO DNA INSIDE THE CELL.

Membranes are made up of fats among which **a free radical can start a damaging chain reaction**. Once the cell membrane becomes damaged by free radicals, it's unable to let food in or to let waste out. Waste begins to accumulate, gradually taking up more and more space in the cell. As a result the cell's water is squeezed out and the cell becomes dehydrated. **It's the cell's inability to hold on to water that could be at the root of cell aging**.

The antioxidant vitamin E can quench the spread of the chain reaction, hence its importance in our diet. **Repair of the cell membrane with our own antioxidants,** helped possibly by vitamin E, could **increase the ability of cells to retain water and resist aging**. This is one of the reasons why you'll see vitamin E quoted as an anti-aging vitamin.

a particular marker for aging – homocysteine

In 1993 Dr. Bruce Ames, an American biochemistry professor, pulled these various strands together. In his research he stated that the accumulation of DNA damage with age is a **major contributor to aging** and to the diseases associated with aging including cancer, heart disease, and brain diseases such as Parkinson's disease and Alzheimer's, as well as the failure of intellectual powers that we know as senility.

Dr. Ames went on to propose that this DNA damage could be partially blocked **by eating the right antioxidant foods,** thus slowing down deterioration in numerous ways.

How to boost your own **ANTIOXIDANT POWER**

Useful antioxidants are found in our food: **vitamins C and E** and **beta-carotene**, the yellow/orange pigment in carrots, apricots, and any yellow/orange fruit or vegetable. When a molecule of vitamin C meets a free radical it becomes oxidized, rendering the free radical harmless. The oxidized vitamin C molecule reverts to its original state by an enzyme called **vitamin C reductase**.

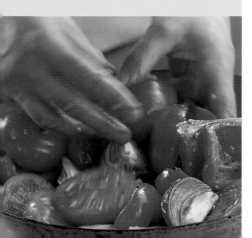

reducing levels of homocysteine

For instance, as we get older we produce more of a substance called **homocysteine**, levels of which can be measured in the blood. Homocysteine makes the blood clot more easily and is thought to be a factor leading to heart attacks. Indeed, many heart attack patients have high levels of homocysteine while they have normal levels of cholesterol. Certain foods containing **folic acid**, like green leafy vegetables, **quickly reduce homocysteine levels** and so modify the "aging factor" of homocysteine and the threat of heart disease.

RENEWABLE *cells*

THE HUMAN BODY HAS AN AMAZING ABILITY TO RENEW ITSELF AND NEW CELLS ARE GROWING TO REPLACE OLD ONES ALL THE TIME, DAY AND NIGHT.

Certain tissues can repair themselves better than others. Bone marrow, for instance, produces **new crops of red blood cells continuously** in order to keep pace with the shelf life of a blood cell, which is less than a month. If our bone marrow didn't replace these dead red blood cells, we'd be anemic in no time. Similarly, the lining of the intestine is **constantly renewed** so that the absorption of foodstuffs remains efficient. However, **as we get older this cell renewal process slows down** and in old age the absorption of nutrients is **much less efficient** than it was in youth.

The skin is the most obvious organ in the body where we can actually watch replenishment going on. **Our skin is literally replaced every 12 months or so.** Cells in the lower layer of the skin, the dermis, divide to form a new layer of skin which migrates to the surface as though on a conveyor belt. The same process renews collagen and elastic fibers, **keeping the surface of the skin smooth for many years,** particularly if it isn't subjected to the harmful effects of sunlight.

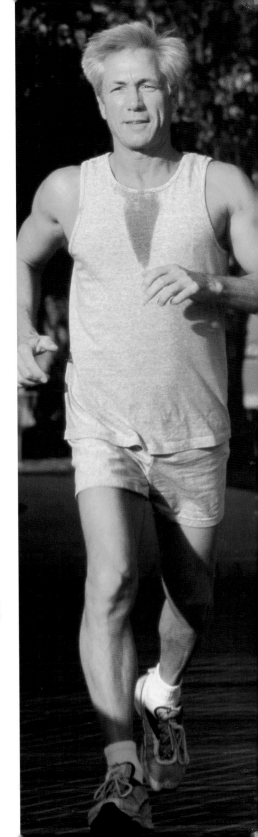

can cells last forever?

So why can't this process of renewal and repair continue forever? The answer's rather surprising: we have a built-in limit in our talent for producing new cells, after which we lose the knack. No cell can keep going indefinitely. The cutoff point is called the **Hayflick Limit,** after Dr. Leonard Hayflick, who first discovered it. **A cell can only renew itself a limited number of times,** somewhere between 40 and 50 it turns out, and after that even the most vigorous cell stops replacing itself. When this happens in the skin, the changes are only too obvious. The face literally drops, with wrinkles, sagging, and dewlaps.

why do cells stop multiplying?

But what makes cells multiply a given number of times and then stop? We know it isn't because cells are programmed to stop; aging isn't programmed into our cells and organs. It's attractive to think that the limit has some useful purpose, to protect us perhaps against unchecked cell renewal – cancer. So as we get older, accumulated damage triggers a mechanism that stops cells from dividing and intervenes before cancer can develop.

decline isn't inevitable

That sounds pretty serious doesn't it? And it suggests that a decline in vigor and strength is inevitable – but it isn't. First of all, we rarely push an organ to its limits. For most of our lives we're unaware of the reserve we have in our bodies to do more if an emergency strikes. **Indeed the capacity of our vital organs is far beyond our everyday needs** and even when we lose capacity there's sufficient slack to keep us going for many decades. For instance, the coronary arteries can be three-quarters blocked before symptoms appear.

changing capacity

What we may notice as we get into our sixties and seventies is that our **excess capacity gets less and less**. So when we're called upon to push the body, we're forced to **draw on our reserves** earlier and earlier.

One of the most prominent signs of getting older is that we lose the physical tolerance we had in youth. At 20 we might have been able to play three vigorous sets of tennis, only rarely getting out of breath or feeling tired. **At 60 we still may be able to play three vigorous sets of tennis,** but we need a

"eat less and

warm-up period to take the body **gradually to its reserve capacity**. I notice the older I get, the longer the warm-up period I need. The body also needs to cool down so that exertion doesn't result in aches, pains, and stiffness — something that never occurred in our twenties and thirties.

SIGNS OF GETTING OLDER

- Being less **active**
- **Increase** in weight (including middle-age spread)
- Less **stamina**
- Aches and pains
- Fatigue
- Inability to sleep
- Loss of **memory** and impaired intellectual function
- Loss of **get-up-and-go**
- Declining **sex** drive

could we live longer by simply eating less?

It is within your power to raise the odds substantially on extending your life. It's very simple: **you eat less**. We've known for some time that **restricting calories extends life span**. Putting animals on a near-starvation diet makes them live up to 50 percent longer than normal. Now we know the same rule applies to primates. **On a low-calorie diet:**

- the body temperature drops
- insulin levels drop
- levels of the steroid hormone DHEA stop declining.

In an ongoing study on aging that has been carried out for more than 40 years in Baltimore, men with lower body temperature, lower insulin levels, and higher levels of DHEA tend to live longer. And the Okinawans, who eat 25–30 percent fewer calories than we do, exhibit the same three markers for longevity and also live to a ripe old age. **Could we all perhaps get closer to those three golden markers by restricting our calories?** It's worth thinking about. (For more details on this, see page 34.)

live longer"

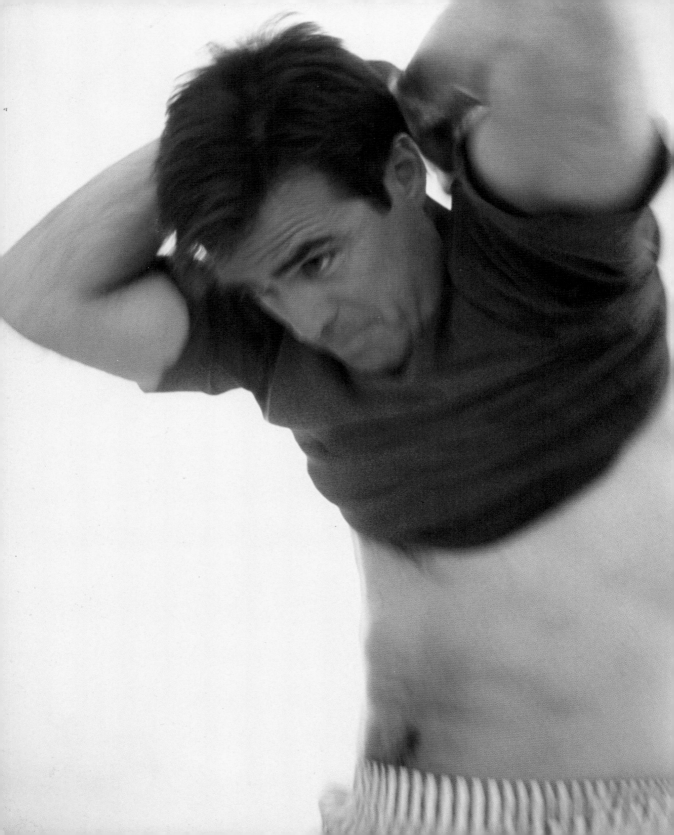

CELL*repair*

CONSISTENT AND MODERATE EXERCISE, SAY 30 MINUTES EVERY DAY, RESULTS IN THE REGULAR FLOW OF LITERALLY THOUSANDS OF HORMONES THAT HAVE BOTH AN IMMEDIATE AND A LONG-TERM EFFECT ON CELL REPAIR.

Endorphins – **our natural painkillers** – are an example of hormones with an immediate effect. Closely related to opium, **they don't only give us an immediate postexercise high but one that may last for eight hours**.

Other hormones act as growth factors and stimulate cells to repair and replenish themselves. They too exert their effect in the short and the long term. **The immediate pulse of these hormones spreads like a tonic to every cell in the body,** increasing efficiency and productivity. Research has shown that some of these growth factors promote the growth of new cells, healing defects and renewing our powers.

exercise and brain cells

Most recently it's been shown that exercise releases a growth hormone that causes **new cells to grow in the brain**. This is quite a revolutionary idea. In the past it was thought that brain cells couldn't repair and renew themselves, hence the devastation of a stroke. But exercise promotes neurogenesis, the growth of new brain cells. This goes some way to explaining the phenomenon that I noticed a year or so after starting a regular exercise regime. My memory was returning, but returning in a surprising way. **Not only could I remember everything better,** but I could also bring memories to the "surface" much more easily than I had been able to in the last 10 or 15 years.

Furthermore, **my cognitive functions improved to a level** I hadn't enjoyed for many years, since I was a junior doctor taking postgraduate exams.

As well as the obvious physical benefits, exercise lifts your mood, treats depression, and reduces tension and stress. I can't do without it. (See chapter 5 for more on this.)

Increase in **SEX HORMONES**

Some other exercise growth factors are much more familiar. They're the sex hormones – estrogen in women and testosterone in men. Exercise transforms DHEA in the adrenal glands to estrogen, meaning that a woman of any age can supplement her own internal production of estrogen by a session on an exercise bicycle. The growth-promoting properties of estrogen are well known, one of the most dramatic being on bone. Estrogen promotes bone health by triggering bone-building cells. Lack of estrogen allows bones to deteriorate and become brittle and prone to fractures. Osteoporosis sets in within a few years of menopause when estrogen levels fall. HRT (see page 51) provides a logical antidote.

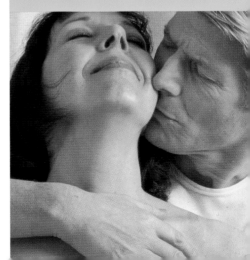

THEN WHY DO WE AGE AT ALL?

So far I've been outlining the way we age, **the how**. But what about the reasons for aging? What about **the why**? Why has evolution allowed us to age?

The latest theory of why we age hinges on the evolutionary idea that human beings are simply vehicles to pass on genes from one generation to the next. From the gene's point of view, *the rest of our body is totally disposable.* The old name for the body is the *soma* and the theory of aging propounded by Professor Tom Kirkwood, gerontologist from the University of Newcastle, is called the **disposable soma theory.** It goes like this:

In order to keep our genes healthy, cell division to make the building blocks of new life (ova in women and sperm in men) must be very accurate.

To maintain this high degree of accuracy, an enormous amount of energy is needed within the cell and, given that any person has a limited amount of energy available, our selfish genes will make sure that the lion's share of energy goes into reproducing themselves.

So during fertile life, when the "disposable" cells of the body – the muscles, bones, joints, and brain – are being repaired, there's less energy left over and renewal gets sloppy. Accidents happen in the DNA of our tissues (breast, prostate, colon) and defects in cells occur.

These defects cause aging and mutations (cancer), so sooner or later the soma is going to die.

In other words, once the genes have been passed on to a future generation, the soma is no longer needed, so the body conserves energy and makes the cells of the soma in a more economical way: this, after the end of fertile life in effect, is aging. **The continuing 10,000 hits per day on DNA** and the faulty repairs of those hits are what make us grow old, though it's only in the last few generations that life expectancy has increased enough for this to matter.

so could we live forever?

Almost certainly not, because natural selection can't deal with things that go wrong late in life when we've stopped having children. What natural selection can deal with is something that harms **young** people **before** they've been able to pass on their genes to the next generation. As far as genes are concerned, mutations such as cancers and diseases of old age hardly matter. The result is that natural selection is quite good at getting rid of harmful mutations in young people and quite bad at clearing out harmful mutations in the elderly. These go unchecked and cause us to age. According to Professor Kirkwood's theory, we age

◆ **because** genes treat bodies as disposable, they invest just enough in maintenance to enable the body to reproduce itself and no more.

◆ **because** the body is designed to favor the interests of the young at the expense of the old.

◆ **because** natural selection cares nothing for harmful mutations later in life.

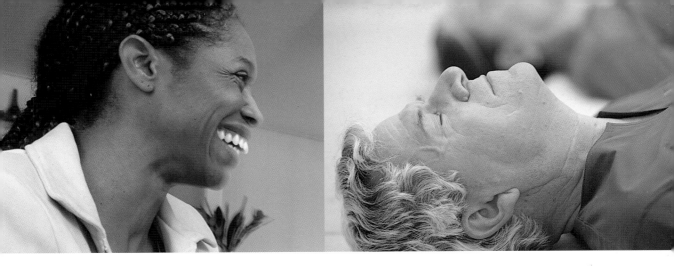

PERSONALITY *types*

THE STRESS-RESISTANT PERSONALITY LIVES LONGEST. YOU'VE PROBABLY NOTICED THAT PEOPLE WHO LIVE TO 100 ARE OFTEN STRONG-WILLED TYPES WITH YOUTHFUL, GET-UP-AND-GO ATTITUDES.

These same people score highly when it comes to self-confidence and resilience, both of which help them cope with major stressful events in their lives. These hardy individuals have an **optimistic outlook on life**, an inner sense of control, emotional stability and adaptability, and little hostility, self-consciousness, or social unease. They are rarely anxious or depressed.

Actively coping with stress or quickly getting over life's emotional setbacks seems to be very important for successful aging. **We all know people who bounce back from emotional trauma,** including poverty, war, and other hardships, with amazing resilience. These people make it their business to stay in close touch with friends and family – a known antidote to stress.

Strong social networks and close family ties are important for both physical and mental well-being. Social ties can actually strengthen the resilience of the immune system, increasing a person's resistance to disease, including cancer. Nonetheless, a fair amount of independence may be one of the reasons why the oldest folk can be active and self-supporting to a very old age.

adaptability is the key

Stress accelerates aging and it may do so by causing shrinkage of the hippocampus in the brain, the main area for memory. It's the negative responses to stress that do the harm in causing premature aging. There's convincing evidence that **adapting to stressful life events through coping contributes a lot to successful aging.** The key to this talent for adapting is simply not to perceive events as stressful. So it's important how we react to everyday modern stresses – excessive noise, traffic jams, rude people, and time constraints.

The quality of *"unflappability"* seems to be crucial and the philosophy *"if you can't do anything about it, don't worry"* is a good one

People who reach a healthy old age handle emergencies better than the average person: they react with less hostility and aggression and have learned to accept change as an inevitable part of life and not to take frustrations personally.

Accepting change is essential if we want to live to a healthy old age. People who live to 100, including holocaust survivors, those growing up in extreme poverty, or those who were orphaned and widowed at a young age, are much better than most at managing stress. Despite their loss, grief, and hardship, their coping skills and philosophical approach help them to get on with their lives.

be optimistic

Optimism is the most important personality trait to have if you wish to live a long life. A recent study on men with AIDS showed that those who were optimistic about their future lived nine months longer than those who weren't. In other words, optimism about our health may actually influence our life expectancy. **Optimism has a positive effect on the immune system too.** Men undergoing coronary bypass surgery recover more quickly if their outlook is optimistic – they walk earlier, express greater life satisfaction, and are less likely to experience a subsequent heart attack. The opposite is also true. The belief that we're powerless to influence situations – something known as learned helplessness – describes a loss of willpower that promotes stress-induced illness. **An emotionally stable, flexible personality helps us to stay healthy far into our senior years.** Strength of will and assertiveness are an added bonus.

could drugs stop us from aging?

The likelihood of our being able to take one vitamin, one magic supplement, or even a handful of both to stop aging is remote. The research team working on aging in mice, for instance, fed compounds such as vitamin E and Q10 to mice and found little effect on life span.

It's unlikely because, as Professor Kirkwood points out, no one has yet found a central clock that dictates the rate of aging of the whole body. Different organs wear out at different rates and for different reasons. Even for a single organ there are likely to be several aging processes at work. So the odds of finding one particular vitamin or drug to retard aging in all organs aren't as good as the prospects of finding interventions that work on individual organs.

And that's where genetics might help. As cells and tissues grow old, strange things happen to the thousands of genes that keep them going. Some genes simply stop giving out instructions. Others that have been silent since birth suddenly spring to life. This switching on and switching off of genes is the most fundamental part of aging. In one study a team looked at more than 6,000 genes in the muscle cells of 5-month-old and 13-month-old mice. The activity of 58 genes more than doubled in the older mice while another 55 genes were half as active.

With this knowledge **it should be possible to find drugs and perhaps nutrients to slow down the aging of individual organs.** That will help enormously in testing the value of overly hyped anti-aging potions now available.

so what can we do now to live longer?

The outlook is pretty good — we have **no** death genes and **we aren't programmed to die**.

We age primarily because our DNA and cell membranes are chemically eroded by free radicals, generated by our own metabolism and as side effects of the way we live. That means we have substantial control over how much damage those free radicals can inflict on our bodies and therefore how fast we age.

We can turn down their generation in our cells with diet — not just what we eat but how much we eat. **And we can limit much of the external damage by defining our lifestyles.**

It's never too late to change; it's never too late to start. Alterations to your lifestyle take effect immediately. Below is a brief rundown of a few useful changes to carry out, more details in the chapters to follow.

MIRIAM'S **ACTION PLAN** FOR LONGER LIFE

lower free radical damage by cutting your calorie intake. Eating fewer calories increases life span and lowers levels of free radicals in the blood. People who live to 100 have fewer free radicals in their blood at that age than 70-year-olds!

include more antioxidant foods and herbs in your diet, especially vegetables and legumes like soy (see chapter 6).

get regular, gentle exercise I'm convinced exercise — not necessarily intense — is the key to a long life. Walking and gardening are fine (see chapter 5).

cultivate positive attitudes Strong social networks and a strong spiritual life will increase your life span through a resilient immune system, a sense of well-being, and satisfaction with life (see chapter 10).

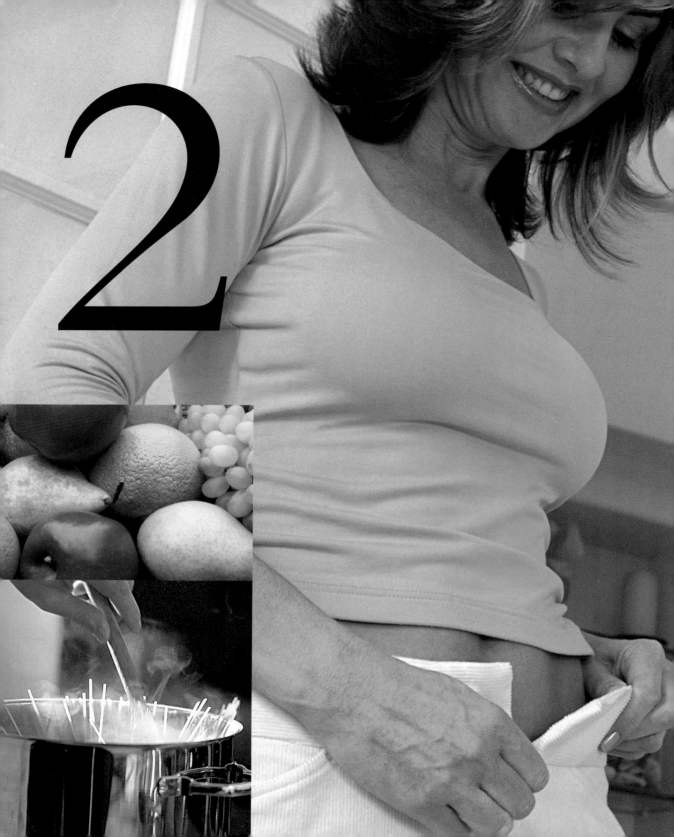

2

FAT IS OLD

It may be unpalatable to the majority of us, particularly as we watch our middle-age spread spreading, but being fat is aging. If you're fat, *you're old well before your time* and this applies in a profound sense as well as a superficial sense. First of all, you **look old**. *Leanness* (not necessarily slenderness or slimness) is a **youthful feature**. Being fat simply makes you look older than you are. What's more, if you're fat, *you move in a way that is aging* – you lack mobility, speed, and agility. You can't get out of a chair easily or run for a bus without getting out of breath. You huff and you puff whenever you have to make a physical effort.
Make no mistake, that's OLD.

CONSEQUENCES *of* OBESITY

OBESITY DAMAGES THE VITAL ORGANS. FOR ONE THING, THERE'S AN ENORMOUSLY INCREASED STRAIN ON YOUR HEART, WHICH HAS TO PUMP BLOOD AROUND THOSE EXTRA POUNDS OF WEIGHT.

More deleterious is the fact that if you're overweight, your blood pressure rises, thereby working your heart harder. The chances are you'll also have prematurely narrowed arteries and place yourself at risk for a heart attack. **Then there's your digestive system, which cannot work efficiently if you're overweight,** your overloaded joints which make you a candidate for arthritis, as well as back problems which restrict activity and curtail your enjoyment of life.

fat and diabetes

Being fat **cripples your metabolism.** The pancreas, the gland that produces **insulin**, is overworked in people who are obese largely **because eating too many calories exhausts insulin supplies.** High calorie intake results in high blood sugar, something that can only be normalized by an increased output of insulin. A pancreas that is stressed for years becomes either exhausted or unable to keep pace with the continuously high blood sugar. This is **adult or mature-onset type 2 diabetes.** Obesity in children and teenagers is epidemic so we now have "adult" type diabetes in children under ten.

We've known for some time that **simply lowering the caloric intake is sufficient to cure type 2 diabetes** in those people whose pancreas can still produce a little insulin. Calorie restriction is the only treatment required.

It's important to bring type 2 diabetes under control because **diabetes is truly aging – it shortens your life.** Untreated diabetes promotes many diseases we associate with aging, such as cataracts, kidney disease, and heart disease.

the key – insulin resistance

Not only does a high calorie intake result in obesity, it also leads to something called **insulin resistance.** Insulin has many functions, but one of its main jobs is to help cells take in sugar from the blood to use for the various body functions that need energy. As we get older our cells become less efficient at using insulin to process blood sugar – they're less sensitive to the action of insulin – they're "resistant" to it. When cells fail to absorb sugar from the blood, sugar levels rise, triggering the pancreas to pour out more insulin. You end up with not only consistently high blood sugar but also high blood insulin.

The higher the blood sugar levels soar, the more insulin your body produces and **the more resistant to insulin you become.** Insulin resistance can push you into type 2 diabetes. Worse, with high insulin levels you crave sweet food. You overeat and binge too, so you can find yourself in a vicious circle where your appetite and your weight are **beyond your control.**

Many researchers believe that high blood insulin levels have far-reaching effects on our vital organs and body chemistry.

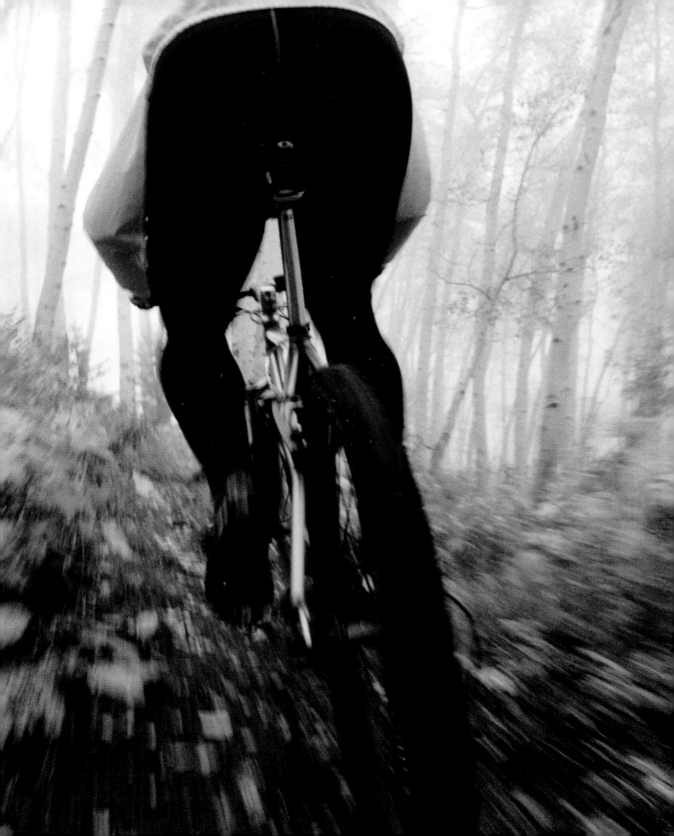

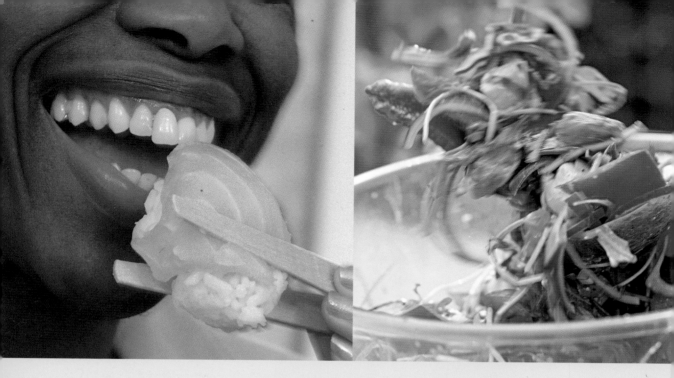

EFFECTS OF **HIGH INSULIN**

on dangerous fats Insulin raises both triglycerides and harmful LDL cholesterol (*low density lipoprotein*). LDL is the kind of cholesterol that causes narrowing of the arteries and brings with it a high risk of heart disease. People with excessive insulin due to insulin resistance tend to have the **densest type of LDL**, the type that most easily finds its way into the walls of arteries, particularly the coronary arteries. High concentration of LDL brings a **three times greater risk** of having a heart attack. Triglycerides are dangerous in themselves, but they also drive down levels of good cholesterol, HDL (*high density lipoprotein*). HDL protects the body from LDL because it helps in the transportation of LDL cholesterol to the liver for destruction.

on blood pressure Many people with high blood pressure also have high levels of insulin and, though we don't know how insulin helps to regulate blood pressure, it's possible it causes blood vessels to constrict, thereby raising pressure.

on arteries Insulin can narrow the arteries by stimulating the growth of muscle fibers in the arterial wall.

on blood clotting Insulin interferes with blood clotting, making it more likely that a clot will form. It does this by interfering with the body's protective mechanism of dissolving blood clots, keeping the blood naturally thin.

KEEP *insulin levels* DOWN

PREVENTING YOUR LEVELS OF INSULIN FROM RISING TOO HIGH
KEEPS YOUR HEART HEALTHY. HERE'S WHAT YOU CAN DO.

CONTROL YOUR WEIGHT

If you're overweight, **losing 20 percent of your weight by sensible eating and exercise could help you avoid insulin resistance**. The heavier you are and the less active you are, the more insulin resistant you're likely to be. As a rule of thumb, being 40 percent over your ideal weight suppresses the ability of your insulin to clear blood sugar by about the same amount.

WATCH YOUR SHAPE

Your tendency to develop insulin resistance – and heart disease and stroke – **increases if your weight is on the upper part of your body** – in other words, when you're **apple shaped** rather than pear shaped. Your waist measurement (rather than the waist-hip ratio) is the best indicator of this tendency – anything over 32in (81cm) in women and 37in (84cm) in men is a danger signal – **and it means you're getting fat.**

DON'T EAT SUGARY FOODS

Sugary, refined carbohydrates increase the load on your insulin system. Your blood sugar soars and your insulin rises. Don't forget that sugar is found in fruit, fruit juices, and honey, and too much of these will overload your system.

AVOID ANIMAL FAT

Insulin can raise levels of dangerous fats in the blood so it's best to eat mainly **healthy fats** – vegetable and fish oils.

EAT LITTLE AND OFTEN

After big meals your **blood sugar rockets** and your insulin with it. Insulin levels are much higher if you eat a few large meals rather than many small meals. Eating most of your calories on too few occasions leads to a yo-yoing of your blood sugar. The more **small meals** you can eat a day (say, six), the steadier your blood sugar will be and therefore the steadier your insulin levels.

SPICE OF LIFE

Cinnamon, cloves, turmeric, and bay leaves seem to **stimulate insulin efficiency** so that your body doesn't have to make as much insulin.

DRINK ALCOHOL IN MODERATION

Alcohol **stimulates insulin activity** so you need less insulin to keep your blood sugar stable. Moderate drinkers have a lower blood sugar, half as much insulin, and higher healthy HDL cholesterol when compared to nondrinkers. This could be why **moderate drinking** has a protective effect against heart disease. Young red wine seems to protect you more than fine old red wine.

EAT VITAMIN- AND MINERAL-RICH FOODS

Vitamin E and chromium **increase insulin's ability to do its job.** Vitamin E is found in oats, seeds, and whole grains. Broccoli, lobster, and mushrooms contain chromium.

the chromium story

Chromium-plated watches and kitchen appliances are perhaps the only way we're even aware of chromium. It is, however, very important to your body and to your health. **There's evidence that chromium helps to control insulin and blood sugar.**

Chromium keeps insulin at normal levels and working efficiently. When you're chromium deficient, your body tends to compensate by manufacturing more insulin and your insulin levels will rise. If your chromium is low, you need about ten times more insulin to process the sugar you eat and we know that high insulin levels are dangerous. Indeed, **some experts think that chromium deficiency leads to insulin resistance.** Eating chromium-rich foods is one way to help prevent insulin imbalance.

what chromium does

Essentially, what chromium does is make insulin more efficient so you need less of it to keep your blood sugar steady. High calorie, sugary foods increase your need for chromium because they tend to wash chromium out of the body. So eating a third of your calories in the form of sugar causes three times the loss of chromium as eating 10 percent of your calories as sugar.

The role of chromium is an "adaptogen": **it normalizes blood sugar no matter what the imbalance.** Studies show that if you have high blood sugar, chromium tends to bring it down, but if you have low blood sugar, chromium tends to bring it up. This useful **balancing act** probably results from chromium's ability to normalize insulin. Possibly because of this effect on insulin, chromium lowers unhealthy LDL cholesterol and raises healthy HDL cholesterol. **It stimulates the immune system too.**

High insulin levels may have an aging effect by lowering the output of DHEA, which is thought by some to be an anti-aging hormone. Chromium opposes this. DHEA is a hormone that dwindles dramatically as we age, in parallel with the increase of insulin resistance. At 75 we only have 10 percent of the DHEA we had at 25. **As DHEA improves brain function,**

WHAT CHROMIUM-RICH FOODS MIGHT DO FOR YOU

- **Lower** insulin levels
- **Control** appetite
- **Stop** bingeing and craving sweet foods
- **Lower** triglyceride levels
- **Lower** unhealthy LDL cholesterol
- **Raise** healthy HDL cholesterol
- **Discourage** atherosclerosis and heart disease
- **Normalize** blood sugar

- **Reduce** your risk of adult-onset type 2 diabetes
- **Boost** your immune system
- **Increase** production of the anti-aging hormone DHEA
- **Normalize** your weight
- **Increase** your energy
- **Increase** lean body mass

memory loss, immunity, muscle fatigue, and osteoporosis, and perhaps may help to block cancer, chromium may augment all these anti-aging affects through its promotion of DHEA.

chromium-rich foods

There are many foods that contain chromium. Make sure that you include some in your diet. They are broccoli, barley, brewer's yeast, shrimp, lobster, liver, whole grains, mushrooms, and beer.

LOSING*fat*

YOUR BODY DOESN'T LIKE YOU BEING FAT. THAT DOESN'T MEAN YOUR BODY DISLIKES YOUR FAT THIGHS, YOUR FAT UPPER ARMS, OR YOUR FAT STOMACH. YOUR BODY IS UNAWARE OF WHERE YOUR FAT IS. ALL THAT YOUR BODY CAN KNOW ABOUT IS YOUR TOTAL FAT.

All the fat in your body is connected, so that fat at the top of your arms is the same to your body as the fat on your thighs or around your stomach. Your body makes no distinction, which is why it's impossible to spot-reduce. **The only way in which your body can lose fat is to lose total fat.**

how do I know I'm fat?

• Stand in front of a mirror without your clothes on and jump up and down. You'll know all right.
• Increasing clothes size.
• Rising weight.

Relying on weight to assess our level of fatness can be misleading. These days we can measure body fat reliably by a method called **bioelectrical impedance or BIA** and this measurement has superseded the BMI index. Healthy body fat levels for men should be 10-20 percent of body weight and 15-30 percent for women. Few of us should be above that, even as we age, because high total body fat is dangerous whatever our age.

Scientists used to believe it was normal and acceptable to gain weight (fat) as we aged. We now know that to be false. **The truth of the matter is that health risks climb steadily as our body fat rises and there's no way around that simple rule**. Far more important than the superficial features of being fat is the fact that even as little as an additional 10 pounds (4.5 kilograms) of fat can increase your risk of coronary heart disease, diabetes, many cancers, and other medical problems which aren't specifically related to your weight. **You can't be fat at any age and be healthy**.

the dieter's friend

Carbohydrates are the body's perfect fuel, and the dieter's best friend. They "burn clean" – they don't leave any "dirty" waste. And if the body doesn't get enough of them you feel miserable and depressed. Deprived of carbohydrates, as in a high protein diet, the body breaks down fat reserves and its own muscle. Unfortunately, fat and protein don't burn cleanly. They produce toxic substances called ketones and aldehydes that make your breath smell – like Juicy Fruit gum – if levels get too high. Ketones and aldehydes are also produced by starvation:

GOOD CARBS,
bad carbs

Not all carbohydrates are created equal – some carbohydrates increase blood sugar more than others and they are said to have a **high glycemic index**. That doesn't mean carbs make you fat, just that high GI foods elevate your insulin levels too much.

High GI foods result in a high, sharp blood sugar peak followed by an insulin peak, which increases the tendency for not only insulin resistance and diabetes but also cravings, binges, overeating, and obesity.

Low GI foods result in slow, shallow blood sugar peaks, no rebound insulin peak, no tendency to insulin resistance, good appetite control, less overeating, and normal weight.

Good carbs = unrefined carbs = low GI foods: fruit, vegetables, whole grains, whole wheat products and whole cereals, particularly oats. So good carbs combine the lowest calories with the highest nutrition.

Bad carbs = refined carbs = high GI foods: any food containing sugar and highly refined foods – cakes, cookies, ice cream and chocolate as well as alcoholic drinks.

on a low-carbohydrate diet **your body thinks you're starving** and goes into hibernation.

This happens if you eat less than 5 ounces or 150 grams of carbohydrate a day, roughly equivalent to 600 calories. Any high-protein or high-fat diet will do this to you. No one wants to lose muscle, so it's essential to eat carbohydrates. But it's better to eat "good carbs" - the kind that don't result in a sharp rise in blood sugar. These **good carbs** don't destabilize your blood sugar (rapidly followed by your insulin) because they release sugar into the bloodstream at a slow enough rate for your insulin system to cope comfortably. A welcome side affect of this steady blood sugar is that your appetite comes under control, cravings are a thing of the past, you don't binge, and you're unlikely to be fat.

The best way to keep your total body fat down is to combine a high complex-carbohydrate diet with an active lifestyle. Your body is happy, you feel good, you stay lean and free of the diseases that we associate with old age but that are due, mostly, to excess total body fat.

weigh less, live longer

Eat more, weigh less – that's the secret of a longer life. The trick is to lower your calorie intake by eating more low calorie foods that give you all the nutrients you need.

A low-calorie diet prolongs life in many animal species – sometimes by as much as a third – and in you too if you adopt it as a way of life. Taking in fewer calories will be automatic if you eat complex carbohydrates, plenty of fiber, and fill up on low-calorie, antioxidant-rich, minimally-processed whole food.

There's a lot of evidence that eating fewer calories every day can slow down your biological clock, **delay aging,** and save you from the diseases that come with age. What's more, it's **never too late** to cut calories and begin staving off aging.

the evidence

Let's take the animal evidence first. Since the mid-1930s it's been known that if you restrict the food intake of laboratory mice, you

What's more, it's never too late to cut calories and begin staving off aging

can lengthen their lives by as much as a year, the human equivalent of 30 extra years. Lowering calorie intake by restricting your diet means undernutrition, not malnutrition, because you get all the essential nutrients, but with a much reduced energy intake. As long as all the essential nutrients are there it makes no difference how you restrict your food, but cutting down on fats and proteins is easiest because they contain the most calories. So cutting down energy intake by 30-50 percent would seem, in animal experiments at least, **to extend the life span by about a third.**

benefits

A longer life isn't the only benefit. Animals that have a calorie-restricted diet are **healthier**, they have more **stamina and endurance**, age more slowly, and develop cancer more slowly. Inside each body cell, key maintenance and repair functions are boosted. Calorie-restricted rodents show the greatest extension of life span when **food is restricted early,** soon after weaning. But even when started in adulthood, dietary restriction has a significant effect on life span, suggesting it's never too late to start.

The Okinawans exhibit all the benefits of reduced calorie intake, including improved blood sugar control and less insulin resistance, **younger, leaner bodies, and increased mental sharpness.** How much calorie restriction is there among the Okinawans? Well, they eat 10-20 percent less than the Japanese who eat about 20 percent less than Americans. This means that the Okinawans eat about 40 percent fewer calories than we do and this is thought to be one of the prime reasons for their incredible life expectancy.

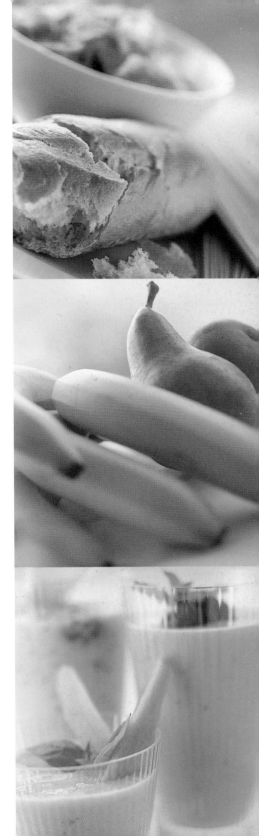

Extraordinary things happen to us when we limit our calorie intake as the Okinawans do.

We produce fewer free radicals which damage and age cells.

Our anti-aging defenses **strengthen**. Underfeeding animals dramatically boosts levels of internally produced antioxidant enzymes, including the powerful superoxide dismutase, catalase, and glutathione peroxidase. These enzymes are **several times more powerful** at neutralizing free radicals than anything we can take as supplements to repair aging damage in cells. Furthermore, they're many times better at flushing carcinogens out of the body than any "cancer-protecting" pill. Hence, the cancer protecting properties of a low calorie diet.

The immune system is given a boost. Calorie-restricted animals have an immune system **one-third stronger** than normal animals and calorie restriction delays the drop in immune response that occurs with age. So the potency of scavenger white blood cells lasts longer in underfed animals.

Our blood sugar and insulin levels drop. When we undereat there's a dramatic drop in blood sugar peaks and insulin peaks.

BENEFITS OF EATING LESS

Here are some of the anti-aging effects seen in Okinawans that were first noted in monkeys fed 30 percent fewer calories than usual:

- ◆ **Lower** total body fat
- ◆ **Lower** metabolic rate
- ◆ **Lower** fasting blood sugar
- ◆ **Increased** glucose tolerance (less insulin resistance)
- ◆ **Lower** insulin blood levels
- ◆ **Greater** insulin sensitivity
- ◆ **Lower** blood pressure
- ◆ **More** lymphocytes (a type of white blood cell which fights infections)
- ◆ **Lower** cholesterol

The pay off is this: if you're thin, and a man, **your life expectancy is 40 percent longer** and you're 60 percent less liable to die of heart disease than if you're overweight.

Eating fewer calories **reduces your overall cancer risk** whether it's cancer of the breast, prostate, or colon. It also seems to protect against the spread of precancerous cells – in one study, the proliferation of precancerous cells in the colon was reduced by 40 percent when calories were reduced by one-third.

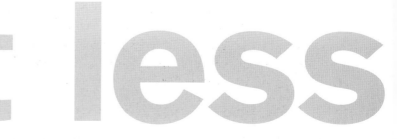

eat less

CUTTING BACK ON CALORIES

To bring you longer life, calorie cutting has to be done slowly, so avoid extremely low-calorie crash diets. This kind of calorie restriction doesn't prolong life. So as a start, an average man might try eating 2,000 calories per day, and a woman 1,800 a day, and lose weight at no more than a pound or so a week. Always check with your doctor before making any changes to your diet.

the sooner you start calorie-restricted eating (once you're fully grown), the better, though starting halfway through your life still has substantial benefits.

you've got to make every calorie count, so eat foods that are high in nutrients but low in calories. The ideal foods are fruits and vegetables, which have the highest concentration of antioxidants, vitamins, and minerals, with the fewest calories.

stop when you first feel full The other useful habit to get into, and one which is a way of life for the Okinawans, is to stop eating when you feel the first sensation of fullness. This will reduce your calorie intake by 20–30 percent.

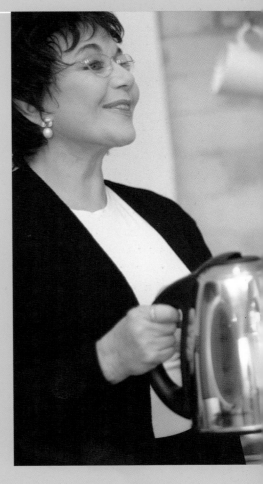

the other trick is to eat slowly We know that it takes the stomach 15–20 minutes to realize it has food in it and then to send a message to your brain that it's starting to feel satisfied. After that your appetite will decrease. The modern habit of eating food quickly on the run means that you can eat an excess of calories in the time it takes your stomach to realize that it's being fed, and therefore miss the cutoff point. So start with a glass of water, sipped slowly, and eat slowly so that you only eat a little in that first half hour. Your stomach and brain will then take over and you'll become sensitive to that feeling of fullness, the signal to stop eating.

chromium can mimic the effects of calorie restriction by increasing sensitivity to insulin, driving the blood sugar level down, and keeping blood insulin levels low. When insulin levels are high we're prone to overeating and bingeing, particularly on high-calorie, nonnutritional foods like candy and ice cream. So paradoxically, when you reduce your calorie intake, you'll also reduce your appetite, thereby making weight control easier.

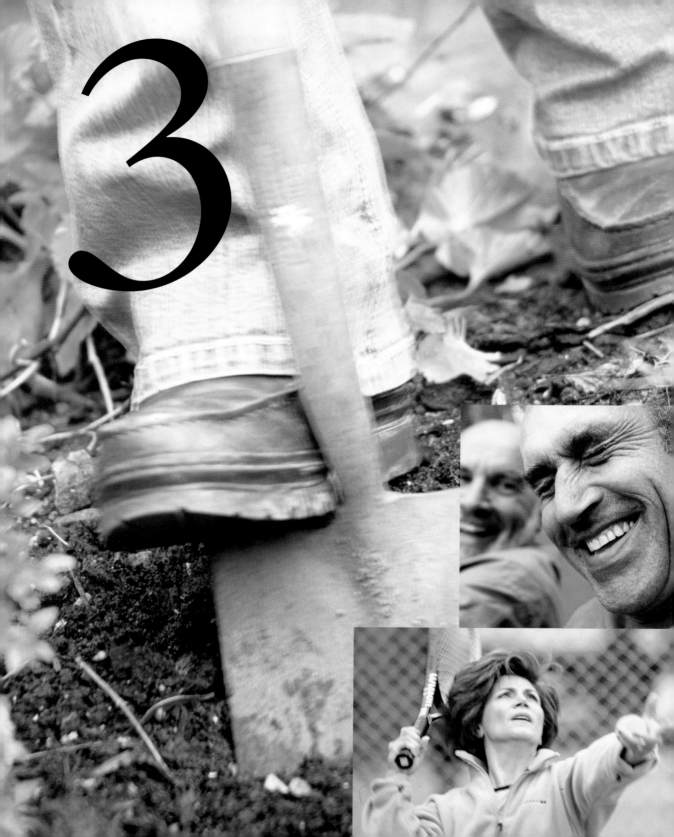

FIGURING OUT
YOUR
50s

The fifties can be tricky, a time for taking stock. During our fifties **the pace of life may slow a little.** We become more personally aware and reflective. We examine our priorities and *grow more tolerant*, with an increasingly *mellow and philosophical* outlook. There may even be a **gradual reversal of roles** in men and women: men may begin to lose some of the drive to be top dog in their job and look to social and leisure activities; women are likely to *be seeking self-expression*. For women, **menopause** is the most significant biological and psychological event, but for both genders *fewer sex hormones* means less youth.

So you think you're having a **MIDLIFE CRISIS?**

Check these statements based on a list from Ross Goldstein, a California psychologist.

1 The future looks as positive as it ever has

2 My life is as rewarding as I expected

3 Security is getting more and more important

4 Compared to earlier, my life lacks adventure and excitement

5 I seem to be getting more not less flexible

6 There doesn't seem to be much satisfaction in life

7 I feel time's running out

8 I wish I could make all the tension and stress go away

9 I'm surer of who I am than when I was young

10 Balancing work and family gets harder and harder

11 I just can't accept my age

12 I'm so tired of struggling to be successful

13 Work is as satisfying as ever

14 I'm worrying about my health more

Scoring
Two points for yes to 3, 4, 6, 7, 8, 10, 11, 12, 13, and 14
Two points for no to 1, 2, 5, 9, and 13

TOTAL SCORE
0–8	No crisis
10–16	You'll take slowing down in your stride
18 or more	You need to make changes in your life

THE *hormone* SLIDE

MENOPAUSE LITERALLY MEANS THE LAST MENSTRUAL CYCLE AND IT SIGNALS THAT A WOMAN'S REPRODUCTIVE LIFE IS OVER.

Menopause can't be kept at bay because eventually women run out of eggs, usually around the age of 50. Men, it should be noted, don't run out of sperm after 50 – sometimes not even at the very end of their lives.

Today **the average menopausal woman is in excellent health** and may live as long after her menopause as the whole of her fertile life before. Indeed, some women are so healthy that with medically assisted fertility techniques **they have given birth to healthy children** way after the age of menopause.

Menopause brings a very abrupt cessation of ovulation and with it the **disappearance of the life-enhancing hormone estrogen**. Indeed, estrogen levels plummet and the sudden change is difficult to adjust to. As a result, the well-known symptoms of menopause emerge.

so is there such a thing as a "male menopause"?

In spite of many claims to the contrary, **there is no such thing as a male menopause**. Men become increasingly prone to lower sex drive and impotence – the failure to produce and maintain an erection – but they don't show the same specific shutdown of sex hormones as do women. So when the "male menopause" or "andropause" is mentioned what do people mean? Mostly it's a slowing down of a man's sexual power.

Even now, little is known about what's called male menopause. All we know for certain is that it's **not the equivalent of female menopause** – there is no sudden shut down of sex hormones. We still don't know when it occurs or if it truly exists, and if it does, whether the experience is similar to a woman's. Do all men experience a "menopause"? If they do, what are the symptoms? And, drawing a parallel with women, would men benefit from hormone replacement therapy too? What would happen to men if hormone replacement therapy were widely used? What would the success rate be? And would there be any harmful or long-term effects?

There are very few answers to any of these questions because so little good research has been done. **Male menopause doesn't have the same drama as a woman's** – the decline of hormones is more **gradual**, taking perhaps two decades – nor does it occur during exactly the same years. In a way, it's more insidious than a woman's, and better thought of as enveloping **all the changes going on in a man's body and mind** as his genital system begins to **wane** over quite a long time. For this reason the word used to describe this phase of a woman's life – the climacteric – is sometimes applied to men. Another word, andropause (a reference to the male sex hormone androgen), is also quoted, though it's a misnomer because there is no "pause," no sudden cessation of hormones.

Whatever happens to a man in his fifties, it has little basis in dramatically changing hormone patterns. His midlife crisis – and in some men it is a crisis – is largely a reaction to feeling **less able and less attractive** and a reassessment of how life is progressing with respect to earlier goals. It has its roots in his waning sexual potency, which is why some men seek **reassurance** in new, young sexual partners.

men – the crisis years

Almost all men between 40 and 50 are going through the most competitive stages of their careers. Tensions brought on by competition at work aren't eased by financial pressures at home. A man in this situation may find that he spends more time following his professional career than with his family. This leaves less time for a loving relationship with his partner, and stress may lead to a gradual lessening in sexual activity.

Other contributory factors include **mental and physical fatigue, overindulgence in food or alcohol**, and **insecurity about performance**. One way of handling this is to withdraw from having to perform and this can lead to total avoidance of sex

Why, as a man grows older, is there a SEXUAL DECLINE?

A study was made by pioneering research team Masters and Johnson. They discovered that definite factors affect a man's sexual responsiveness.

Monotony – being in a sexual rut.

A close second is a man's **preoccupation** with work.

Fatigue, mental or physical, contributes to a decline in sexual response.

The older man's penchant for **eating and drinking** too much plays its part.

Illness, mental or physical, in either partner may lead to a further decline.

FEAR that his performance doesn't come up to scratch may be greater than at any other time in a man's life, especially during a time of stressful career decisions.

Monotony is the factor quoted most often and most constantly as leading to a loss of interest in sex and sexual performance. The end result may be having sex out of a sense of duty. Overfamiliarity with a partner is often blamed; the female may no longer be stimulating to her man and vice versa. Neither partner sees the necessity of making themselves sexually interesting and that triggers boredom.

in the relationship. Physical or mental illness can lower or even eliminate sexual drive. All these problems need to be discussed with a partner.

fear of failure

There is no doubt that "fear of failure" plays a very important part in the aging man's withdrawal from sexual activities.

Once a man has noticed that his potency is declining, or he experiences even one occasion when he's unable to achieve sexual satisfaction through impotence, he may **withdraw voluntarily from any kind of sexual activity.** This is mainly because most men are unable to face the ego-shattering experience of repeated episodes of sexual inadequacy. Most men are unable to accept the fact that a lessening of sexual drive and lowering of sexual performance are parts of normal aging. They make all sorts of excuses and will blame many different kinds of external factors rather than face the truth that their bodies are maturing.

why does testosterone wane?

Research shows that while a man in his early twenties can produce around 6 milligrams of testosterone a day, by the age of 50 the level **can have dropped by two-thirds or more.** Just why this happens to some men isn't clear. **One theory** is that production of the hormone drops because of age-related wear and tear in the testes.

A second theory on why testosterone wanes is that as men get older, increasing amounts of testosterone are being diverted to repair the physical effects of age, reducing the amount of free testosterone in the body. **Triggers that reduce testosterone** are said to include **stress, weight gain, drinking too much alcohol,** and **lack of exercise,** as well as **aging.**

Though the jury is still out, research is suggesting that HRT for certain men may work. **Carefully judged testosterone treatment could be effective, possibly safe.** Early studies would lead us to believe that a combination of testosterone and Viagra is even better. When testosterone is

SO – HOW WILL YOU KNOW?

If you're a man on the brink of a midlife crisis this may be a picture you recognize:

- Your **hair** is thinning
- **Libido** is waning, erections failing, and **energy** lessening
- **Stress** is unrelenting
- **Children** are leaving home
- Friends have had **heart attacks**
- **Parents** have died

If this scenario fits you, you're probably in the throes of a midlife crisis. Is this male menopause? Or andropause? Well, it extends over a much longer period than the usual midlife crisis. It could be that a midlife crisis in the early fifties ushers in a sexual crisis in the late fifties.

WHAT TO EXPECT OF TESTOSTERONE?

In a British report Dr. Malcolm Carruthers alleges you could expect the following benefits:

◆ **Increase** in vitality and well-being
◆ **Increase** in drive and assertiveness
◆ **To be happier,** less irritable, easier to live with
◆ **To cope better** at work and at home
◆ **Increased** hair growth on your body
◆ **No further** head hair loss
◆ **Possible** enlargement of penis
◆ **Possible** increased sensitivity of the genital area

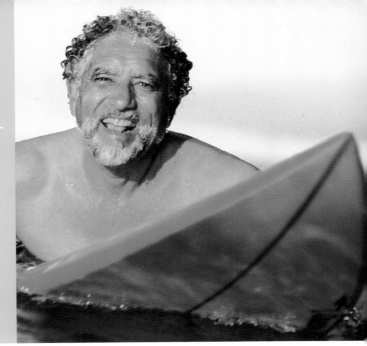

given alone, erection problems clear up in two-thirds of cases. But when they take Viagra too, the rate increases to more than 95 percent.

are hormones the solution?

In 1970 it was suggested that a man who finds his potency declining may be showing signs of **low levels of testosterone**, which could amount to a deficiency. But until studies had shown there was a general requirement by the body for testosterone replacement therapy, men had to be treated on an individual basis, based on rigorous monitoring.

There are endocrinologists in many parts of the world who make a special study of "male menopause" and who are using **hormone replacement therapy** for their male patients. However, the whole area still awaits clear definition and guidelines. Until then, HRT for men will remain a highly specialized, controversial field, not generally prescribed.

In this respect, **women are better off than men**. It may be because women are honest and brave enough to declare that their bodies are deficient, whereas men, particularly in the sensitive area of sexual activities, have yet to come to terms with their changing bodies.

is testosterone the answer to a man's prayers?

Testosterone has been called the king of hormones – hormone of kings – because:

• **It's responsible** for the sex drive in men and women.

• **It affects the health** of men and women through life. Even in women it contributes to bone and muscle strength, stamina, mental vigor, drive, and determination.

• **It's been called the "success" hormone** because most High-T-Guys (high-testosterone men) attempt to control and influence other people, express opinions assertively, get angry

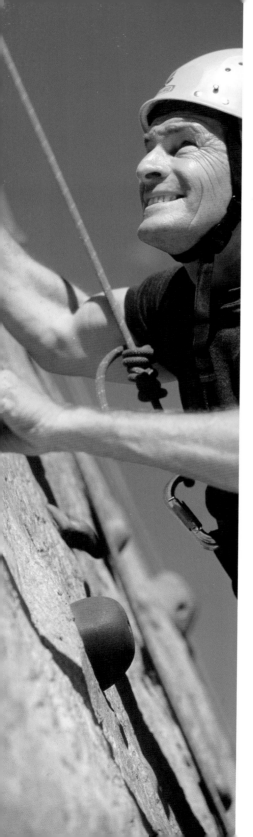

often, and try to dominate social situations. No man would want to be without it.

So is it simply a matter of replacing it? Not quite. In addition to all its life-affirming qualities, testosterone is responsible for some scary side effects on the body: it raises cholesterol, so is a risk factor for coronary heart disease and strokes. And it's implicated in prostate problems. Testosterone can therefore only be given as replacement therapy in carefully judged doses by specialists.

PLUS – the bad news is that 85 percent of men with symptoms would **NOT** qualify for testosterone replacement therapy because tests would show that their own testosterone was adequate for their body's needs.

how can testosterone be given?

Injections Several promising new injections are available with an extended action lasting between two and four months.
Pills Testosterone undecanoate is available in oil-filled capsules which need to be taken two or three times a day.
Pellets Six to ten pellets at a time are injected into the fat of the buttock under a local anesthetic. They last around six months, then a man will feel he needs a top-off.
Patches A skin patch is available in Britain for men who need testosterone replacement therapy.

effects of male HRT

A detailed study is being performed in Britain which will look at the effect of male hormone replacement therapy on 100 volunteers aged 45–55 (incidentally too small a number to give definitive results or guidelines for general treatment). Half the men will receive injections of male hormones and the other half none. What we still need is convincing evidence on the effects of male HRT, and it is hoped that the study will provide this.

Nonetheless thousands of men are being treated for the effects of hormone deficiency. At a world conference on male aging, eight out of ten experts said **they were in favor of prescribing testosterone replacement therapy to men** to relieve symptoms.

MENOPAUSE

A WOMAN'S MENOPAUSE CAN HAVE BOTH INSTANT AND LONG-TERM AGING EFFECTS.

Instant effects are the symptoms of estrogen withdrawal, such as hot flashes, night sweats, fatigue, loss of intellectual capacity, dry vagina, loss of sex drive, and urinary symptoms like cystitis. **Long-term,** and much more serious, is the effect of estrogen withdrawal on health – osteoporosis, arterial disease, heart attacks, strokes, and Alzheimer's, all potentially fatal. All of these conditions can interfere with long life, but more important, they can make the later years of life uncomfortable and restricted. In other words they make us old – if we let them.

keeping young the Okinawan way...

Many in the West, including myself, advocate the use of hormone replacement therapy, both to treat the immediate symptoms of menopause and to avoid the long-term ill health that occurs later. We now also have a new group of drugs called SERMs, or Selective Estrogen Receptor Modulators, that give **protection against osteoporosis and heart disease**, though they don't treat the initial symptoms of menopause like HRT.

However, among the Okinawan woman there are **virtually none who use HRT**. They claim they don't need it. They experience menopause **naturally** and without drugs, with fewer complications such as hot flashes, hip fracture, or heart disease, and it's illuminating to see how they do it. It would seem that there are several aspects of their lifestyle that make menopause easier to deal with. They are mainly diet related – for example, they eat many **flavonoids derived from soy products** – but not smoking, and getting light exercise, are also important.

Okinawan women get natural SERMs through their diet, mainly from the large quantities of soy and flax they eat. Soy contains phytoestrogens (plant estrogens) called flavonoids. The other important phytoestrogens are lignans derived from flax and grains. All plants, but especially beans, peas, onions, and broccoli, contain natural SERMs, though not as much as soy and flax.

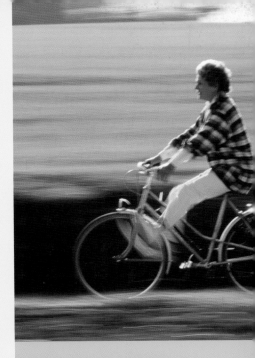

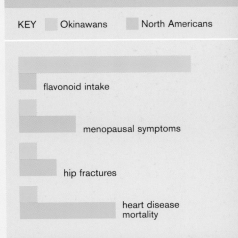

NATURE'S SERMS
and their possible effects

KEY   Okinawans   North Americans

flavonoid intake

menopausal symptoms

hip fractures

heart disease mortality

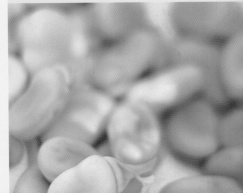

natural DHEA

Okinawan seniors also have a higher level of sex hormones, including natural DHEA, estrogen, and testosterone, than similarly aged Americans, suggesting that Okinawans are physiologically younger. The lifestyle that accounts for this youthfulness includes the Okinawan diet, a low-calorie intake, and exercise. Of course these hormones decline as Okinawans age, but they seem to do so more slowly.

DHEA has been reported to **protect against heart disease, memory loss, depression,** osteoporosis, certain cancers, and diabetes. We now know that DHEA levels decline in parallel with age so it may be the **best marker** of biological age we have. Measuring DHEA levels in people may be akin to looking at a horse's teeth or counting rings to find the age of a tree. The fact that **Okinawans have higher DHEA levels than North Americans of the same age** may be the best proof yet that the Okinawan lifestyle slows the aging process and promotes long life.

Seventy-year-old Okinawan women have **estrogen levels three times higher** than their Western counterparts. It's possible to speculate that the higher estrogen levels are a sign that **Okinawans are physiologically younger than Westerners.**

And Okinawan men have higher testosterone levels than similarly aged North American men. Indeed, the level of testosterone of 100-year-old men in Okinawa is hardly different from that of 70-year-old North Americans, and some Okinawans of 100 years are **still sexually active**, suggesting that it is the underlying process of aging that explains sexual decline.

In the West, growth hormone was thought to be another **anti-aging hormone**. Dosing leads to more muscle mass, decrease in body fat, and an increase in bone density, plus greater well-being and alertness. But these effects are only seen in men who are low in growth hormone levels to begin with — it doesn't show any results in men with normal growth hormone levels.

Yet again exercise contributes, this time with **youth hormones**. Every time you exercise, you convert the androgens produced by the adrenal gland (on top of the kidneys) into estrogen. Walking, even gardening, **bumps up your internal estrogen** and this process continues after menopause, in fact until the end of your life.

SEX HORMONES
in Okinawans and North Americans

	DHEA	Testosterone	Estrogen
	(relative amounts in the body)		
Men (age)			
Okinawan (70)	3	450	36
American (70)	2	300	21
Okinawan (100)	1	300	12
Women (age)			
Okinawan (70)	3	13	26
American (70)	1	17	6
Okinawan (100)	1	39	4

HOW TO *cheat* BONE AGING

EVERY WOMAN OVER THE AGE OF 55 COULD BE A VICTIM OF OSTEOPOROSIS OR BRITTLE BONES.

Estrogen keeps bones strong and healthy. Without it they get brittle and snap. A woman who doesn't take hormone replacement therapy can **lose a third of her bone mass** within three years of stopping her periods. That's painful, but worse, **it can be fatal** – one in four women who go into the hospital with a hip fracture due to osteoporosis never come out – they die there. And osteoporosis isn't an exclusively female problem – men can suffer from it too.

Osteoporosis means "bone that has many holes," making it weak and fragile. When we're young, worn-out bone gets broken down by cells called osteoclasts and repaired by cells called osteoblasts. In youth this fine balance of removing and building bone keeps our skeleton strong and solid. But for 15 years after menopause, the pace at which bone is removed is faster and so osteoporosis develops, leaving it vulnerable to fracture.

Osteoporosis is a progressive condition that makes bones more likely to break, particularly the hips, wrists, and backbone, and can lead to curvature of the spine. **Osteoporosis is responsible for 200,000 fractures each year**, commonly to the hip, wrist, and spine.

women at risk?

Women at high risk of developing osteoporosis should take hormone replacement therapy

YOU ARE AT RISK IF:

- you have a positive **family history**
- you start off with a **low bone density** from an early age, say from dieting a lot
- you've had amenorrhea – lack of periods
- you've had a **hysterectomy** with removal of the ovaries
- **you smoke**
- you've taken **steroid** medication

(HRT) immediately after menopause for five years. Then if symptoms aren't bothersome, they can go on to take a Selective Estrogen Receptor Modulator (SERM).

prevention pays ...

In 1998 it was estimated that the cost of treating a fractured hip was $7,500, and for people who go on to need long-term residential nursing care after breaking a hip there's an additional bill of $30,500 per year. Far better to prevent osteoporosis from developing or to halt its progress once it has developed.

... with health benefits

- You'll **avoid** bone and joint pain.
- Your bones **won't fracture**.
- You won't get a **dowager's hump**.

gray hair – take care

Researchers have checked out whether **premature gray hair** may indicate bone thinning. At the University of Auckland in New Zealand a study of more than 400 normal postmenopausal women showed gray hair before the age of 40 was indicative of thin bones. So premature gray hair could be an **invaluable risk marker** for osteoporosis.

keeping young bones

DIET

• The first line of defense against osteoporosis is **increasing calcium intake through diet.** Eat calcium-rich foods, including dairy products and canned fish with bones, such as sardines. Calcium supplements can be prescribed. To maximize benefits, calcium should be taken with other treatments such as vitamin D and HRT.
• Milk and dairy products contain calcium but can also be high in fat. **Choose skim milk and low-fat products.**
• If the body lacks vitamin D, it won't be able to absorb the calcium. **Vitamin D is in oily fish** such as sardines, herring, and mackerel, fortified cereals, bread, and margarine. Cod liver oil capsules are also a good source.

EXERCISE

• You may have put off exercising for years but you simply can't when you reach menopausal years (40 years onward). The evidence is irresistible.
• People who get exercise twice a week **have denser bones** than those who get exercise once a week who, in turn, have denser bones than those who never get exercise at all.
• There's a **significant improvement** for women who exercise for half an hour three times a week.

REDUCE your chance of BRITTLE BONES

There's EXCELLENT evidence that these will help protect you

◆ Get plenty of physical activity
◆ Eat foods containing calcium and vitamin D
◆ Take HRT to keep estrogen levels high

◆ Don't let yourself get too thin
◆ Don't smoke

And there's evidence that these may POSSIBLY protect you

◆ Eat green leafy vegetables
◆ Eat foods containing magnesium and natural SERMs (e.g. soy)

◆ Keep alcohol consumption low
◆ Keep red meat consumption low
◆ Keep salt intake low

DRUGS TO KEEP YOUR BONES YOUNG

hormone replacement therapy is a good way to prevent and treat osteoporosis. Taking HRT also helps **relieve distressing menopausal symptoms** such as hot flashes, night sweats, headaches, and vaginal dryness. There are more than 30 forms of HRT available in pills, patches, implants, or gels.

testosterone is a treatment for men who are deficient in the male sex hormone, but it **can also increase bone density** in men with osteoporosis who have normal testosterone levels. It's available as injections or implants.

anabolic steroids can increase bone and muscle mass, though *nandrolone decanoate* is the only anabolic steroid currently licensed for treating osteoporosis, and injections are carefully monitored due to side effects.

bisphosphonates are nonhormonal treatments for osteoporosis, which work by switching off the cells that break down bone, allowing **bone-building cells to work more efficiently**. There are three bisphosphonates available in the UK, *alendronate* (Fosamax), *etidronate* (Didronel PMO) and *risedrinate* (Actanel).

calcium and vitamin D Most people should be able to obtain adequate calcium from their diet but supplements are an alternative for people who find this difficult. Calcium alone has a limited effect as a treatment for osteoporosis, but combined with vitamin D it's particularly helpful for the elderly and housebound, who cannot obtain natural sunlight and may have a poor diet.

calcitriol is an active form of vitamin D given to postmenopausal women who have osteoporosis in the spine. Calcitriol **improves the absorption of calcium from the gut**, since calcium cannot be absorbed without vitamin D.

calcitonin is a hormone made by the thyroid gland, which prevents the cells that break down bone from working properly, improving the action of bone-building cells. Currently, calcitonin is only available as injections and only in one form. Because *calcitonin* has **a pain-killing effect** it can be useful to use for a short time following a spinal fracture.

SERMs (Selective Estrogen Receptor Modulators) are a new generation of synthetic hormone replacement, which **reduce the risk of osteoporosis** and heart disease, but do not increase the risk of breast or endometrial cancers. One form, *raloxifene*, is licensed for the prevention and treatment of osteoporosis in postmenopausal women.

HRT has both immediate and long-term benefits

A WORD *about* HRT

HRT (HORMONE REPLACEMENT THERAPY)
IS SELF-EXPLANATORY. IT REPLACES THE
FEMALE HORMONE ESTROGEN WHICH THE
OVARIES STOP MAKING AFTER MENOPAUSE.

In terms of its age-defying effects, HRT has both immediate and long-term benefits. The immediate effect is to relieve menopausal symptoms, including hot flashes, night sweats, dry vagina, inability to concentrate, tearfulness, anxiety, and depression.

longer-term effects

If anything, these are **even more important** because HRT will prevent brittle bones, protect against ovarian cancer and colon cancer, prevent the development of Alzheimer's disease, and just about **halve the rate of untimely death** as compared to women not taking it.

With the advent of the latest forms of HRT there is no need to have a monthly bleed and even though HRT marginally increases the risk of blood clots and pulmonary embolus, the decreased risk of fractures offsets this increase.

the latest perspective on HRT

In July 2002 a US study was published suggesting an increased risk of invasive breast cancer (by 26 percent), heart attacks (by 29 percent), and strokes (by 41 percent) on long-term HRT. Several points need to be made to clarify the report's findings:
• When we assess the risk of breast cancer, we do so against a baseline of 1.0 – every woman has a risk of breast cancer of 1.0. That means the risk of getting breast cancer for every woman is 1.0 per 1,000 women over 10 years.
• If, for some reason, that risk goes up to 1.50 per 1,000 women over 10 years that increase is reported as a 50 percent increase.

So, in simple terms, the 26 percent increase in risk of breast cancer in the US study means that the risk went from one woman in 1,000 to 1.26 women in 1,000 over a 10-year period, which by any accounting is not a huge jump.

results

These results are not a surprise. British studies in 1997 and 1998 revealed similar figures and we didn't panic then.

We didn't panic for good reason: the increased risk is no more than **the increased risk you impose on yourself** if you're overweight, put off your first child until you're over 30, drink too much alcohol, or have no children at all. There's no need to panic now.

We must remember that not every form of HRT carries the same risk, so these results apply only to the kind of HRT pills used in the US study. **There are** many different forms of HRT available – a lot women favor skin gels and patches. These treatments don't affect the body and breasts as much as the oral medication but still offer the same benefits

benefits of HRT

The benefits of HRT confirmed in this study are:
• A 37 percent reduction in **bowel cancer**
• A 33 percent reduction in **hip fracture**
• A 24 percent reduction in **all fractures**
Add to this the emerging evidence that HRT can probably prevent Alzheimer's.

And there's proof that HRT is 98 percent effective in treating menopausal symptoms such as hot flashes, night sweats, and vaginal dryness.

It keeps women's genital organs healthy, including the bladder, and therefore protects against cystitis.

Then there's the sound sleep, strong muscles, increased stamina, and mental tonic effect, all benefits of HRT

the latest research

In February 2003 a British study of 13,000 women stated that women with diabetes should not take HRT, and found no increased risk of heart disease on HRT but no protection either. **In March 2003** a US study reported no improvement in quality of life on HRT, though the authors admitted there were limitations to the study.

ALTERNATIVES TO HRT

If you're worried about HRT, and I wouldn't blame you if you were, keep in mind there are alternatives with no increase in breast cancer risk.
◆ **Tibolone** will relieve menopausal symptoms and has few adverse effects on the breast.
◆ Another kind of drug, called **SERMs**, doesn't help menopausal symptoms but strengthens bones and protects you from heart disease.

living with the risk

I personally have decided not to sacrifice the benefits of HRT and to live with any perceived risk. I'm reassured that, despite the frightening headlines, the researchers state that, for each individual woman, **the risks of HRT are still very low.** It's only when you lump thousands of women together that they become a concern. I will live with that, in exchange for **vigor, an active brain, a certain fearlessness, and a zest for life.**

KEEPING UP **APPEARANCES**

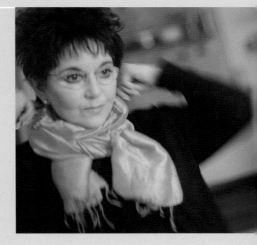

Many women become overly conscious of the signs of aging in their faces and bodies during menopause. It's very important to feel comfortable with the way you look – not only will your confidence improve, but also **your whole outlook will benefit**. A feeling of self-esteem is never more important than as you get older, and looking after your appearance is a good way of promoting *self-worth*. Your body will look better if you eat a good diet and get exercise. You can make the most of your skin and hair if you take good care of them.

Paying attention to your figure will mean that your clothes are more flattering.

There's no secret formula for looking good. You have to think carefully and logically about **how to make the most of your good points** and successfully conceal your bad ones. There's no need to buy expensive cosmetics and clothes. It's much more important *to look natural and feel comfortable*. The wonderful thing about reaching menopause is that there are no prescribed roles for you to play, and no set rules that you have to follow.

Shapelessness and poor posture can give the impression of age. A **relaxed, upright posture** and a **supple figure** can make you look much younger. Make sure that you stand with your feet parallel, your pelvis straight and your spine vertical. Your shoulders should be *relaxed* rather than hunched. You will not only improve your appearance by paying attention to your posture and gait, but you will also help maintain the health of your spine and back muscles.

don't give up on fashion

Avoid seeing your age as a constraint on what you should and shouldn't wear. If you're interested in clothes, try to be fashionable – it keeps you *looking* young and, more important, *feeling* young. It also tells the world that you are not living in the past. It has a stimulating effect on you, forcing you to look at yourself in a new light.

Scan the fashion magazines and keep a look out for **new fashion trends**, be it in the width of the shoulder, where a belt is placed, or the shape of a silhouette or sleeve. As an older woman, avoid exaggerated trends, but in any outfit try to include at least one fashionable feature that will bring your image up to date. **Make the most of your assets**. If you have a *good bust line*, show it. If your *waistline is trim and attractive*, display it. If your *ankles and legs are good* make sure your hemlines aren't too low.

MANAGING *your* MENOPAUSE

HRT ISN'T FOR EVERYONE, BUT THAT DOESN'T MEAN YOU CAN'T HAVE THE MENOPAUSE YOU'D LIKE. THERE ARE MANY DIFFERENT ROUTES TO CHOOSE FROM AND YOU CAN MANAGE YOUR MENOPAUSE YOURSELF BY PICKING FROM A NUMBER OF COMPLEMENTARY THERAPIES, RANGING FROM YOGA TO AROMATHERAPY.

Tuning in to COMPLEMENTARY therapy

Any medicine that heals or relieves discomfort without having any harmful side effects is, in my opinion, good medicine. Although HRT is the major treatment advocated by the medical establishment, complementary medicine **offers natural alternatives**, though I must emphasize that very few have been shown to be better than a placebo (a dummy pill). Anecdotal success stories, though, can't be the basis of general recommendation.

Complementary medicine argues that our bodies have a **life force**, which becomes disturbed when diseased but then reasserts itself if the body stops being abused and is nourished correctly.

Just like the best conventional medicine, the best unconventional medicine is holistic – it treats the **whole person**, rather than an isolated symptom. The naturopath is sceptical of symptomatic remedies because they fail to treat the root cause of the illness. Here's a rundown.

NATUROPATHY

[Note: There is no clinical evidence of effectiveness.]
Many types of complementary medicine are based on naturopathy.

Its principals are as follows:
• The patient is treated, not the disease.
• The whole body is treated, not just part of it.
• The underlying factors causing the disease must be removed.
• Disease is a disturbance of a life force, demonstrated by tension, rigidity, or congestion somewhere in the body, for example the muscles.
• The patient's own life force is the true healer.

• The body must have a "healing crisis" in which the life force cleanses the body by eliminating accumulated "toxins." The use of drugs in conventional medicine, while superficially curing the disease, drives it deep within the body, leaving behind a chronic condition for the future.

Naturopaths consider nutrition to be the anchor of health, and treatment usually involves fasting (one of the oldest of all therapeutic methods) and other dietary constraints. You should drink pure water and eat food that is organically grown, unprocessed, and, as far as possible, uncooked. **Animal protein should not make up more than 25 percent of the diet.** Food supplements from natural sources rather than vitamin supplements are recommended. Wheat-germ oil, kelp, and royal jelly can be particularly helpful during menopause.

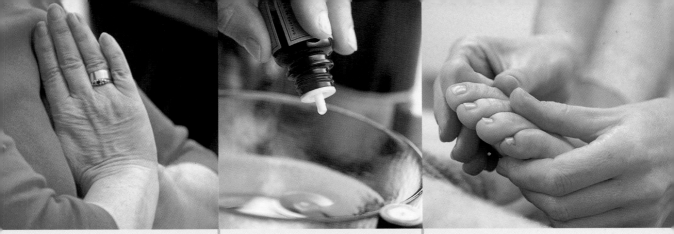

Naturopaths also believe that health depends on adopting a healthy and well-balanced attitude of mind by practicing relaxation exercises, yoga, meditation, and psychotherapy.

AROMATHERAPY

[Note: There is no clinical evidence of effectiveness.]
This is a relatively recent addition to complementary medicine, although its roots go back through the centuries. Human beings have **a highly developed sense of smell** and we can react to an odor within a split second. Babies bond with their mothers through scent and lovers are attracted by **each other's pheromones, or chemical secretions**. Smells can be mood enhancing and they may relieve pain and illness.

The oil essences that are used in aromatherapy are pure distillations from plants, and are very concentrated. In a dilute form, they can be inhaled and absorbed through the lining of the air passages. The essential oils can be used singly or blended, and have different properties; some are antiviral, some affect blood pressure, and some are general healers.

Massage using essential oils is relaxing and enjoyable, and beneficial in reducing many stress-related conditions. Essential oils are actually absorbed through the skin during massage or bathing and through the lungs when inhaled. Oral doses are not generally used, except in the case of garlic, which may be taken in capsule form.

The emphasis in aromatherapy is on treating minor ailments and promoting **health and well-being**, both physical and mental. For this reason, aromatherapy has achieved a wide popularity.

AROMATHERAPY REMEDIES
said to be helpful for menopausal symptoms

Essential oil	Symptom
Cypress, geranium, rose	Heavy periods
Avocado, wheat germ	Dry skin
Juniper, lavender, rosemary	Muscle and joint pain
Lavender, peppermint	Headaches
Basil	Fatigue
Neroli, lavender	Insomnia
Lemon grass, ylang-ylang	Premenstrual symptoms
Clary sage, rose	Depressed mood

The methods of inhaling essential oils are as follows:
• On a compress (although you should be careful not to apply undiluted essential oils to the skin because they are highly concentrated).
• Heating diluted essential oils on an oil burner.
• Inhaled as a vapor. Add three drops of essential oil to a bowl of steaming water and then cover your head with a towel and breathe in deeply. This method is good for skin problems.
• Inhaled on a handkerchief or pillow.
• Added to warm water in a bath. This method is good for nourishing the skin and relieving tension. It is one of the easiest ways of using essential oils – you should spend at least 15 minutes in the bath to derive the full benefit from the treatment.

• Applied to the skin as massage oil. The essential oil is diluted with a base oil such as sweet almond oil or soy oil. About 20 drops of essential oil should be added to 3.3fl oz (100ml) of base oil.

HOMEOPATHY

[Note: There is no clinical evidence of effectiveness.]
This is a form of natural healing based on the principle that a substance that produces the same symptoms as an illness will, in a very dilute form, help to cure that illness. Homeopathic remedies are derived from mineral, animal, or vegetable matter.

The homeopathic view of menopausal problems is that they are a **manifestation of existing imbalances** that can only be treated with regard to the mental and physical make-up of the individual. Women are encouraged to **prepare** for menopause by looking at their **overall health**, including exercise, stress management, and diet, and developing a positive attitude before it starts.

When consulting a homeopathic practitioner, not only are your symptoms assessed, but also **your personality and constitution, likes and dislikes** – all of this information is noted and used to form the basis of a decision as to which treatment should be given. For example, sepia may be a suitable remedy for someone who is irritable, moody, or dejected.

If you would like to use homeopathy to treat your symptoms it is a good idea to consult a homeopathic practitioner. If you decide to treat yourself, keep in mind the following:
• You should stop taking a remedy as soon as your symptoms start to improve.
• If your symptoms are not relieved after six doses, increase the potency or seek advice since you may have chosen the wrong remedy or the wrong dose.
• Store homeopathic remedies in

HOMEOPATHIC REMEDIES
said to be helpful for menopausal symptoms

Remedy	Symptom
Lachesis	Hot flashes
Pulsatilla	Insomnia, PMS, joint pain
Sepia	Dry vagina, prolapse, flashes, thinning hair
Sulphur	Dry itchy vulva and skin
Bryonia	PMS, mastalgia
Belladonna	Hot flashes and night sweats

a cool, dark place away from strong odors.

• Some substances, such as coffee, peppermint, menthol, and camphor counteract the effects of homeopathic remedies and should be avoided while taking a remedy.

• Some homeopathic pills are coated in lactose so avoid them if you are allergic to lactose.

• Homeopathic remedies should be discontinued when symptoms are relieved and recommenced as symptoms recur – not taken continuously.

HERBALISM

[Note: Some have evidence of clinical effectiveness.]
Herbalism is one of the oldest healing methods. Treatments matured through centuries of hit-or-miss practice until particular herbs were linked to particular ailments.

Over the centuries, developments in conventional medicine began to cast doubt on the efficacy of natural remedies, but since the 1950s herbalism has enjoyed renewed popularity and can sometimes be compared favorably with modern drugs, which may create allergies or spread resistant strains of bacteria.

GUIDELINES for taking herbs

◆ Always use herbs in **moderation**.
◆ **Discontinue** use if you start to experience side effects.
◆ Give each herb a week or two to **assess its efficacy**
◆ Start by taking a herb **in tea form**. Increase the amount from half a cup a day to several cups a day, over a period of a week.
◆ Don't take herbs for longer than a few months **without a break**.
◆ If you are taking medication, you should **check with your doctor** before you take a herbal remedy (see pages 185–89).
◆ **Don't defer seeking medical advice** because you are taking a herbal remedy and **always tell your doctor** what you are taking.

Like homeopathy, the goals behind herbal treatment are to remove the **cause of the symptoms** rather than merely the symptoms themselves, and to improve the patient's general standard of health.

However, herbalism does offer **an attractive alternative to other forms of treatment** in that it may allow the patient to experiment with a variety of herbs without the complication of serious side effects. It's also recognized that herbal remedies can work as **a complement to conventional medicine**. Herbs can be very effective in relieving menopausal symptoms.

There are many herbs that can help to relieve both the physical and emotional symptoms of menopause, but three in particular are **sage, vitex agnus-castus, and black cohosh**. Sage may help alleviate hot flashes, and you can take it in tea form, made from fresh or dried sage. Simply boil the leaves with a cup of water and strain. Sage tea does have quite a strong taste, and while some women find it calming to the stomach, others find it unpalatable. If you prefer, try taking sage in pill form, available from most herbalists.

The herb vitex agnus-castus (also known as vitex or chaste berry) has long been associated with menopausal disorders and it may **help to normalize hormone levels**, acting as a natural type of HRT. Some herbalists recommend the following combination of herbs to treat hot flashes: blackcurrant leaves, hawthorn tops, sage, and vitex agnus-castus. This may be drunk in an infusion three times daily for six weeks.

Black cohosh has estrogenic properties and can help if you are feeling weak and tense. It also has antispasmodic and sedative properties and will **help to alleviate pre-menstrual tension, pains, and bloating.** Black cohosh works well in combination with vitex agnus-castus.

ACUPUNCTURE

[Note: There is some clinical evidence of effectiveness.]
The name comes from the Latin and means "to pierce with a needle."

Acupuncture reputedly originated when it was noticed that Chinese soldiers wounded in battle by arrows, not only recovered from the arrow wound, but also **gained relief from other ailments.** From this observation, the technique of inserting needles into the body for therapeutic purposes evolved. Acupuncture has been used in China for 5,000 years.

The basic theory behind acupuncture is that **a life or energy force** flows through the body along channels called **meridians**, which are quite distinct from the lines followed by nerves. This life force must flow unimpeded if bodily health is to be maintained.

When we become ill, the energy flowing along a particular meridian may be affected at a site considerably distant from the sick part of the body. The acupuncturist aims to **restore the flow of energy** in the affected meridian by the use of copper, silver, or gold needles superficially inserted into the flesh at specific points along the meridian. These needles are so fine that they can hardly be felt as they enter the skin.

Depending on the position of the selected point, the needles may be inserted vertically, at an angle, or sometimes almost horizontally. The needle is then rotated, moved up and down, or used **to conduct heat or a mild electric current.** This is thought to set up some kind of current along the meridian line. It passes to the central nervous system and has an

effect on the organ or area that is malfunctioning by reestablishing **the flow of energy** through the meridian.

Acupuncture is one of the few Eastern practices that is widely accepted in the West, although its applications are not nearly so widespread here. In China, major operations, including heart transplant surgery, may be performed using acupuncture as the only form of pain relief.

MASSAGE

[Note: There is some evidence of effectiveness but not in the long term.]
Many claims are made about the virtues of massage. Some are false, some plausible, and some indisputable. For example, massage does not help to break down fat, but it may relieve emotional tension, and it definitely speeds up local circulation and improves **nourishment of tissues.** During a massage, parts of the body are treated in a specific order. **The direction of massage is always toward the heart,** assisting the return of venous blood (containing waste) to the heart and cleansing oxygenation in the

lungs. The patient lies down and the masseur massages each foot and leg in turn. Next comes the abdomen, the arms, wrists, hands, and fingers, and then the back of the body.

Swedish massage involves **vigorous massage strokes**, such as beating with the sides of the hands from the base of the spine to the neck and back again. Although massage is generally a very safe therapy, you should avoid vigorous massage if you have any sort of skin disease, or if your skin has been injured.

Neuromuscular massage consists of pressing with the fingertips, and was adapted from an Indian technique in the 1930s by Stanley Leif, an osteopath who wanted to find a way of relaxing patients' muscles before osteopathic manipulation. Specific motor points in the muscles are deeply massaged in an attempt to damp down the output to the sensory nerves in the area, and break the vicious circle of pain and muscle spasm from which we can sometimes suffer. Once muscular tension has been relieved using this technique, the muscle will be less likely to spring back into its previous tense position.

YOGA

[Note: There is no clinical evidence of effectiveness for treating ailments.] This is probably the best known of all meditation and movement therapies. Yoga's holistic approach encompasses **stretching movements, mental relaxation, and deep breathing** and can help you to deal with menopausal symptoms very effectively.

The form of yoga that has been embraced by the West is Hatha yoga, which has been practiced in India for 6,000 years. The basic goal is to encourage **a healthy mind to exist in a healthy body** and bring both into harmony.

Yoga consists of a series of postures, called *asanas*, which promote a relaxed and supple body and a peaceful state of mind. **Anyone can take up yoga,** whatever their age — you simply do as much as you find comfortable. Many people find that it helps them to overcome specific problems, such as smoking or excessive drinking. Some studies have shown that yoga can **help to reduce high blood pressure** and alleviate menstrual problems.

Yoga promotes good posture and mental tranquillity, which may alleviate backache, mild depression, and sleeping problems. Yoga can be practiced by all, but if you suffer from severe back disorders, dizziness, heart trouble, or any other serious medical conditions, it is wise to **consult your doctor** before starting.

GUIDELINES for practicing yoga

- Breathe **deeply and rhythmically** through your nose.
- Some yoga positions can feel uncomfortable at first — try not to force yourself into a difficult position.
- Work **slowly** at becoming supple.
- Hold a posture for as long as it is comfortable. Aim for 30 seconds initially in standing and sitting postures.
- Wear **comfortable loose clothing** and keep your feet bare to stop yourself from slipping.
- Don't practice yoga for at least four hours after a large meal.

BE *positive*

A POSITIVE ATTITUDE IN YOUR FIFTIES CAN LAST THE REST OF YOUR LIFE. THE FIRST STEP IN DEVELOPING A POSITIVE ATTITUDE IS TO LOOK BACK AND ASSESS WHAT YOU HAVE ALREADY ACCOMPLISHED.

This can reassure you and give you the impetus you need to make decisions about the future. You may find yourself debating two alternatives: trying to continue living and working as you have always done; or starting to make changes, perhaps reducing your workload. It's important as we get older to learn how to **enjoy leisure time** and to find new and varied diversions.

• **Find out what excites you and motivates you**. Stop spending time on things that don't interest you, household chores for example. You

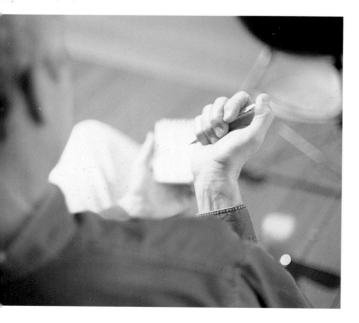

have as much potential as when you were young but now you are better equipped to harness it.

• **Make a list of things you "must" do in the rest of your life**. Some women break out of their usual lifestyle after many years as a wife, mother, and family caretaker to indulge an entrepreneurial spirit. They branch out on their own, perhaps opening a store or running a small business. You may remember your mother claiming that she was growing old in her fifties. If you're still alive at 85, as my mother is, **35 years is a long time to be old** – and an intolerable length of time to be inactive.

• **Make the most of each month, year, and decade**. Repeat this to yourself every day. If you feel you lack energy, get angry, particularly if you feel you've **stifled your anger** and held back in the past. Use it as fuel. We can benefit even more from joining a group of women of a similar age and sharing our experiences.

• **If you think your goals and vision seem impossible or idealistic**, read about women who have accomplished things in the second half of their lives. At the age of 42, the ballerina Margot Fonteyn, partnered by Rudolph Nureyev, then 23, was aware that everyone would be judging the way they looked together. She responded by making sure that she was strong enough to keep up with him. She did this by filling her repertoire with her most difficult roles so that her stamina, strength, discipline, and most of all, her courage would never drop below her already high standards. **Find yourself a role model** for continuing a productive and creative life. Forget your weaknesses, **list all your strengths** – and then go out to make your ideas reality.

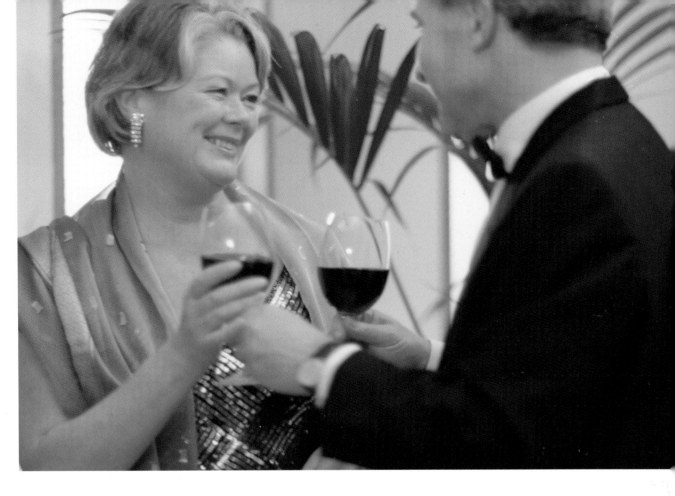

the empty nest

If a large part of your adult life has been invested in your children, it can be hard to cope with the silence and emptiness when they've all left home. A great part of yourself seems to have vanished into thin air. Particularly vulnerable are women who have defined their role in life in terms of **pregnancy and motherhood**. For such women the empty nest can take away part of their identity, and in some cases can make them feel purposeless and bring a sense of loss.

When their children leave home, some women may undergo an **emotional** and **intellectual** trauma similar to bereavement.

They have to find a new focus to their lives and the empty nest can spur major reassessment. Being aware of the eventuality means that a woman can prepare herself, perhaps by starting new activities and making career moves.

Because Western culture celebrates youth, many women **fear growing older**, without the clear role that motherhood gave them. I well remember the youngest of my four sons leaving home: no more nurturing, no more caring for them, no more mothering. Despite the fact that I hadn't defined myself only as a mother and had a flourishing career, **my parenting role** was integral to my understanding of myself and my

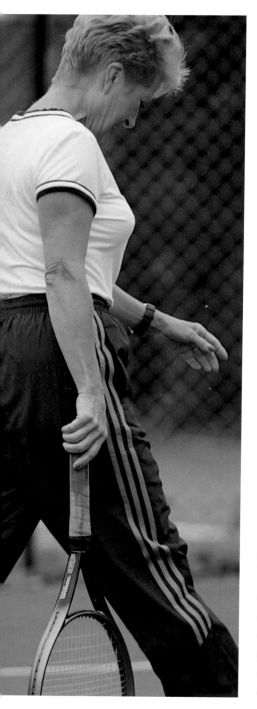

self-image. I suffered a double bereavement it seemed – loss of my sons and loss of role and it took a year or so to adapt to the loss of being an active mother.

The grieving was misplaced however. **No one stops being a parent. My role was simply different**. I entered a new parenting role, less hands on, more cheerleader and supporter – and all the better for that. **My role as a mother grew up** and I with it. And of course, back then I completely overlooked the advent of grandchildren.

taking advantage of your inner resources

Menopause is sometimes incorrectly stereotyped as the start of a gradual decline into old age, when your body loses its feminine qualities and becomes sexually redundant. Women know from experience that this is far from the truth. With care, your body remains one to be proud of, your mental resilience continues to be great, and you still have a valuable role to play in society.

think positively!

While health and vigor during menopause years depend a great deal on eating a good diet and exercising, these are not the only resources you have to draw upon. **Rest, relaxation, and a variety of leisure activities will help you to keep active and mentally alert**. You also need self-affirming thoughts to maintain your self-confidence. Never allow yourself to think that you are unattractive, lackluster, or out of touch. **The strong interaction between your mind and body** means that you can make your menopause more difficult with negative thoughts. In other words, if you believe you're sick, you can start to behave like a sick person.

If you repeat some of these statements like a mantra each day, you will gradually become convinced of their truth. **Positive thoughts and attitudes will maintain your self-esteem.**
• My body is **strong and healthy** and can become **healthier** each day.
• My female organs are in **good shape**.
• My body chemistry is **effective and balanced**.

- I eat **healthy**, nourishing food.
- I'm learning to **handle stress**.
- I'm calm and **relaxed**.
- I work **efficiently** and competently.
- I have the **freedom** and confidence to enjoy life.
- I can be happy and **optimistic** at this time of my life.
- My life **belongs to me** and it brings me pleasure.
- I devote **time to myself** each day.
- My friends and family are **more enjoyable** than ever.
- I'm going through menopause **more easily and more comfortably** with each passing day.

avoid high-stress foods

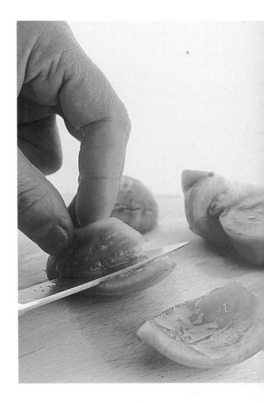

High-stress food substances, such as sugar, caffeine, and alcohol, which contribute to various menopausal problems, contain few nutrients and, in some cases, may be addictive. The chart below outlines some low-stress substitutes that can be used. If possible, you'll find it's best to avoid black pepper, monosodium glutamate, and very hot spices (which worsen hot flashes), or **cut your intake of these foods** by half.

REDUCE high-stress foods in your diet

High-stress foods	Low-stress substitutes to try
4oz (135g) white flour	4oz (135g) whole-wheat flour, less two tablespoons
1 square chocolate	1 square of carob or 1 teaspoon powdered carob
1 tablespoon coffee	1 tablespoon decaffeinated coffee
½ teaspoon salt	½ teaspoon of one of the following: potassium, salt substitute, yeast extract, basil, tarragon, oregano
4fl oz (125ml) wine	4fl oz (125ml) light wine
8fl oz (250ml) beer	8fl oz (250ml) light beer
8fl oz (250ml) milk	8fl oz (250ml) soy milk, nut milk, or grain milk
5oz (150g) sugar	One of the following: ¼ cup molasses, ½ cup honey, ½ cup maple syrup, ½ cup barley malt, 2 cups apple juice

VITAMINS and **FOODS** that will see you through your fifties

Vitamin	Source	Complaint
Vitamin A (retinol and fibro-carotene)	Carrots, spinach, turnips, apricots, fresh liver, cantaloupes, sweet potatoes	Excessive menstrual bleeding, cervical abnormalities, cystic disease and breast cancer, leukoplakia, and other skin conditions
Folic Acid (Vitamin B complex)	Green leafy vegetables, nuts, peas, beans, liver, and kidney	Cervical abnormalities and cancer, osteoporosis, diabetes mellitus
Vitamin B3 (Niacin)	Meat and poultry, fish, legumes, whole wheat, bran	Hyperlipidemia (high concentration of blood fat), hypoglycemia (low blood glucose)
Vitamin B6 (Pyriodoxine)	Meat and poultry, fish, bananas, whole-grain cereals, dairy products	Cervical abnormalities, cancer, diabetes mellitus
Vitamin B12 (Cyanocobalamin)	Poultry, eggs, and milk, B12-enriched soy produce (no vegetable contains B12)	Anxiety, depression, mood swings, fatigue
Vitamin C (Ascorbic acid)	Citrus fruit, strawberries, broccoli, green peppers	Excessive menstrual bleeding, cervical abnormalities, chloasma
Vitamin D (Calciferol)	Sunlight, oily fish, fortified cereals and bread, fortified margarine	Poor calcium absorption leading to an increase in the risk of osteoporosis
Vitamin E (Tocopherol)	Vegetable oils, green leafy vegetables, cereals, dried beans, whole grains, bread	Hot flashes, anxiety, vaginal complaints (e.g. dryness), chloasma and other skin conditions, atherosclerosis, osteoarthritis

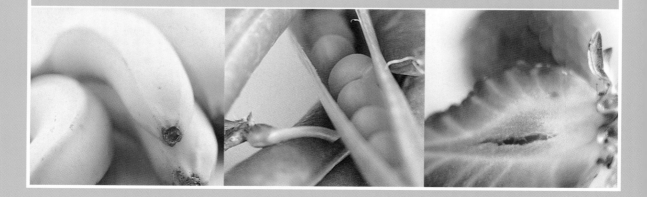

MINERALS to freshen up your fifties

Mineral	Source	Complaint
Calcium	Milk and milk products, dark green leafy vegetables, citrus fruit, dried peas and beans	Osteoporosis, hyperlipidemia (high concentration of blood fat), hypertension
Magnesium	Green leafy vegetables, nuts, soy beans, whole-grain cereals	Osteoporosis, fatigue, diabetes mellitus, coronary artery disease
Potassium	Orange juice, bananas, dried fruits, peanut butter, meat	Fatigue, heart disease, hypertension, anxiety, depression
Zinc	Meat, liver, eggs, poultry, seafood	Osteoporosis
Iron	Nuts, liver, red meats, egg yolk, green leafy vegetables, dried fruits	Excessive menstrual bleeding
Iodine	Seafood, fish, seaweed	Hypothyroidism
Chromium	Meat, cheese, whole grains, breads	Hypoglycemia (low blood glucose)
Selenium	Seafood, meat, whole-grain cereals	Breast cancer
Manganese	Nuts, fruit and vegetables, whole-grain cereals	Atherosclerosis
Bioflavonoids	All citrus fruits, especially the pulp and pith	Hot flashes, excessive menstrual bleeding, vaginal problems, anxiety, irritability, and other emotional problems

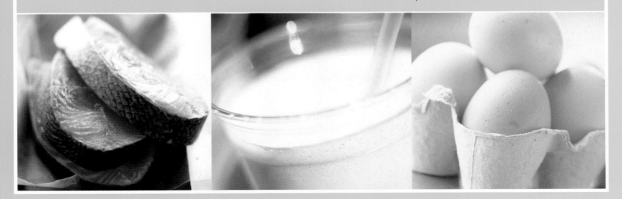

UNWIND

If you're relaxed, you will be better able to deal with problems and conflicts at home and work, and you'll find personal relationships easier to manage. Relaxation can often help you to deal with menopausal symptoms such as hot flashes, too.

deep muscle relaxation

This technique may take a little time to learn, but it will help you cope with stress, lower your blood pressure, decrease your chance of getting headaches, and make you sleep better.

1 Find a peaceful place, lie on your back or sit in a comfortable chair and close your eyes.

2 Begin by tensing your right hand (or left, if you are left-handed) and then letting it go loose. Now imagine that your hand feels heavy and warm. Repeat with your right forearm, upper arm, and shoulder, then move on to the right foot, the lower leg, and the upper leg. Do exactly the same thing with the left side of your body. By the time you've finished, your hands, arms, and legs should feel heavy, relaxed, and warm. Give yourself a few seconds for these feelings to develop and to get used to the sensation.

3 Now relax the muscles around your hips and waist. Let the relaxation flow up to the abdomen into the chest. A good trick is to try to imagine the surface under you pushing up into your back, so that you get a sensation of heaviness. You will find your breathing starts to slow down.

4 Now let the relaxation go up into your shoulders, jaw, and facial muscles.

5 Pay special attention to the muscles around your eyes and forehead – tense them and then let the frown melt away. Finish by imagining that your forehead feels cool and smooth.

6 If you can, you should practice this twice a day for 15–20 minutes each time. However, even as little as three minutes will be sufficient time to give you a sense of well-being. The best time to practice is just before mealtimes or an hour afterward. Once you've mastered deep muscle relaxation, you're ready to go on to deep mental relaxation.

deep mental relaxation

This is designed to clear your mind of stressful thoughts, anxieties, and tension. You can retreat or escape to this whenever you want to. Find a place where you know you will not be disturbed and lie down or make yourself comfortable in a chair. Close your eyes and start by breathing deeply several times.

1 Allow thoughts to freely associate in your head.

2 Stop any recurring thoughts by simply saying "no" to them under your breath, and repeating "no" until they go away.

3 With your eyes closed, imagine a tranquil scene such as a clear blue sky and a calm blue sea. Whatever you imagine, try to see the color blue, since this is very therapeutic.

4 Concentrate absolutely on your breathing – make sure that it is slow and natural. Follow each breath as you inhale and exhale.

5 By now you should be feeling calm and rested. You may find it helpful to repeat a soothing work or mantra, such as "love," "peace," or "calm." Think of a calming sound like "ah," and say it silently to yourself in your mind when you're breathing out.

6 Remind yourself to keep the muscles of your face, eyes, and forehead relaxed, and imagine that your forehead is cool and smooth.

When you've mastered both deep muscle and deep mental relaxation, they are fairly easy to combine. Practice them twice a day until you've become competent.

PEACEFUL*nights*

IN OUR FIFTIES WE START TO NOTICE A CHANGE IN OUR SLEEPING PATTERNS BECAUSE OUR NEED FOR SLEEP DIMINISHES AS WE GET OLDER.

While a newborn baby needs anything up to 15 or 16 hours a day, a child of eight or so probably doesn't need any more sleep than an adult. In young adulthood most of us can function on six or seven hours of sleep a day. However, by the time we reach our seventies it is quite common for us to sleep soundly for only about two hours and to **doze intermittently** for the rest of the night.

Sleep researchers believe that **our need to sleep is not entirely physical.** There are almost certainly chemical components so it isn't a tired body that drives us to sleep, **it's a tired brain.** Think of the brain as a battery: 16 to 18 hours of wakefulness run the battery down and **it needs to sleep to recharge.** When we've had enough sleep, our brain cells are charged with granules containing chemicals **necessary for efficient intellectual function.** When we're tired, however, brain cells become depleted of these granules. During sleep the granules reappear.

As a general rule of thumb, our need for sleep runs parallel with our growth rate. Our sleep needs start to trail off from around seven or eight hours a night by roughly **an hour every decade,** until we may need as little as only four hours per night in our sixties.

body clock

An internal clock with a regular 24-hour rhythm governs all our body functions. **For each individual, this rhythm is slightly different,** but it does conform to a general pattern. It is largely determined by blood levels of cortisol, the life-giving hormone which is secreted by the adrenal gland. By about midnight the blood level of cortisol is sinking rapidly **to reach its lowest ebb** between the hours of two and four in the morning.

Subsequently, the adrenal glands start to pick up and cortisol floods the body sufficiently to trigger waking somewhere between the hours of six and nine in the morning. **Early-morning people** have an early cortisol peak. **Night-time people,** who are slow to wake in the morning and don't really get going until midday, have a later peak.

we need less sleep

OUR CHANGING CLOCK

As we get older our 24-hour body clock can speed up or slow down.

◆ Our sleep is **lighter** with less dreaming so we wake more often during the night.

◆ **Too little of a hormone,** ADH (antidiuretic hormone) is produced during the night so we want to urinate in the night when previously we didn't.

◆ We feel **sleepy** during the day and need **catnaps** which blunt our need for sleep at the normal time.

◆ We can sleep for several hours early in the evening, which can prevent sleep entirely later on.

estrogen and sleep

Lack of estrogen contingent on menopause means women have to manage without its tranquillizing and hypnotic effects – **we get withdrawal of our natural sleeping pill** – with attendant wakefulness. In addition, sleep is controlled by two centers in the brain. One is sensitive to **external factors** like darkness, habits, and social and domestic cues – other people saying that they are tired and going to bed – and **internal cues**, like physical or mental fatigue, and these send us to sleep. A second center keeps us asleep; this is triggered by chemical reactions in the body and brain cells, which occur toward the end of the day.

Estrogen assures that both these mechanisms keep working during our fertile years, but both are disrupted by the estrogen deficiency of menopause. As you'd expect, **HRT goes a long way toward correcting sleep patterns**.

dealing with insomnia

If you find yourself habitually lying awake at night next to a snoring partner, don't lie there fuming, allowing resentment to build up. It's better to **be constructive about insomnia** and take advantage of it. Get out of bed, go downstairs, and make yourself a cup of tea. Find a book to read or do some job which you have been waiting to do for ages. It is never a good idea to lie in bed feeling resentful if you can't get to sleep. **Try to think positively about the few hours you have gained** and make the best use of them.

Many people with insomnia **sleep much more than they think they do**. Studies show they tend to wake more often than normal sleepers. It's the quality, rather than the quantity of sleep that's the problem in insomnia. If you can fall asleep, even for an hour, you benefit because the essential part of sleep consists of Slow Wave Sleep. This is the only time the brain is **totally at rest** and it occurs largely during the first half of a night's sleep.

as we get older"

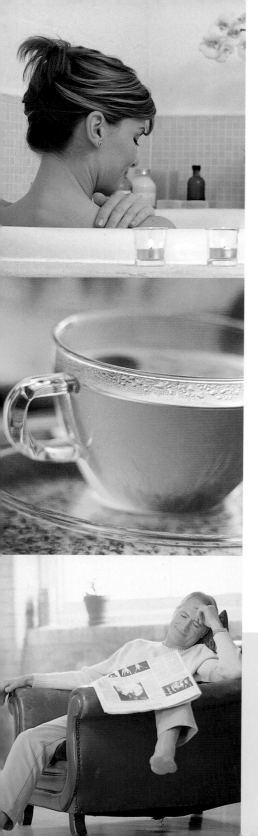

the causes

The most powerful cause of insomnia is resentment. No one feeling resentful or angry can sleep. But the most common cause of insomnia is **worry about a problem**.

Other causes are physical, such as sleep apnea (see page 73) and restless legs, but noise and light stop you from sleeping too. **Insomnia can also be a symptom of psychological illness**. For example, anxious or depressed people may find it difficult to fall asleep.

sleep enemies

• **Stress** When we're stressed the production of adrenaline increases, heightening alertness and making sleeping difficult.

• **Depression** Feeling low affects hormone levels and the sleep cycles of Non Rapid Eye Movement (NREM) and Rapid Eye Movement (REM) are often unbalanced.

• **Anger** Bearing a grudge or plotting revenge can prevent sleep completely. Save formulating a smart reply to your critical boss for daylight hours.

• **Caffeine** Coffee has an accumulative effect and there's hidden caffeine in things like carbonated drinks and chocolate.

• **Smoking and heavy drinking** These cause insomnia and ruin sleep quality. It's been shown that smokers sleep less deeply than nonsmokers. **Cigarettes** raise the heart rate, blood pressure, and adrenaline levels, hindering sleep. **Alcohol** wreaks havoc with hormones controlling sleep and, after an initial snooze, causes hours of wakefulness.

• **An overactive thyroid may cause insomnia**. Foods that help regulate thyroid activity include brussels sprouts, broccoli, and kale.

seeking treatment

• Your doctor will treat an **obvious physical or psychological cause** for your insomnia.

• For **long-term insomnia** with no obvious cause, EEG recordings of brain-wave patterns and an assessment of breathing, muscle activity, and other bodily functions during sleep may reveal the extent and pattern of the problem.

HELP YOURSELF TO HAVE
SWEET DREAMS

1 Your bedroom should be a peaceful sanctuary for sleeping. Oil squeaky hinges, and make sure windows open and close efficiently. Put up heavy curtains to keep out the light. Your bed should be firm. If it's past its prime, put plywood under the mattress.

2 Eat well during the day. Carbohydrates such as whole-wheat bread, whole-grain cereals, and pasta are important for good sleep. High-carbohydrate foods help produce the calming hormone serotonin, which regulates sugar in the body. Low sugar levels can lead to bad sleep.

3 Make sure the last meal of the day is satisfying. Lettuce, banana, and avocado are good late-night snacks since they contain the natural sleep-inducing chemical tryptophan.

4 Get exercise in the day, even if it's just a walk, since any form of exercise promotes sound sleep. Inactivity is a major cause of insomnia, because the unused energy stops us from sleeping.

5 Read or watch something relaxing during the last hour before bed to help you unwind.

6 Take a relaxing bath with essential oil of lavender added. While you're there, drink a warm glass of milk with a little honey. Milk also contains tryptophan, and honey is an ancient remedy for insomnia. If milk doesn't work for you, try an herbal tea like camomile or valerian.

7 Dim bedroom lights and put a few drops of a calming essential oil like jasmine in an incense burner.

8 Turn around the alarm clock so you can't worry about not being asleep.

9 Sleep will come more easily if your pulse rate is slow and blood pressure is down. Lie fairly still and control your movements by taking deep, slow breaths and concentrating on your breathing. Then concentrate on relaxing your body, starting with your forehead by relaxing a frown, then relax the muscles of the jaw, chin, and neck. Make your arms feel limp.

10 Become aware of the pressure of your body lying on the bed, then gradually work down your legs until they are completely relaxed, including your toes. Many people are asleep before they get to their feet.

11 Empty your mind and think about a favorite thing. When another thought creeps in, concentrate on the favorite thing again.

12 Try to establish a bedtime and a waking time and stick to them.

• **Keeping a log of sleep patterns** may also be helpful.
• **Sleep clinics for insomniacs** are few and far between, but you could ask your doctor to make inquiries for you.
• **Sleeping pills or tranquilizers** may be prescribed as a short-term measure, but only for severe cases and generally as a last resort. There are several over-the-counter remedies but as they all have side effects, they should all be used with caution and not for prolonged periods. Always let your doctor know you are taking them.
• **Complementary remedies** Health writer Bonnie Estridge gives high marks to ayurvedic massage and homeopathy as cures for insomnia, and if you have the money you may like to do your own test.

snoring isn't a joke

It could be a **warning sign** you should take seriously. Snoring is a noise caused when floppy tissue at the back of the throat, like the uvula, blocks the upper air passages.

Turbulent air flow creates quite violent vibrations of the soft palate or other structures in the mouth, nose, and throat. Depending on how flappable these structures are, vibrations can produce snorting sounds of such resonance that the decibels can be heard throughout the house and curtail the sleep of anyone who's in it.

Most causes of snoring are easily remedied and there's a good chance that **simple treatment** or a **change in lifestyle** will improve things. But other causes are more complex and need specialist investigation and treatment.

WHAT MAKES US MORE LIKELY TO SNORE

◆ Obstruction by the tongue if it drops back
◆ Small or collapsing nostrils
◆ Deviated nasal septum, say from a sports injury
◆ Overnight mucus congestion
◆ Large, floppy soft palate or uvula
◆ Enlarged nasal bones in the nostrils and nasal polyps
◆ In children, enlarged adenoids and mouth breathing

Smoking, being overweight, consumption of alcohol, use of sleeping pills, poor sleeping position, and reaction to house dust and dust mites also make us more likely to snore. **Avoiding these factors may reduce the likelihood of snoring.**

is snoring dangerous?

Snoring itself isn't serious but it can be a symptom of a more serious disorder, **sleep apnea**, in which the snorer stops breathing several times an hour during sleep. The point is that people with sleep apnea are prone to irregular heartbeats, possibly even heart attacks. And periods of low oxygen might be bad for the brain too.

The most vulnerable person is a man over the age of 45 or a woman who's gone through menopause and isn't taking hormone replacement therapy. **So if you're a middle-aged snorer, ask your doctor to check you over.**

what is sleep apnea?

Sleep apnea is caused by loose tissue at the back of the throat leading to loud snoring and closing of the airways as air is sucked in. The person appears to stop breathing (apnea) and, even though they may not completely wake up, the sleep pattern is disturbed. Sufferers get up feeling unrefreshed and continually tired. More often than not, they're unaware of their condition. Heart attacks are a hazard of sleep apnea, so if you suffer from it see your doctor.

There are three types of sleep apnea:
• Obstructive Sleep Apnea (OSA), caused by a blockage in the upper airway
• Central Sleep Apnea (CSA), where incorrect signals are transmitted from the brain
• Mixed Sleep Apnea (MSA), a combination of OSA and CSA.

Common symptoms of sleep apnea are:
• loud snoring
• feelings of choking and shortness of breath
• restless, unrefreshing sleep
• excessive daytime sleepiness
• personality changes
• morning headaches

what can be done?

Several hospitals have sleep apnea and snoring clinics, which can investigate the cause of snoring and diagnose sleep apnea. Your doctor can refer you for special tests to diagnose the cause of your snoring and recommend treatment, including lifestyle changes and surgery.

MAKE THE MOST
OF YOUR FIFTIES

See your fifties as a run-up to the rest of your life. That way you'll achieve the perspective of putting in place (or planning to put in place) the many adjustments your sixties, seventies, eighties, and nineties are going to demand.

If you can see your fifties like this they become **really exciting** – like preparing for a long vacation – except that unlike any other vacation you have few constraints, and those you have can be dealt with if you keep a **positive, optimistic, and determined frame of mind**.

To start, just make a list of all the things you are free to do now that you never were in the past. Say to yourself, I can:
◆ **forget** the children
◆ go **slowly** if I want to
◆ spend more time than I used to on **myself**
◆ have **treats** with the girls/guys
◆ go on an **around-the-world trip** for three months
◆ spoil my **grandchildren**… and so on.

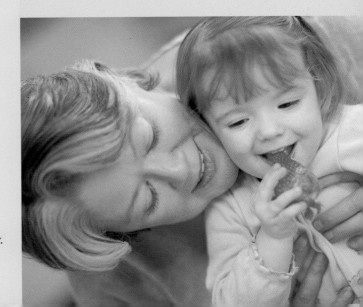

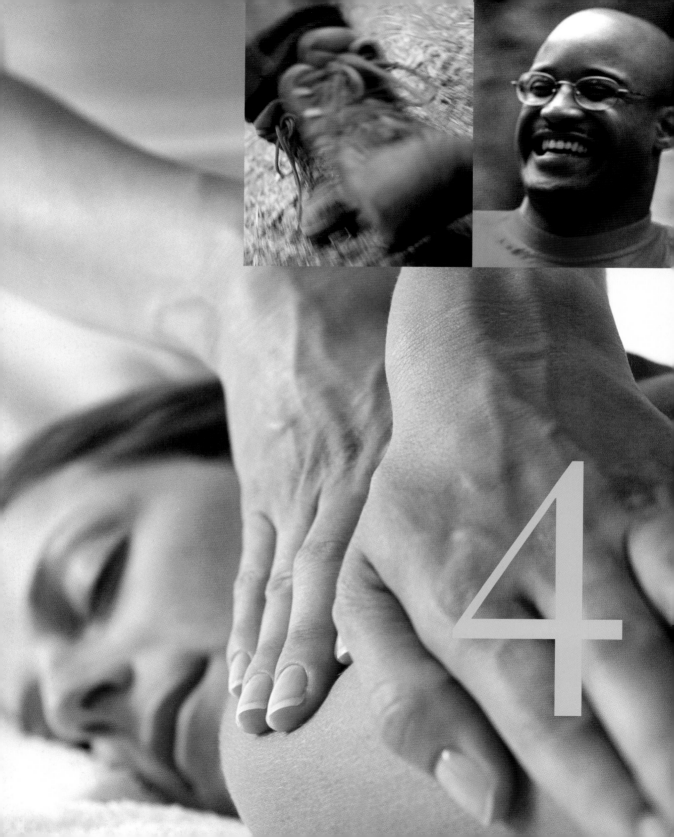

4

HOW TO
CHEAT
AGING

It's not possible to outwit our *genetic inheritance*,
nor the fact that our genes treat the body as disposable.
But we can **cheat** a bit because we have the means to
stretch our **life span potential** to its maximum. *Cheating
aging* really means subverting the progress of diseases that
beset our organs as we grow older. That requires **almost
tireless vigilance** and a bit of effort. It means observing
and listening to our bodies for early signs of change and
testing regularly for chemical markers of future problems.
That of itself means taking the long view and **planning for
a long, active life**. With a number of painless lifestyle
changes to *help us avoid life-threatening conditions* like
heart disease and cancer, that's what we can all aim for.

What happens inside your body as you live longer   ... how to prevent it ...

Organ	Change	Age-related diseases	What you can do to defy age
Teeth	Jawbone shrinks and gums recede	Teeth loosen, sensitive dentine exposed	Good oral hygiene, see hygienist every 6 months
Bones	Soften, thin and become brittle – osteoporosis	Fractures, collapsed vertebrae, dowager's hump	Do weight-bearing exercise 3–5 times a week, good diet
Joints	Wear and tear, destruction, inflammation	Arthritis, polymyalgia rheumatica	Don't become overweight, good posture, keep active
Arteries	Narrow due to clogging up from fatty lumps in walls	Atherosclerosis most serious in heart strain	Keep weight normal, low animal fat diet, fish oils, don't smoke
Heart	Overworked because of high blood pressure	Angina, coronary heart disease, heart attack	Exercise 3–5 times a week, low animal fat, fish oils, don't smoke, keep weight normal
Brain	Brain tissue dies from poor blood supply, clot, or hemorrhage	Loss of memory, Parkinson's, Alzheimer's, stroke	As for arteries, exercise for new brain cells, learn a new language
Lungs	Loss of elasticity, breathing problems	Chronic obstructive pulmonary disease (COPD), emphysema	Don't smoke
Immune system	Less responsive, more easily exhausted, less sensitive	Proneness to infections and cancers	Good diet, regular exercise
Eyes	The lens becomes more opaque, the retina less sensitive	Cataracts, age-related macular degeneration (ARMD)	Wear sunglasses in bright sunlight, don't become over-weight and go on to Type 2 diabetes, watch blood pressure
Ears	Less sensitive, more sensitive	Hearing loss, Ménière's disease	Protect from loud noises especially in youth, don't wear headphones
Digestive system	Digestive enzymes fewer, less stomach acid, food less well absorbed	Gas, bloating, anemias	Drink a lot of water with meals to stimulate stomach acid
Skin	Loss of collagen and elasticity, abnormal pigmentation	Thinning, wrinkles, age spots	Stay out of sun, use sunscreen on face, neck, and backs of hands every day
Hormonal system	Sudden cessation in women, gradual decline in men	Menopause, impotence in men	Get regular exercise, eat soy foods

... and how to avoid it

Screening	Drugs and procedures
See dentist every 6 months	Use orthodontics, cosmetic dentistry
Bone density scans at 60	Fish oils, HRT, SERMs, bisphosphonates
When symptoms occur	Green-lipped mussel extract, COX-2 inhibitors, NSAIDs, joint replacement
Cholesterol profile	Statins (see page 81), bypass surgery
BP every 2 years, cholesterol profile, ECG if symptoms arise	Drugs (see page 86), bypass surgery
As for arteries and heart, early Alzheimer's screen when symptoms arise	As for arteries and heart
Chest x-ray	
	Yearly influenza vaccine
Check every 2 years, check blood pressure as above	Lens replacement, laser surgery
Check every 3 years	Hearing aid
Endoscopy when symptoms arise, check for helicobacter, check out persistent indigestion	Antibiotics for helicobacter
Check out any pigmented spot that enlarges	Retinoic acid, cosmetic procedures
	HRT

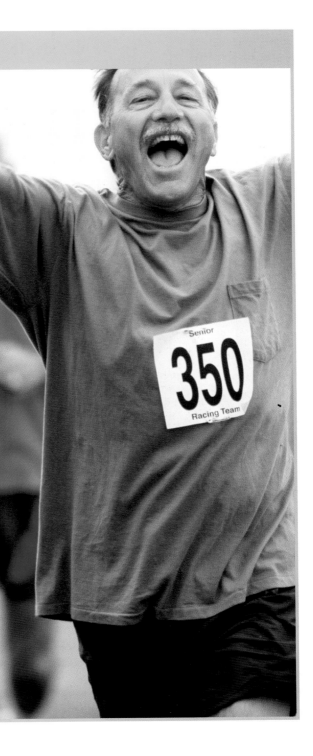

FIRST*steps*

A GOOD FIRST STEP TO CHEATING AGING IS TO TRY TO AVOID CERTAIN DISEASES AND CHANGES IN THE BODY THAT ACCOMPANY GETTING OLDER. STAYING ACTIVE IS THE FIRST GOAL.

Staying **gently active** all day should become your goal. The reason why we have to stay active is that the power of our muscles declines as we get older, so many people in their seventies are operating at their limit.

At the University of Newcastle upon Tyne, Professor Doug Turnbull has carried out research showing that **vigorous exercise might actually slow down** the cellular changes that cause aging in muscles. Veteran athletes who continue running into old age accumulate less DNA damage in their muscle fibers than the rest of us — meaning that, in absolutely real terms, they have **younger muscles**. But maybe that's because you can't be a veteran athlete if you don't have young muscles.

sex as exercise

Sex is one of the most pleasant ways of getting regular exercise and the **use it or lose it** principle applies to sex as much to any other aspect of aging. **Sex can get better and better** as we get older. The news is good — research among 80- and 90-year-old women showed that their **desire for sex** was as great as ever, but they were frustrated by the paucity of partners!

mental exercise keeps your mind young

And exercising the mind **keeps the body young**. Regular mental exercise like doing crossword puzzles and playing chess **slows down memory loss**. There is also some evidence that education beyond school can delay the onset of Alzheimer's. One of the best ways to put your mind through its paces is to **keep learning** and tackling new situations — that

taking vigorous exercise can

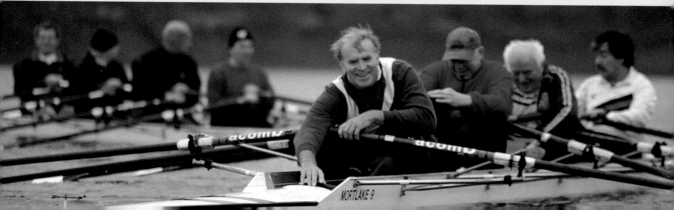

keeps the brain young. Just reading this book is probably adding a year or so to your life.

effects of physical exercise

Physical exercise increases the **adaptability** of the heart and lungs, thus compensating for the decline in function that occurs with age. It also opens up "spare" arteries to the heart muscle, ensuring that blood will reach the tissues even if one gets blocked off. Exercise **reduces the likelihood of a heart attack** and lowers blood pressure, thereby reducing the risk of stroke.

The elastic limits of exercise are enormous. Testimony to this are the geriatric marathon runners – the oldest competitor in the 2002 London Marathon was a **90-year-old woman** who completed the 26-mile race in 11 hours 34 minutes. This kind of fitness isn't achievable by all of us unless we are fanatical about exercise so it's better to concentrate on realistic goals – moderate fitness should be our aim.

DEFYING AGE

As Dr. James Le Fanu says in his book, *How to Live to 90*, there are three ways we can set about defying the diseases that make us old.

1 **Change your lifestyle** to incorporate the healthy habits recommended in this book. These could extend your life.

2 **Have regular tests** and screening to spot the early signs of the diseases we think of as "old."

3 Where appropriate, **get prescription drugs** from your doctor to prevent diseases or to treat the early stages and halt their progress. An example would be a statin drug to lower cholesterol.

what changes as we get older

We're all aware of the three major age-related diseases – **heart disease, stroke,** and **cancer.** The chances of suffering from one of these

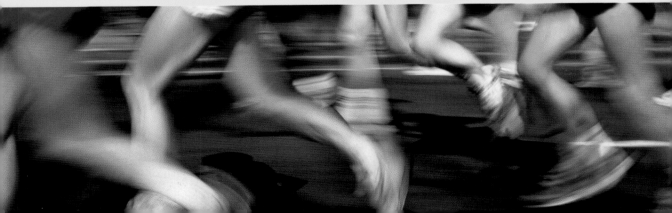

slow down muscle aging

diseases increases with each decade of life – though it doesn't have to. The basic defect which underlies both heart disease and stroke is what occurs in **the lining of our arteries.**

Arteries are one of the most stressed organs of the body, subject to the pressure of each heartbeat – that's your blood pressure – and in particular, to the turbulence of blood flow which results from 80 beats per minute for 70 years. It's not surprising that our arteries show signs of wear and tear when we get to 60 or 70.

The main sign is a condition called **atherosclerosis** when the arteries become narrowed by lumps of fat deposited just under the surface. A distorted artery carries insufficient blood to the tissues, depriving them of oxygen, and this happens in all our organs as we age if the arteries narrow down. In the case of heart muscle, this effect produces pain (**angina**); in the brain it causes lapses of memory, concentration and lowered mental agility. If a clot develops in an artery at the site of damage or next to a fatty lump the dramatic consequence is a heart attack or a stroke depending on where the clot lodges.

Few of us in the West can avoid atherosclerosis altogether. It's virtually a consequence of our diet, even a healthy one. However, if you don't get exercise and lead a sedentary life, if you smoke or have high blood pressure that isn't treated, the development of atherosclerosis accelerates and **causes you to age faster.**

HEALTHY*heart*

IF WE MEASURE CARDIAC OUTPUT – THE RATE AT WHICH THE HEART PUMPS BLOOD AROUND THE BODY – WE FIND LITTLE CHANGE WITH AGE IN HEALTHY PEOPLE WHO GET EXERCISE.

But the heart itself changes quite a lot. Stiffening in the walls of the arteries results in a gradual increase in blood pressure, which the heart has to fight with each beat. To keep output constant the heart has to **work harder** and the left ventricle, the chamber that pumps the blood around the body, grows bigger. Each heartbeat

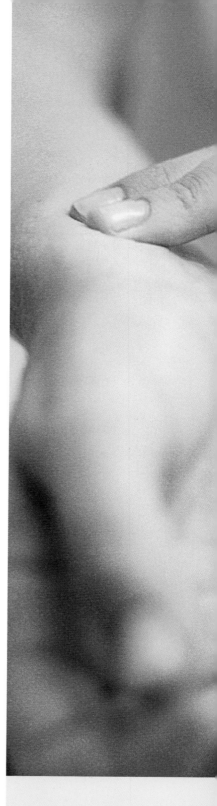

HEART checks

Cholesterol

One of the most crucial factors for arterial health is a low ratio of *dangerous cholesterol* (LDL) to *good cholesterol* (HDL). The thing to remember is that the more LDL you have in your body, the more HDL you need to neutralize it. Some people have such a healthily high level of HDL that no matter how much LDL they accumulate they never have high cholesterol levels. That's why high HDL protects you from heart disease. A high level would be more than 6·0 and a level lower than 3·5 would be in the danger zone.

Homocysteine

Homocysteine is a byproduct of eating protein – mostly from meat sources – but as long as we eat a diet rich in B vitamins such as folic acid, vitamin B6, and vitamin B12, we can convert homocysteine to a harmless byproduct. If we're short of those vitamins, homocysteine levels rise and bring a higher risk of arterial disease, leg ulcers, blood clots (deep vein thrombosis), and possibly dementia, including Alzheimer's disease.

Blood pressure

Because high blood pressure is such a potent risk factor for strokes, it's the most important heart check (see page 83).

costs the heart more and more energy. Eventually overall efficiency of the heart declines and may even drop significantly. **That's why a low blood pressure is healthy** and why your doctor is so pleased to find that your blood pressure is in the normal range – he knows your heart isn't being overworked.

As the heart fights poor nutrition (narrowed arteries) and increased workload (rising blood pressure) we begin to see two distinct features of heart aging:

• **Loss of reserve power** – that's the spare capacity to handle unusual demands like running for a bus.

• **Loss of the ability to take on more work** – the heart can't adapt anymore to cope with its increasing workload, or it takes longer to adapt. In other words it needs a longer "warm up" period to reach peak efficiency and go into overdrive – something I've noticed myself in my daily exercises. It's the most dramatic aspect of heart aging.

keep your arteries and your heart young

A pretty certain rule is that if you **keep your arteries young**, your heart will stay young. In particular, if you keep your coronary arteries – those that supply the heart muscles – young, you cut down your chance of a heart attack and of developing high blood pressure and the symptoms of heart disease like angina.

drugs to prevent your heart and arteries from aging

The latest generation of drugs which lower cholesterol – the **statins** – are considered by many doctors to be **true miracle drugs**. It's now clear that they help prevent heart attacks and strokes too.

In addition, statins probably **reduce a person's risk** of developing diabetes and Alzheimer's disease. In people with certain organ transplants they lower the rate of rejection. Eventually, they could have a role in treating some cancers.

Experts believe more people should take them. Just recently it was suggested that tripling the numbers of Americans taking statins could **reduce heart attacks by a third**. But the ability to

Keep your **HEART AND ARTERIES** healthy

There's EXCELLENT evidence that these lifestyle factors will help

- Eating fish (contains omega-3 fat)
- Keeping weight normal
- Having a low cholesterol ratio (LDL to HDL)
- Having low homocysteine levels
- Diet low in saturated fat

- Physical activity
- Not smoking
- Having good social support
- Keeping depression at bay
- Being able to switch off and relax

There's GOOD evidence that these lifestyle factors will help

- Eating foods that contain flavonoids and folic acid
- Eating vegetables and vitamin E-rich foods
- Moderate alcohol intake

- Eating monounsaturated fats
- Normal blood pressure

There's evidence that these lifestyle factors may POSSIBLY help

- Eating foods rich in vitamins B3, B6, and B12

reduce a person's risk of heart attack and stroke is only one of the things statins can do. In one study of 6,000 men with high cholesterol but no diagnosed heart disease, those assigned to take a drug called **pravastatin** were 30 percent less likely than average to develop diabetes.

And that's not all. People over 50 taking statins have **one-third the risk of developing dementia** compared to those who have normal cholesterol levels and aren't on the drug.

Originally, statins were extracted from fungi. They all work by inhibiting, but not completely blocking, the way the body makes cholesterol – essential to cell membranes and the starting material for many hormones. **The good news** is that statins have been taken for long enough

by so many patients that it's unlikely there'll be unpleasant side effects turning up.

aspirin

Aspirin has been around for decades, but only now are all its healing effects becoming apparent. They are so many and varied that aspirin is being rightly named **a wonder drug**. For people who've had a heart attack or a stroke, **aspirin reduces the risk** of having another as long as the blood pressure isn't high. Only a small dose (75mg) of aspirin is needed every day to protect you from one of these medical emergencies. Taken for a couple of days prior to a long flight it will also protect you from deep vein thrombosis (DVT) – also known as "economy class syndrome" – provided your blood pressure is normal.

Aspirin works because it's a mild blood thinner and prevents clots from forming, so shouldn't everyone take aspirin? Most doctors would say that **only people at high risk** or who have a strong family history of heart attacks should take regular daily doses of aspirin because even a moderately high blood pressure increases the risk of hemorrhagic stroke. These days those same people should probably take 75mg of aspirin prior to taking a long flight to prevent a deep vein thrombosis. Aspirin also appears to **protect against** colon cancer.

keeping your blood pressure young

You can help control your blood pressure by watching your **weight**, getting regular **exercise,** and making sure that your **salt consumption is low**. If these lifestyle approaches fail, you can use medication from your doctor. One of the best things you can do for your children is to **make sure that they never acquire a taste for salt** – or sugar for that matter – by never adding it to food and never having it on the table at mealtimes.

We know that an increased blood pressure is a major factor for strokes and heart attacks. And it can be dealt with by simply going to your doctor once every two years to **check your blood pressure**. Having taken it, your doctor will judge your future blood pressure readings against this initial one.

I'm not in favor of quick checkups of blood pressure. Don't just dash into a clinic, for example, unless you can lie down for 15 minutes before the reading is taken. No blood pressure reading is valid unless you rest before it, nor should one reading alone be considered final. **Three consecutive readings at weekly intervals is the minimum.**

The reason for my being so particular about keeping your blood pressure normal is that the hazards of having high blood pressure are considerable. But however high it may become, **it can be easily treated** and kept within the normal range. Treatments are extremely simple – for instance, the use of diuretics to get rid of excess fluid. These alone can reduce the risk of stroke by something like a third.

If you have mild to moderately high blood pressure (140/90) the first line of attack is **to alter your lifestyle.**

YOUR BLOOD PRESSURE AND YOUR LIFE SPAN

Your chances of a long life	Blood pressure (taken on three separate occasions)
Optimal	Under 120/80
Average	Over 120/80 but under 130/85
Below average	Over 130/85 but under 140/90
Must be treated rigorously	Over 140/90

KEEP *blood pressure* LOW

THERE ARE SEVERAL EASY THINGS YOU CAN DO TO LOWER YOUR BLOOD PRESSURE. NONE IS TOO IRKSOME AND NONE WILL COST YOU EXTRA MONEY. AND THERE'S THE BONUS THAT YOU'LL IMPROVE YOUR OVERALL HEALTH.

The most important measures are as follows:
- **avoid** being overweight
- **keep** your alcohol consumption down
- **reduce** your salt intake or cut out salt alltogether
- **exercise** regularly, a minimum of three times a week for about 30 minutes
- **stop** smoking

KEEP THE WEIGHT OFF

There's a strong link between being overweight and having high blood pressure. If your weight's above normal for your height, you should **try to lose the extra pounds** and bring your blood pressure down. You don't need to aim for an ideal weight. Try to be **within the healthy range** for your height. If you can't lose weight by yourself, your doctor may refer you to a nutritionist for advice on different ways to change how and what you eat. You don't have to give up eating all the food you enjoy. Some people find a dieter's group or club very helpful to give them moral support.

Even if you're not overweight:
- **eat fish**, white meat (for example, chicken without the skin), cottage cheese, low-fat yogurt, low-fat milk.
- **aim** for seven pieces of fresh fruit and vegetables a day – eat seasonal vegetables and fruit when you can; when fresh vegetables are expensive eat frozen ones instead. A diet containing plenty of fruit and vegetables increases potassium intake, and this can help lower your blood pressure too.
- **broil** food instead of frying it when possible.
- **don't** eat butter, cheese, and whole milk, fried foods and snacks, cakes, cookies, and chocolate, fatty meat.

REDUCE SALT INTAKE

A HIGH intake of salt affects your blood pressure. Salt can also increase the amount of fluid that you retain in your body.

Fresh food contains very little salt. Most of the salt we eat is in processed foods, or in salt added to food while cooking or at the table. So try to reduce the amount of salt you eat.
- **Look at labels** on food you eat. If sodium chloride (NaCl), sodium bensoate, or monosodium glutamate are included in the list you may be eating extra salt without knowing.
- **Cut down** on processed foods. Salt is hidden in many processed foods – canned or packaged soups, breakfast cereals, bread, canned or processed fish, chips, nuts, burgers, and prepared meals.
- **Look** for low-salt bread – some supermarkets do sell it.
- **Cut down** on hard cheese, bacon, ham, sausages, and corned beef which all contain a lot of salt as do smoked meats and cheese.

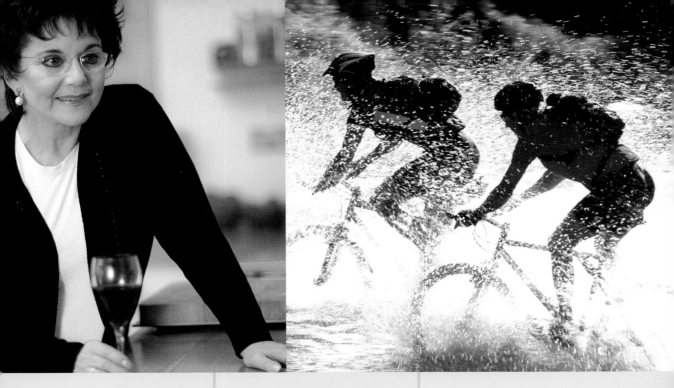

• **Use salt very sparingly** in cooking, if at all. If you feel that you can't do without salt, you might try a salt substitute (after checking with your doctor). Rock salt and sea salt are not salt substitutes.

It's better to **avoid the taste of salt altogether.** You'll find that your sense of taste adjusts so that you no longer like the taste of salt, especially if you add herbs such as basil and thyme that release the natural salts in food to your cooking.

KEEP YOUR ALCOHOL LEVELS DOWN

Drinking a moderate amount of alcohol is harmless unless you're trying to lose weight, but high alcohol intake **increases your chance** of developing high blood pressure.

• Limit your alcohol to no more than 21 units per week. One unit is equal to a small glass of wine OR ten ounces of ordinary-strength beer, ale, or lager OR a single measure of liquor.

• Try to spread your units evenly over the week and avoid a big drinking session.

• A lot of alcohol the night before can raise your blood pressure significantly the next day.

• Talk to your doctor if you're drinking more alcohol than you should and finding it difficult to cut down.

EXERCISE

Exercise can help reduce your blood pressure and keep your weight down. **It's also a good stress reliever.** Stress isn't a cause of high blood pressure although many people believe it is.

What type of exercise should you do? **Any vigorous activity** like walking, swimming, cycling, jogging, dancing, or gardening is good for you. The important thing is to **choose an activity that you enjoy** – if you don't like a particular form of exercise you'll find you won't do it regularly enough. Exercise doesn't need to be too strenuous either. You should **start slowly** and build up the amount of exercise that you do. Start by walking briskly. You don't have to jog unless you want to. Walk the dog; use the stairs, not the elevator and **keep mobile!** Try to do at least 20–30 minutes three times a week. For some people, it isn't advisable to lift heavy weights or to take part in strenuous activities such as playing tennis. Check with your doctor if you're thinking of taking up a new sport that is very taxing. **If you haven't done any exercise recently, speak to your doctor first.**

STOPPING SMOKING

Giving up smoking won't lower your blood pressure, but it lowers your risk of getting high blood pressure by minimizing the chance of blood vessel damage that can lead to a heart attack or stroke. **It's so important that you stop smoking, I suggest you make a plan and prepare yourself to stop. If you have an action plan, prepare well and you'll succeed.**

Many smokers wonder if aids to quit smoking work and if they should try them. Most experts agree, and I am with them, that there's no substitute for will power, but it's worth trying nicotine gum or skin patches, hypnosis, acupuncture, and going to smoking cessation clinics. Your doctor or pharmacist can give advice on how to stop smoking and on aids to help you.

GET A DOG!

This is probably the best single thing you can do to keep your blood pressure down and your heart healthy. There are many studies that show **pets are good for your health** and help you to live longer:

• An Australian study has shown blood pressure and cholesterol are lower in pet owners.

• Pet owners are more likely to be alive one year after a heart attack .

• Under test conditions women's hearts responded better to stress when their dogs were nearby than when alone or with a supportive woman friend.

• A dog's companionship is healing – of those who suffer bereavement, dog owners see their doctors less often than people without a dog.

DRUGS TO LOWER your blood pressure

Mild blood pressure may not need medical treatment, merely **changes to lifestyle**, such as lowering your salt intake, getting regular exercise, and losing weight. The simplest form of drug treatment is a water pill or *diuretic* but, as a side effect, this may reveal hidden diabetes and cause impotence in men. The third line of drug treatment involves an array of treatments to lower blood pressure, which once started should continue and be monitored for the rest of your life to keep your blood pressure down.

◆ Have your **blood pressure** checked every two years.

◆ Don't start treatment unless it's been found to be high on at least **three** separate occasions.

◆ After a couple of years discuss the possibility of **stopping treatment** to see if your blood pressure remains normal.

STOP *your brain from* AGING

IN OLD AGE PEOPLE FIND IT EASIER TO REMEMBER THE DISTANT PAST THAN THE RECENT PAST. BUT THE AGE-RELATED ASPECT OF FORGETFULNESS IS REALLY QUITE MODEST.

We do lose a number of brain cells as we get older, but **a minuscule amount in proportion to the number that remain**. A more significant cause of declining mental function is likely to be oxygen deficiency due to the stiffening and narrowing up of arteries.

Opinions and attitudes can also become more rigid, so that the acceptance of new ideas or information can become progressively more difficult. But as long as **mental skills are exercised continuously,** they shouldn't decline to any significant degree. It's not, however, so easy to master complex new skills.

Although intellectual deterioration is considered to be a result of aging, it's actually a physical process that begins around the age of 16. For most of our adult lives, we don't notice any deterioration, mainly because we gain new experiences and knowledge, which compensate. This is why **an alert mind** and a willingness to embrace new ideas, opinions, and situations will keep us **mentally young**. It's important to **keep thinking and planning for yourself**. Age itself shouldn't bring any marked intellectual decline.

how you can defy aging of your brain

Mental fitness can be as easy to maintain as physical fitness, and we must strive to maintain a basic state of mental health so that we can **rise to challenges**, cope with emergencies, and have the resilience to survive stressful situations in the long-term. As we get older, we have to deal with emotional trauma, such as the loss of parents and possibly our partner.

Self-knowledge requires **supreme realism**: we have to learn that we aren't unique in suffering, that difficult times come and go, that adversity is normal, and that some failures are inevitable. As we grow older, we should leave behind preconceptions and prejudices, and constantly be prepared to **change our attitudes**. We need to work with our emotions in a constructive and helpful way, and yet still be affectionate and tender with ourselves.

staying mentally fit

We can learn a lot by observing the qualities of people whose **mental and emotional resilience** we admire. The following qualities result from emotional openness, flexibility, and self-reliance:
- **Independence** and recognition of others' independence, privacy, and peace.
- **Lack of self-pity**, so that when a problem arises it's looked at objectively.
- The attitude that **nothing is hopeless** and problems are there to be solved.
- A sense of **inner security** rather than security gained from controlling others.
- Being prepared to take on **responsibility** for your own mistakes.

- Having a few **close relationships** rather than many superficial ones.
- A sense of **realism about the goals** you can set yourself.
- Being **in touch with your emotions**, and feeling free to express them.

Just as a muscle becomes weak and wastes away if it's not exercised, so your brain will slow and become feeble if you don't think. The **best mental exercise is work**. Research on Japanese octogenarians showed that those who kept going into their offices, even for an hour a day, had greater mental powers and lived longer than those who had retired at 60 and given up disciplined thinking.

So the first tip to **maintain mental fitness** is daily intellectual work. It helps if your efforts are judged by your peers, but work of any kind provides mental stimuli. Interaction with other people forces you to assess what they're saying, and respond with questions and comments. Your brain has to assimilate information and your cognitive processes remain active.

keep thinking

As we get older, it can become more difficult for us to form new brain connections, so we have to make certain that old and well-established connections are continually used. The only way to do this is through **thinking**. Thinking is not a passive process – it means engaging in, questioning, and absorbing what is happening all around us.

For example, arithmetical "exercises" are encountered in daily life and you can engage in them more actively. Anticipate your supermarket bill by adding up the cost of your shopping as you put things in your basket, or estimate how much change you'll receive. Try to judge the size and quantity of objects and then measure them to check on your judgement.

Try to add to your vocabulary by noting down each new word you see or hear on a daily basis. Keep a dictionary handy to check on meanings, and use the word in subsequent conversations. Read a daily newspaper article or watch the television news and discuss the main events of the day with a friend.

Think of your brain as a **muscle that needs exercising**. One of the best brain exercises is learning something new – a new language is exactly the kind of challenge your brain needs to stay agile. Tackling a new language can be daunting but becomes less so if you know how your brain would prefer to go about it, so try the **learning questionnaire** opposite.

Think about taking evening classes. The range of courses available to adults is huge – there are craft courses that take up a couple of hours a week or you can take full-time courses in academic subjects such as history or literature.

maintaining memory

As we get older, our long-term memory gets clearer; it's our short-term memory that may suffer. If you are worried about being forgetful, there are several exercises and techniques that will aid your short-term memory.
- When you read a book or a magazine article, **summarize the plot** or the points made in it to a friend. Refer to names, places, and dates.
- When you're going shopping, try to collect as many items as you can without referring to your shopping list.

DISCOVER YOUR LEARNING STYLE

Following your own style is important if you want to keep learning right to the end of your life. Find out your learning style from this questionnaire – it will point the way to how you can keep your brain young. Choose one answer to each question.

1 When studying an unfamiliar subject, you:
a prefer to gather information from diverse topic areas
b prefer to focus on one topic

2 You would rather:
a know a little about a great many subjects
b become an expert on just one subject

3 When studying from a textbook, you:
a skip ahead and read chapters of special interest out of sequence
b work systematically from one chapter to the next, not moving on until you have understood earlier material

4 You are best at remembering:
a general principles
b specific facts

5 When asking people for information about some subject of interest, you:
a tend to ask broad questions that call for somewhat general answers

b tend to ask narrow questions that demand specific answers

6 When browsing in a library or bookstore, you:
a roam around looking at books on many different subjects
b stay more or less in one place looking at books on just a couple of subjects

7 When performing some tasks, you:
a like to have background information not strictly related to the work
b prefer to concentrate only on strictly relevant information

8 You think that educators should:
a give students exposure to a wide range of subjects in college
b ensure that students mainly acquire in-depth knowledge related to their specialities

9 When on vacation, you'd rather
a spend a short amount of time in several places
b stay in one place the whole time and get to know it well

10 When learning something, you would rather:
a follow general guidelines
b work with a detailed plan of action

11 Do you agree that, in addition to specialized knowledge, a person should know some math, art, physics, literature, psychology, politics, languages, biology, history, and medicine?
If you think people should study four or more of these subjects, score an **a** on this question.

SCORE
Add up your **a** and **b** answers.
If you marked six or more of the questions with an **a** you're a big picture person. You learn best in an unstructured way, not bothering about details at first, jumping about from place to place and working on several topics at once.
With six or more of **b** you're a detailed person who works systematically and logically. You absorb material thoroughly before moving on and you love the sense of mastery you feel with each step.

TESTING FOR **ALZHEIMER'S**

As Alzheimer's disease is diagnosed more and more, many families worry that a parent or relative is in the early stages of this condition. Trying this test, sensitively, might give you an idea of whether or not you need to check with the doctor.

TEST 1: How good is his memory and concentration?

Ask the following questions. If he gets any answers wrong, make a note of the points scored. Score 0 for correct answers.

1 What year is it now? *Score 4 points for a wrong answer*

2 What month is it now? *Score 3 points for a wrong answer*

Now ask your relative to repeat this memory phrase aloud: Mary Smith, 20 Market Street, Springfield

3 About what time is it? (within 1 hour). *Score 3 points for a wrong answer*

4 Count backward from 20 to 10. *Score 2 points for one mistake; score 4 points for 2 or more mistakes*

5 Say the months of the year in reverse order. *Score 2 points for one mistake; score 4 points for 2 or more mistakes*

6 Ask your relative to repeat the memory phrase again. *Score 2 points for each mistake to a maximum of 10 points*

TEST ONE SCORE: The score can range from 0 (no mistakes) to 28 (all wrong). A score greater than 10 may indicate Alzheimer's.

TEST 2: How independent is he?

This test helps you measure how dependent on others your relative has become. The higher the score, the more dependent. For each question, select the answer from the following list that best describes the current situation and add up the points.

3 points: dependent
2 points: needs help
1 point: does (or could do) by himself but with difficulty
0 points: does (or could do) by himself with no difficulty.

Assess your relative's capability on the following activities and score accordingly

1 Writing checks, paying bills, etc.

2 Completing tax returns or papers, handling business affairs

3 Shopping alone for clothes, household necessities, or groceries

4 Playing game of skill, working on a hobby

5 Heating water, making cup of coffee, turning off the stove

6 Preparing a balanced meal

7 Keeping track of current events

8 Paying attention to, understanding, discussing TV, or a book or magazine

9 Remembering appointments, family occasions, holidays, medications

10 Traveling out of neighborhood, driving, arranging to take a bus

TEST TWO SCORE: A score higher than 9 may indicate Alzheimer's.

TOTAL SCORE: Add the scores of tests one and two to make the total. A total of higher than 20 points may indicate Alzheimer's.

• If you walk into a room and forget why you've gone into it, go back to the place that you came from and don't leave until you have remembered the reason for going there.

• If you've lost something, **track it down by a process of elimination.** Write down the last six things you did prior to losing it and where you were for each activity. If necessary, **draw a grid** on a piece of paper with what you were doing along one side and where you were along the bottom. The item you've lost lies in one of those squares; just check each one out.

HELP YOUR MEMORY

If there are several things you want to remember to do, try using a mnemonic. For example, tasks such as ironing a shirt, making a phone call, and typing an e-mail can be abbreviated into a single word. Take the first letters of each task, and make them into a word, for example "PIT" (Phone/Iron/Type), which will act as a memory aid.

your most powerful anti-aging tool

It used to be thought that the brain could not repair itself, that it couldn't grow new brain cells to replace those that died. We now know this is not the case: **exercise releases hormones that stimulate the growth of new brain cells** and cell connections. So exercise reverses some of the effect of aging of the brain. Some new research points the way to **keeping our memories fresh.** It may be that your memory isn't going, you've just forgotten how to use it. Here's how researchers have figured out you can reclaim it.

American researchers monitored brain activity in old and young adults while they memorized words. The younger group performed better and a specific region of their brain lit up as they did the task.

That didn't happen in the older subjects, but when they were told to think of the word's meaning at the same time, the brain was activated and their **performance improved dramatically.** Researchers speculate that younger people spontaneously employ this memory strategy, but as the brain ages it stops using it automatically.

drugs to halt dementia

There is no cure for dementia, but drugs such as donepezil may slow the loss of mental function in mild to moderate cases.

HRT (and possibly **aspirin** and NSAIDs) will protect against the development of Alzheimer's as well as helping you to retain your memory, keep emotionally stable, concentrate, assess new information, and make decisions – **all expressions of a youthful brain.**

There isn't a routine test at present that will pick up or warn of Alzheimer's, though scans will detect brain shrinkage in established Alzheimer's patients. The test opposite can act as a useful screen before consulting a doctor, but be very careful not to pressure or upset your relative if you decide to try the test.

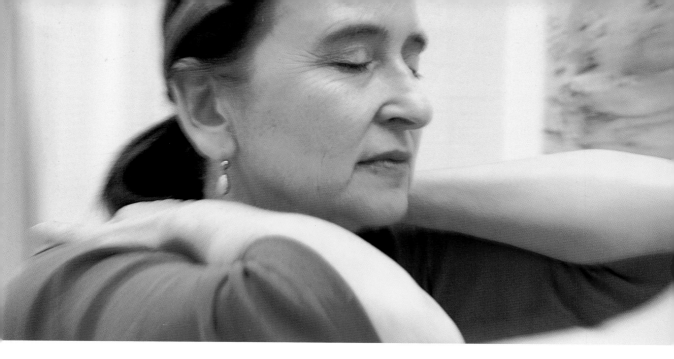

HOW*our joints*AGE

ANY FORM OF ARTHRITIS LIMITS MOVEMENT AND MOBILITY. IT CAN CUT DOWN OUR ENJOYMENT OF LIFE AS WE GET OLDER.

There are two main types of arthritis: **rheumatoid arthritis**, which can occur at any age and has an immunological basis, and **osteoarthritis,** which we traditionally think of as the aging of joints through wear and tear. It typically shows up after 60. It's this type of arthritis that we can all try to avoid.

Osteoarthritis is a thinning, wearing down, or roughening of the cartilage that covers the ends of the bones at the joints. This damage may be complicated by chemical changes in the cartilage which can cause a joint to become inflamed, painful, and stiff.

Arthritis is one of the oldest diseases known. Paintings done by early man more than 40,000 years ago illustrate an arthritic relative who is stooped and walks with bent knees. Arthritis occurs in all races and at all ages. Just as most functions in the body begin to show measurable decline around the age of 30, early signs of joint degeneration begin to appear. Everyone over 35 has some tiny degree of osteoarthritis, but we can do a lot to halt its progression. It also occurs in animals – the *Diplodocus* dinosaur at the Natural History Museum in London has arthritis in its tail!

why do we get arthritis?

Nobody knows exactly why osteoarthritis occurs, but it does become more frequent as we get older and has been described as part of the normal aging process that affects us all.

HOW TO CHEAT OSTEOARTHRITIS

Quite often the initial changes in osteoarthritis are symptomless, so it's essential that you embark on a life-long program, certainly from your twenties onward, of taking care of your joints.
The main factors that keep joints healthy, mobile, and young would come under the heading of lifestyle.

◆ **Destress your joints** by not becoming overweight; remember all your weight eventually is borne by your knees and ankles.

◆ **Put** your joints continually through their full range of movement by playing sports and keeping active.

◆ **Protect your spine** by paying attention to posture.

◆ **Nurse your back** by lifting heavy weights correctly (with your thighs) and always sitting with good lumbar support.

◆ **Fit, firm, strong muscles** protect joints, so strong abdominal muscles act as a supportive splint for your back and will do so all your life if you make time to exercise muscle groups.

◆ **Avoid** sports that injure joints – for example soccer, which damages knees.

It's unusual for it to show before middle age, unless there's previous injury or prolonged stress to a joint. Other factors, such as being overweight and having bad posture, will worsen the condition. It occurs most frequently in those joints that are subjected to the **most stress**: knees, hips, ankles, feet, hands, and spine.

The main symptoms of arthritis are painful, creaky joints. Even small joints like those of the fingers and toes are affected as well as the bigger, weight-bearing joints, which take the most wear and tear during life. One of the most familiar places for osteoarthritis is in the final joints of the fingers and thumb – this shows up after menopause. As a sort of defense against arthritis, the body quite often builds up little pieces of bone around the joints, so you often can see the pea-sized swellings at the side of the joints that are characteristic of osteoarthritis. They're called **Heberden's nodes** after the man who first described them.

Far and away the most common weight-bearing joints to be involved are the knees and hips. In the knee you can often hear a grating sound as the rough cartilages grind together. Later on there may be so much pain that the range of movement of the knee is limited. Then there may be loss of stability in the knee joint too. I've often heard people say that their "knee lets them down" and this causes them to fall. Just as the joints build bone to form Heberden's nodes in the fingers, so they do in the knee and it may become swollen and deformed and fluid may collect.

Osteoarthritis of the hip is probably the most disabling type of arthritis because the pain and stiffness interfere so crucially with everyday life. It makes getting out of a chair very difficult, climbing on and off a bus very slow, walking up and down the stairs an act of endurance, and getting in and out of the bath quite hazardous. Sometimes it's difficult to pinpoint osteoarthritis

"Start caring for your joints from your 20s onward if you want to lessen your chances of arthritis"

in the hip because pain isn't always felt there — it's often referred down to the knees. The arthritis progresses in exactly the same way as in the knee.

do supplements work?

Some people swear by supplements such as chondroitin sulphate to curb stiffness in joints, but good medical data to support such claims are scant.

Since 1974 New Zealanders have been using green-lipped mussel for its anti-inflammatory and antiarthritic powers and there does seem to be some reasonable science behind it. This species of mussel contains COX-2 inflammatory inhibitors, well known to the pharmaceutical industry as **powerful anti-inflammatory agents** with few side effects. Research is ongoing at Dunedin University in New Zealand.

drugs to treat osteoarthritis

There's no known cure for osteoarthritis. Relief from discomfort is achieved through the judicious use of anti-inflammatory agents and analgesics.

If your osteoarthritis is going to be a long-term condition, then your treatment and management should also be viewed in the long term. The mainstay of treatment is pain-killing drugs. Some of the newer NSAIDs (nonsteroidal anti-inflammatory drugs) don't have to be taken more than once or twice a day, are very effective in relieving pain, help to increase mobility and strength, and may alter the course of the arthritis. **Physical therapy** is also extremely important in encouraging full movement of the joints, thereby increasing the muscle strength in the limbs and leading to greater stability and mobility. A wider range of movements, particularly for the hip and knee joints, help to distribute forces such as weight bearing over a larger area of the joint's surface and this helps prevent its gradual deterioration.

These days almost any joint that has been damaged by arthritis or injury can be surgically **replaced with an artificial one made of metal, ceramic, or plastic.** The most common operations are on the hip and knee and they can be done whatever your age.

HIP*replacement*

A HIP OPERATION CAN GIVE YOU A NEW LEASE ON LIFE AND ALLOW YOU TO START DANCING AND PLAYING SPORTS AGAIN.

In a **hip replacement operation**, both the pelvic socket and the head of the thighbone (femur) are replaced with an artificial joint. You'll need a general anesthetic and a short stay in the hospital. In the first two weeks following the operation, the new joint is unstable and patients must be careful not to dislocate it.

Hip replacement has been used primarily to treat hips that are worn out by osteoarthritis, making walking difficult and day-to-day life painful. But now we have newer techniques that **prolong the life of artificial hips** and can treat younger patients. Nearly 50,000 hip operations are done in Britain each year, of which more than two-thirds are for severe osteoarthritis and the rest are for a variety of conditions that cause deterioration of the hip joint.

why is it done?

Hip replacement is most often performed in older people whose joints are stiff and painful as a result of osteoarthritis and who find medication isn't effective. It may also be needed if rheumatoid arthritis has spread to the hip joint, making walking difficult, or if the top end of the femur is badly fractured and, after healing, the surface of the bone is irregular.

The operation isn't usually advised for young patients, since their greater activity puts more strain on the artificial joints and it isn't known how long a replacement is likely to last.

self help pre-op

The **best way of helping yourself** before the operation is to **lose weight**. Every pound lost can help because during normal walking the human hip can experience forces equivalent to three to five times body weight. During strenuous activity, this may rise to as much as twelve times body weight. So, a woman weighing 132lb (60kg) may sometimes put pressure on her hips that is equivalent to 1500lb (**720kg**)!

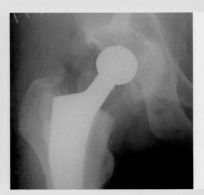

What happens in a hip replacement operation?

In the basic operation, the surgeon cuts off the top of the femur, the thigh bone, which forms the ball-and-socket hip joint. The "socket" part of the joint that sits in the pelvic bone is then enlarged and lined to take the artificial "ball" part of the joint. This socket can be made of metal or plastic; the ball and the shaft are metal. The shaft of the femur is then hollowed out to accommodate the shaft on which the ball sits. It's fixed in place with a special cement that binds it to the bone of the hollowed-out femur.

what kind of artificial hip?

There are at least **60 different artificial hips** available and there are two main types: those which are fixed using special cement, and non-cemented hip replacements. The latter rely either on being fitted very tightly into the bone, or by the use of specially placed holes in the artificial hip into which the new bone grows, fixing the new joint in place. This type is usually used for younger patients who may need another replacement in the future.

recovery period

You'll find the joint remains unstable for a week or two after the operation, and you must be careful not to dislocate the new joint during this time. You'll be advised to sleep on your back and not to cross your legs, and you'll be taught how to get in and out of the bath without disturbing your new joint.

post-op

After surgery, you'll lie on your back with your legs separated by a wedge-shaped cushion to make sure that the new joint remains in the correct position. Walking is allowed after a few days, using a walker or crutches, and gradually most activities are resumed. For example, most people are able to drive after about eight weeks.

are there any complications?

There's a level of risk attached to any surgical procedure and this will have been assessed by your surgeon. However, the likelihood of complications during or after a total hip replacement is small. Infection of the wound or new hip occurs in about 1 percent of cases and in about 3 percent the ball of the joint may dislocate. This is why it's important to restrict certain movements during the healing stage.

A hip replacement operation is usually very successful. There's a 95 percent chance that the operation will leave patients totally free from pain and, in time, regain 75 percent of their normal range of movement.

outlook

Hip replacement can change your life – **it's a remarkably successful operation** that has transformed the lives of many people who suffered from severe pain and stiffness. However, with time, a substantial proportion of artificial joints show signs on X-ray of loosening at the cemented union between the bone and the metal shaft that holds the ball in place.

Surgeons and bioengineers are continuing to develop **newer joint designs** that don't rely on cement to hold them in place. They're also trying to improve the surfaces of the implant materials, so that they grow together with the patient's own bone to reduce wear, making replacement unnecessary.

Hip resurfacing works best in patients who do worse with hip replacement. The diseased or damaged surfaces of the hip joint are removed and a metal cap is fitted over the ball of the joint with cement. This slots into a metal liner in the hip socket using hydroxyapatite, a synthetic bone into which the surrounding bone grows. **Recovery is quicker** and because less bone is cut away from the patient's own hips, it's possible to do a full hip replacement later in life if needed. It isn't suitable for older patients because their bone quality and strength is not so good.

KEEP *cancers* AT BAY

CANCERS AREN'T ONE DISEASE ANY MORE THAN VIRUS INFECTIONS ARE CONFINED TO THE FLU. THERE'S A SPECTRUM GOING FROM BENIGN TO MALIGNANT TO AGGRESSIVE.

Many cancers are slow growing and relatively benign, allowing many opportunities for spotting them early and eradicating them completely.

The first check you can run on yourself to see if you're a possible candidate for a cancer (and take the appropriate action for regular monitoring) is to **find out your family history**. Some cancers do run in families. In some families there may be a clear cancer gene like the BRCA-1 for breast cancer, ovarian cancer, and colon cancer. If your family has such a history or gene you should get expert medical advice. This alone could assure you a long life.

But, in addition there are signs you must never ignore (see below). Of themselves they don't point to cancer but, once they're reported, a doctor will work toward ruling out cancer.

On a brighter note, there's more and more information accumulating that **some easily achievable lifestyle changes** may guard against cancers. Here's a few – take your pick:
• **Look at what you're eating** and how you're eating.
• Eating **certain foods and eating less of everything** could protect you from cancer. The Okinawans consume about 40 percent fewer calories than we do and have many fewer cancers than we do. **Lower-calorie diets protect** because they result in fewer damaging free radicals. The key is to eat a high complex carbohydrate, high-fiber diet, so you get low-calorie, oxidant-rich, minimally processed whole food. You eat more, you weigh less, you stay young, AND YOU PROTECT YOURSELF FROM CANCER.
• Eating a low-calorie diet will mean you have **a low total body fat**, one of the ways in which you can protect your body against cancers from springing up. The link here is thought to be with "cancer-causing" hormones such as **insulin-like growth factor**, which is plentiful if you're fat. If you stay lean you **minimize your exposure** to these insidious hormones.

DON'T IGNORE THESE SIGNS

◆ Any change in a wart or mole
◆ Any ulcer that doesn't heal
◆ A sudden change in bowel habit
◆ Sudden hoarseness of the voice or a persistent cough
◆ Persistent heartburn or indigestion
◆ A lump or thickening in the breast
◆ The sudden appearance of blood or discharge

CANCER-DEFYING HABITS

Here are some simple lifestyle habits to adopt that will help you defy age and reduce your risk of cancer. They're painless – and they'll make a difference.

fruit and vegetables are the key Protect yourself by eating **as many fruits and vegetables as you can** every day. What most health educators recommend is five fruits and vegetables a day. However, the Okinawans eat many more and if you count rice, bean sprouts, nuts, and seeds they get closer to 12 or 13. Fruits and vegetables are high-fiber foods (complex carbohydrates) that don't result in high blood sugar. They don't therefore stimulate the production of insulin and insulin-like growth factor and so may protect against cancers of the breast, prostate, and colon.

healthy fats help Another way of protecting yourself against cancer is to eat *good fats*. This involves a high intake of monounsaturated fats (see page 154) and a high intake of omega-3 polyunsaturated fat to balance out the omega-6-loaded Western diet (see page 159).

substitute soy Foods (mainly soy and flax) containing flavonoids (the flavonols, the flavones, the isoflavones, and the bioflavonoids) all seem to protect against cancer (see page 154). The most recent study from Australia shows that women who eat the **most soy flavonoids** are at significantly lower risk of breast cancer than those who have a minimal flavonoid intake.

ditch the drink If you want to stay free of cancer your alcohol consumption must be no more than *moderate*. Men who are heavy drinkers even increase their risk of breast and esophageal cancer. The link with colon cancer may be through folic acid, which is thought to protect against colon cancer, and which is destroyed by alcohol. Keep well below recommended limits – no more than 3–4 units a day for men and 2–3 for women.

excel at exercise The exercise story isn't finished yet. As I say throughout this book exercise is pivotal in reducing the risk of many diseases, including cancers of the colon and breast. We still don't know why exercise is such a powerful preventive factor. It may act in many different ways, including lowering body fat levels and decreasing circulating insulin levels. Exercise helps the muscles mop up insulin so there's less around to stimulate cancer growth in breast or colon cells. **Exercise may decrease your risk of getting any cancer by as much as half**, and all you have to do is to walk briskly for half an hour or more every day or tend your garden. The key is keeping active.

screening for free radicals

As we know free radicals are highly reactive compounds produced during normal cell metabolism that damage other cells in the body and are thought to be the main cause of aging (see page 13). Changes to your lifestyle such as a low calorie intake, a diet high in antioxidant foods like vegetables, and regular physical activity can limit the amount of free radical damage.

One of the most important research findings is that eating fewer calories increases your life span because low calorie intake also reduces the level of free radicals in the blood. The **plasma lipid peroxide** is the measure of free radicals in the blood and we know from studying the Okinawans that their way of life results in a **lower lipid peroxide** than people of a similar age following a Western way of life.

avoiding breast cancer

Before the age of about 45 the breast is too fibrous for mammography to be a useful tool. After this age however, **regular mammographic screening** should be performed **every three years** for the rest of a woman's life. There's now clear evidence that early detection by screening cuts down the number of women dying from breast cancer.

During her fertile years, frequent breast self-examination makes every woman aware of her breasts so that she's familiar with their shape and texture at various times of the month. She's poised to spot a new lump should it appear and she can seek advice from her doctor right away. In women under 45 with suspected tumor of the breast, ultrasound investigation is often fruitful.

Reduce your risk of **BREAST CANCER**

There's evidence that these lifestyle factors will PROBABLY help you

- Having children, with first pregnancy before 30
- Breast-feeding
- Eating fruit and vegetables
- Eating foods containing vitamin A, carotenoids, fiber, flavonoids, natural SERMs (see page 45)
- Keeping weight normal
- Staying active
- Not smoking
- Low alcohol intake

And these may POSSIBLY help too

- Eating fatty fish (contains omega-3 fat)
- Eating food containing lycopene (tomatoes)
- Eating foods containing monounsaturated fat, omega-3 fat, vitamin C
- Eating a diet low in animal protein and saturated (animal) fats

Interpreting your **PAP SMEAR** results

Results	Next action
Negative	No follow-up; next smear in three years
The mildest inflammation known as mild dysplasia, or CIN I	Another Pap smear in six months
More severe inflammation called moderate dysplasia, or CIN 2	Colposcopy (non-invasive, used for further examination)
Severe dysplasia with or without noninvasive cancer, or CIN III	Colposcopy with or without cone biopsy

avoiding cervical cancer

No woman who is regularly screened will develop cervical cancer. The screening test to prevent cancer of the cervix is the **cervical Pap smear.** Women should have Pap smears within six months of becoming sexually active, then every three to five years until they reach the age of 60.

avoiding prostate cancer

Many of the same risk factors that apply to breast cancer apply to prostate cancer. One growth factor that might link these two cancers, and possibly colon cancer as well, is the insulin-like growth factor (IGF-1) and it's produced in higher than normal amounts in overweight people. Men with a high IGF-1 level were found to be much more likely to get prostate cancer so

Stages of **CERVICAL PRECANCER** and **CANCER** explained

PRECANCER
The mildest stage, known as mild dysplasia or **CIN I**
More severe inflammation, NOT CANCER, called moderate dysplasia or **CIN II**
Severe dysplasia, with or without noninvasive cancer in situ, or **CIN III**

CANCER
Stage 1 Cancer confined to the cervix
Stage 2 Cancer extends beyond the cervix to involve the top of the vagina and/or tissue immediately surrounding the cervix
Stage 3 Cancer extends to the lower part of the vagina and/or the side wall of the pelvis
Stage 4 Cancer extends beyond the pelvis and/or involves the bladder or rectum

Because CIN III takes several years to go on to STAGE I a Pap smear every three years will pick up changes before cancer can spread and action can be taken to prevent that from ever happening.

the message is yet again, **watch your weight and keep total body fat levels down.**

While prostate cancer is endemic in the Western world and Europe, it's much less prevalant in Okinawa, 80 percent less so in fact. **Vegetables seem to protect against prostate cancer** and certain vegetable constituents may inhibit the cancer process: flavonoids in soy; beta-carotene in carrots; lycopene in tomatoes.

PSA (Prostate-specific antigen) is a marker for prostate cancer risk. High total body fat and high alcohol intake adds to this risk factor and **soy foods lower it.** A diet high in flavonoids may even stop prostate cancer cells growing.

prostate cancer screening

This cancer may be silent until it's quite advanced but the possibility of **detecting it early has greatly improved** since we've had a blood test for a chemical marker, the Prostate Specific Antigen or PSA. Any man who notices urinary symptoms such as urgency, dribbling or difficulty starting to urinate should ask his doctor for a PSA test. PSA is prostate specific but not cancer specific. A raised reading, though not always indicative of prostatic cancer, is the signal for further tests to confirm **early diagnosis** and begin treatment while the cancer is still confined to the gland and **potentially curable.**

False positives do arise because PSA may be high simply with benign enlargement of the prostate. Prostate cancer is treated less and less with a prostatectomy (radical surgery to remove the gland in its entirety) and more and more with "watchful waiting."

Reduce your risk of **PROSTATE CANCER**

There's evidence that these lifestyle factors will PROBABLY help protect you

- Eating foods containing carotenoids, flavonoids, vitamins D and E
- Eating soy products, tomatoes (for lycopene), vegetables
- Low intake of meat, milk, and other dairy products
- Low intake of saturated fat

And these may POSSIBLY help too

- Low calorie intake
- Polyunsaturated fatty acids from vegetables, not animal foods
- Low alcohol intake
- Not being overweight

Reduce your risk of **COLON CANCER**

There's EXCELLENT evidence that these lifestyle factors will help protect you

- Physical activity
- Eating vegetables

And there's evidence that these will PROBABLY protect you

- Eating foods containing carotenoids, fiber, flavonoids, and lignans (plant nutrients)
- High folic acid intake
- Eating low GI foods (starch)
- Low alcohol intake
- Not being overweight
- Low intake of red meat
- Avoiding overcooked or processed meat
- Not smoking
- Diet low in saturated (animal) fat

These may POSSIBLY help too

- Eating cereals and foods containing vitamins C, D, E
- Coffee
- Low calorie intake

Reduce your risk of **OVARIAN CANCER**

There's evidence that these lifestyle factors will PROBABLY help protect you

- Breast-feeding
- Taking oral contraceptives
- Taking HRT
- Eating vegetables and fruit
- Having children
- Not being overweight

And these may POSSIBLY help too

- Eating food containing carotenoids and flavonoids
- Eating fish
- Low intake of milk products and saturated animal fats
- Low total fat intake

avoiding colon cancer

Colon cancer is the second most common cancer in most Western countries. It's probably better understood than any other cancer because the lining of the colon can turn from normal to abnormal due to dietary challenges. These challenges damage the colon's genetic machinery. This first stage is called cancer initiation. The abnormal cells then begin to reproduce themselves – this is called cancer promotion. Given an increase supply of growth factors such as insulin (from being overweight) they will grow rapidly and produce a lump called a polyp. Once in this form, a cancer will quickly grow through the wall of the colon and spread to other parts of the body. This is metastasizing cancer.

A very few cases of colon cancer are the result of a cancer gene which may run through a family. Other than that, the good news about colon cancer is that it's associated with **factors that are in your control,** like your **fiber intake** and the quality of your diet. It may be that an enzyme derived from the fiber in food can block a stage of the colon cancer process. Foods that contain high fiber are whole grains, vegetables, fruits, legumes, and whole cereals. By eating them you're **feeding yourself valuable cancer fighting agents**.

screening for colon cancer

Fecal testing by your doctor for traces of blood in your stool can raise the alarm, so you should have this test done every two years or so as part of your routine checkup.

Sigmoidoscopy, when a tube is passed up to your colon, can detect the presence of a polyp which would trigger further investigation.

avoiding ovarian cancer

This cancer is pretty rare but dangerous because it grows silently, so can be quite advanced before it's detected. Then any treatment option may be ineffective. We have screening tools like the blood test for the ovarian cancer marker CA-125, but it's poor at detecting early tumors. Ovarian cancer tends to show up in women who are high risk for breast cancer, so making lifestyle changes similar to those for reducing breast cancer risk can favor prevention.

other cancer screening tests

• **Abdominal examinations** to detect an aneurysm.
• **Pelvic ultrasound** to detect ovarian and uterine cancer at an early stage or before the cancer has formed so that it can be cured.
• **Free radical** levels – one of the main agents of aging.

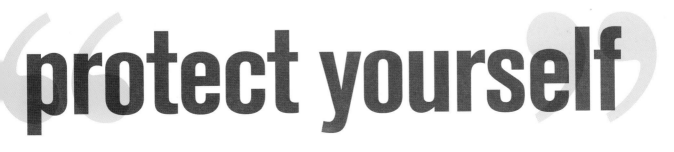

protect yourself

KEEPING *young* EYES

AS WE GROW OLDER, WE MAY NOTICE SOME IMPAIRMENT IN
ALL OUR SENSES – SIGHT, HEARING, SMELL, AND TASTE – AND CERTAIN
PARTS OF OUR EYES SUCH AS THE LENS AND CORNEA BEGIN TO WEAR.
THE RETINA IS NO LONGER AS PRISTINE AS IT WAS, FLOATERS (HARMLESS SPECKS
OF PROTEIN) BECOME MORE NUMEROUS.

The eyes were made to see. Seeing doesn't tire them and they need no more exercise than seeing and looking. Some "seeing work," however, tires the eye muscles, especially if they have to perform one task for hours on end, like reading from a computer screen. Your eye muscles, like any other muscle, **enjoy periods of rest** interspersed with activity.

how to protect your eyes from aging

Give your eyes periodic rests and changes of pace; let them relax between sessions of close work. Give your eye muscles a workout to keep them young and supple.

• **Raise your eyes** from the page or screen and focus on a distant object – it's instantly relaxing.

• We tend to lose our ability to track fast-moving objects so get someone to shine a flashlight on a wall in a darkened room and move it around. Track it with your own flashlight.

• **Playing sports helps you keep your hand-eye coordination.** Just take a ball and bounce it off a wall as you used to as a kid and catch it.

• To **keep your peripheral vision intact**, move your thumb close up and then away from your face. Follow it as you make different patterns with it – crosses and circles – but keep the rest of the room in view.

• Keep your eyes working in sync with one another with this exercise. Thread three beads on to a string 6ft (1.8m) long. Fasten one end to the wall at eye height and hold the other end. Slide one bead close to the wall, the second

4ft (1.2m) from the wall, and the third 16in (40cm) from your nose. Focus from one bead to the next. Close up, the string forms a V. If they're in unison at 6ft (1.8m) and 4ft (1.2m) your eyes make it form an X.

prevention is better than cure

To preserve young eyes the best thing you can do is to **have regular eye checkups** and specialist examinations if necessary. And always visit your doctor if any of the following arise:
• One of your eyes becomes red for no reason
• Your vision suddenly changes
• An eye becomes painful and the pain persistent
• There's a sudden arrival of flashing lights, especially in the corners of your eye(s).

changes in the eyes

With age the eyes themselves tend to change shape – they become elongated or shortened. Both defects can be corrected with glasses and contact lenses. But there are three potential changes to the eyes which we think of as aging.
• **Cataracts**
• **ARMD – age-related macular degeneration**
• **Glaucoma**

Cataracts are opacities within the lens. We now know that unprotected **exposure to bright sunlight** causes the premature appearance of cataracts as does **diabetes** – including type 2 adult-onset diabetes secondary to obesity, and **insulin resistance** with high insulin levels (see page 28). Everyone over the age of 65 will have cataracts to some extent, the clouding of the lens causing haziness of vision and glare. Bright lights may dazzle with halos around the light source. The lens also becomes yellowish, which means that color vision is affected, filtering violets and blues until only reds reach the retina. If you have early cataracts forming you should also read with the light behind you over your right or left shoulder, and in bright sunlight it can help to wear a wide-brimmed hat and tinted sunglasses. Fortunately cataracts can be cured by removing the lens and there are many sophisticated techniques available whereby a new lens can be inserted at the same time as the old lens is removed. For self-help screening and treatments, see the chart on page 76–77.

glaucoma

In this condition the free circulation of fluid within the eye is blocked, impairing vision. **Glaucoma**, which can occur in the forties and fifties, is due to increased pressure inside the eyeball which typically causes a painful, red eye and if not treated, eventual blindness. Fortunately most eye examinations, including those done by opticians, include readings of **intraocular pressure** so that an increase can be spotted early. The measurement is called tonometry. Glaucoma is readily amenable to treatment, preventing any visual damage. You should have any painful, red eye checked by your doctor whatever your age.

Everyone is at risk of glaucoma, but if you have a family history of it, are over 40, take steroids, have had an accident or surgery to your eye or have diabetes, you're at higher risk and should see an eye specialist annually.

ARMD

The **macula** is the center of the retina on which objects are focused in order for us to see clearly. When ARMD starts, blobs begin to appear in

TESTING FOR ARMD YOURSELF

You can test yourself for early signs of ARMD using the Amsler Grid – a grid of squares with a dot in the center. Simple to do, it could alert you to the early stages of macular degeneration so you can seek treatment without delay.

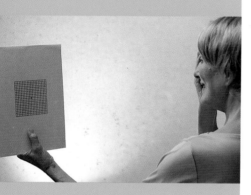

◆ Wear your reading glasses if you need them. Hold the grid about 12in (30cm) away.

◆ Cover one eye and look at the dot in the center of the grid.

◆ The lines of the grid should be straight and the squares the same size. You should be able to see all four corners of the grid.

◆ Now cover the other eye and repeat the test.

◆ If any lines look crooked, fuzzy or broken or you notice any distortion of the grid, check with your doctor.

the center of the visual field, a feature that distinguishes this condition from glaucoma where the first difficulty is usually with peripheral vision.

During your lifetime the center of the retina is constantly bombarded by very strong light rays in order to form a clear image of what you see. In fact the retina sees as a result of **light-activated chemistry** and over the years the byproducts of this chemistry build up as a kind of sludge. A lifetime of retinal chemistry leads to damage in the retinal cells, allowing fluid and blood to leak, causing loss of vision right in the central part of the visual field, in the macula, where light-activated chemistry is greatest. Laser therapy can prevent deterioration but treatment isn't always satisfactory.

There's a lot you can do yourself for ARMD. Make sure you have good lighting for reading and use **low vision aids**, the simplest form being a magnifying glass or mini-telescope that you can carry around in your pocket. There are also magnifying lenses that allow you to read while leaving your hands free.

AND *young ears*

HALF THE PEOPLE WHO GO ON TO GET HEARING IMPAIRMENT NOTICE CHANGES BEFORE THE AGE OF 40 SO YOU MUST TAKE ACTION AT THE FIRST SIGN OF ANY PROBLEMS.

That way you'll avoid social isolation and the risk of limiting your job prospects and denting your self-esteem from feeling more and more on the sidelines. People who are hard of hearing often meet with impatience and embarrassment, and even long-standing relationships can be disrupted.

All of us notice a blunting in our hearing with age because the eardrum stiffens and doesn't vibrate as it used to. Usually only after 60, however, does the transmission of sound across the middle ear get less sharp because of arthritis between the tiny bony ossicles or numbing of the fine auditory nerve endings.

CHECK OUT YOUR HEARING

How will I know if my hearing's going? Check out this test. Answer "nearly always," "half the time," "occasionally," or "never" to each statement.

1 I have a problem hearing over the phone

2 I have trouble following conversation when two or more people are talking at the same time

3 People complain that I turn the TV volume too high

4 I have to strain to understand conversations

5 I miss hearing some common sounds, such as the phone or doorbell ringing

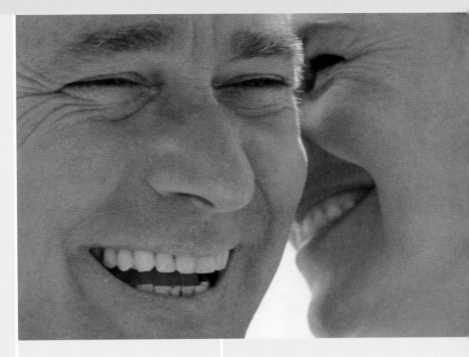

6 I have trouble hearing conversations in a noisy background, such as at a party

7 I get confused about where sounds come from

8 I misunderstand some words in a sentence and need to ask people to repeat themselves

9 I especially have trouble understanding the speech of women and children

10 I have worked in noisy environments (on assembly lines, with electric drills, near jet engines, and so on)

11 I hear fine – if people just speak clearly

12 People get annoyed because I misunderstand what they say

13 I misunderstand what others are saying and make inappropriate responses

14 I avoid social activities because I cannot hear well and fear I'll reply improperly

15 *(To be answered by a family member or friend)* Do you think this person has a hearing loss?

ANSWERS

Nearly always = 3   Occasionally = 1
Half the time = 3   Never = 0

SCORING

0–5: Your hearing is fine
6–9: See an ear specialist soon
10 and above: See an ear specialist immediately

Our ears have evolved to be very sensitive to quiet sounds. Loud sounds, be they sudden or continuous, can cause hearing loss – it's best to avoid them at all costs. Oddly, as the ear ages it can become both less and more sensitive, the former leading to impairment of hearing, the latter to ringing in the ears (tinnitus). This is often a feature of Ménière's disease which your doctor can treat.

lifetime changes

So as you can see there are plenty of ways of defying age and maintaining your well-being. Below is the first of a series of lists, detailing what I have found to be valuable ways of helping yourself stay healthy throughout your life.

HOW OFTEN should general health screening tests be done?

- **Cholesterol** – once if normal; once a year if treatment is needed
- **Chest X-ray** for smokers and ex-smokers – once a year
- **Blood pressure** – every two years
- **Mammograms, Pap smear, and PSA** (prostate-specific antigen) – every three years
- **Physical examination**, sigmoidoscopy (see page 103), and stool blood testing – every five years
- **Eyes** – every year
- **Ears** – every two years
- **Teeth** – every six months

DRUGS of a lifetime

Statins
HRT
Selegiline (for Alzheimer's)
Retinoic acid (for the skin)
Aspirin

FOODS of a lifetime

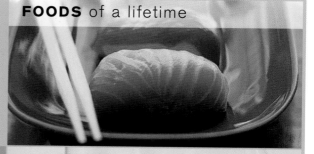

SUPPLEMENTS of a lifetime

HABITS of a lifetime

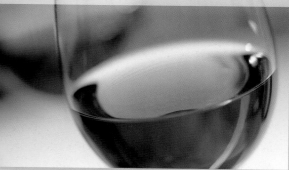

WARNING SIGNS YOU MUST CHECK WITH YOUR DOCTOR

To help prolong your life there are some symptoms you should never ignore whatever your age. They could be early warning signs of something serious and if you heed them they can usually be treated in good time and cured.

the appearance of blood, even streaks, in your sputum, urine, bowel movements or vaginal discharge **must always be checked out by your doctor** who will want to make sure you don't have a tumor.

from the age of 45 never put a new and sudden attack of heartburn, indigestion, or tightness or pain in the chest down to something harmless. Consult your doctor, especially if the symptoms come on after exertion or a heavy meal. **They could signal a heart condition**, even a heart attack, and need prompt attention.

a painful red eye with blurred vision or halos around lights, especially at night or in the dark, **is an early sign of acute glaucoma** and high pressure in your eyeball. Damage to your eye can be prevented with early medical treatment.

hoarseness of the voice that persists for more than a couple of weeks should never be ignored or written off as a viral infection because it **could be the first symptom of a tumor of the larynx**. In its early stages a laryngeal tumor can be cured completely. Hoarseness or a persistent irritable cough can also be a late symptom of cancer of the lung.

a passing paralysis of the face, leg, and hands or temporary loss of vision or memory should never be ignored because it's an **early warning sign of a stroke**. These transient ischemic attacks (T.I.A.) mean that a tiny clot has passed down one of the arteries to the brain or to the retina at the back of the eye, dissolving afterward. A T.I.A. should be treated as a warning sign of a stroke. If you alert your doctor and blood-thinning drugs are given to you, the stroke may never happen.

a headache with a tender spot in your temple just above your eye can mean that you have inflammation in the temporal artery, one of the blood vessels supplying the brain. It needs prompt treatment with steroids and you should **see your doctor immediately** because blindness may sometimes be the result.

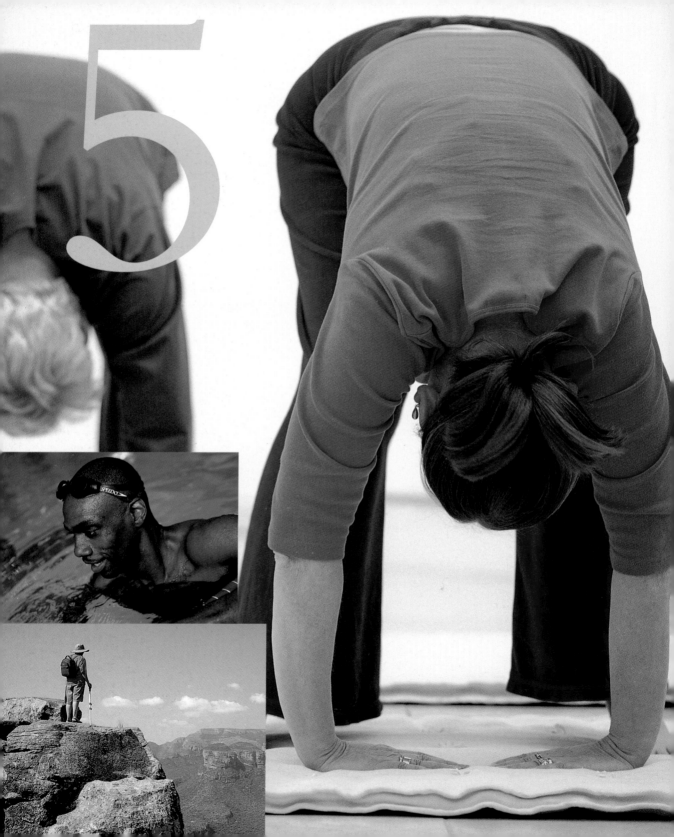

5

ACTIVE
MEANS
YOUNGER

Our bodies really *hate being inactive*. For thousands
of years of our evolution we were running much of the
time – active hunter-gatherers. Every member of the human
race undertook **exercise almost constantly** every day of
their lives while they were awake. The body hasn't so far
evolved to cope with inactivity. *It hasn't had time*.
Over the millennia we've learned to cope very well with
lack of food – indeed we've evolved to withstand starvation
– but our bodies have **no way of coping** with lack of
exercise. These days many of us lead a primarily *sedentary*
life, and *it's a killer*. The body knows of no way to deal
with the sedentary life. All it can do is decay.

WHY *we need* EXERCISE

INACTIVITY CAUSES PROBLEMS BECAUSE OUR METABOLISM IS GEARED TO USE THE ENERGY FROM THE FOOD WE EAT BY BEING AGILE, MOBILE, ON OUR FEET, MOVING AROUND MOST OF THE TIME.

If we're not, there's a great deal of surplus energy and without activity that surplus energy cannot be gotten rid of. It accumulates in the only way the body knows how, as fat. Think of a toddler. Toddlers are called toddlers because they "toddle" most of the time. They run around, they're never still. **They rarely rest.** The toddler is an example of the human body in an ideal state and it's an ideal state not just for two- and three-year-olds, but for as long as we live.

The Okinawans, **the longest-living people** on the planet, have proven it to be so. They're active for most of the day in various ways, though none involves a strenuous workout in the gym. They **keep active with walking, gardening, dancing,** and what we might call the "soft" martial arts like tai chi. They don't do much jogging at lunch hour or cycling in the afternoon, they just keep their bodies **on the move** for quite long periods each day, and that's all the body needs to defy age.

So the message is not more strenuous, high-impact exercise to prolong your life. It's much more appealing – **stay on your feet** for as many hours as you can every day. **Brisk walking** is the closest you have to get to a workout.

HOW exercise staves off age

What aging does to you	The signs of aging	How exercise makes you younger
Loss of muscle strength	We lose 10 percent of muscle mass every 10 years after 65.	Exercise increases the size and strength of your muscles, including your heart. Stronger arms and legs help keep you mobile and able to carry heavy bags.
Loss of bone calcium	Women lose a third to a half of bone density by 90, increasing the risk of bone fracture. One in four women with a fractured hip will die.	Weight-bearing exercise keeps bones healthy, improves balance, and lessens the risk of falling and breaking brittle bones.
Loss of heart/lung efficiency (breathlessness)	Most people lose more than half their cardiovascular fitness between ages 20 and 80.	Exercise stops this. It prevents heart disease and other chronic diseases and increases your life expectancy.

exercise and mental well-being

Physical activity can boost both **physical and mental well-being** and change your outlook on life; it could even prevent problems from starting in the first place. I know from personal experience that regular physical activity **can lift your mood** and help you deal with negative emotions like anger and depression. It brings you a general sense of **optimism** and mental well-being, as well as making you feel in good physical condition.

I've noticed that if I wake feeling a bit down, 30 minutes on my exercise bike **cures the blues**. That's because exercise floods my body with hormones that **reduce tension levels** and feelings of stress and fatigue. There's no time-lag – these changes happen right after a session, even though I don't pedal that strenuously.

No wonder I'm addicted to it. I can't miss a single day.

exercise makes you feel better about yourself

Exercise can make a huge difference to anyone suffering anxiety and low self-esteem and what's more it has only good side effects. Studies have shown that people **feel better about themselves once they start an exercise program**. Changes to body shape, as you begin to lose weight and feel your muscle tone getting better, improve your self-image, which can boost mental well-being. Exercise helps you to see just what you're capable of and gives you a **sense of achievement**. Learning a new skill or achieving a goal, however minor, boosts self-esteem and motivation.

Exercise is an antidepressant: both aerobic activity, such as brisk walking, running,

EXERCISE AND MENTAL HEALTH

Statistics on this are really very convincing.

◆ Among those with mental health problems **57 percent report that exercise improved motivation**, 50 percent have improved self-esteem, and 24 percent are helped with their social skills.

◆ **Exercise helps to relieve symptoms of depression** in 65 percent of those surveyed, stress in 62 percent, anxiety in 56 percent, manic depression in 12 percent, and symptoms of schizophrenia in 10 percent.

◆ In a survey of gym members **64 percent report improved self-esteem**, 64 percent have boosted energy levels, and 58 percent improved motivation; 35 percent have better performance at work, 68 percent think their mental well-being will suffer if they stop exercising, and only 18 percent think it won't.

or cycling, and resistance activity, such as using weights in a gym, can help people who have moderate to severe depression. The **antidepressant effect of exercise** is as powerful as some traditional forms of treatment such as physical therapy and group therapy. More research needs to be done, but it does seem that physical activity can be used alongside other treatments for mental health problems.

Some people with anxiety disorders have found exercise as effective as remedies like meditation or relaxation exercises. Just one session of physical activity can bring temporary **relief to stress and anxiety**, and regular activity may have a long-term effect.

exercise protects you from cancer

Physically active men and women have **half the risk of getting colon cancer** of their sedentary friends. The protection may be due to the favorable effect of exercise on insulin, prostaglandins, and bile, all of which cause overgrowth of the colon lining. Exercise also speeds up bowel movements, cutting down the

length of contact between fecal carcinogens and the colonic lining.

The hormones implicated in breast and uterine cancer are modulated by exercise. Studies show that activity can be responsible for a **30 percent reduction in breast cancer rates** and the more exercise you get, the greater the protection. So physical activity probably **protects against the formation of cancer**. And it may protect against recurrence and survival after a cancer has been detected.

The evidence is most compelling for colon and breast cancer, but moderate activity like walking and cycling should be part of everyone's cancer-protection program.

exercise keeps your heart elastic

You never know when you're going to call on your heart to perform in a superhuman way. If your heart has been allowed to become slack and fat as any unfit muscle will, it won't be able to respond in an emergency. You may be fortunate to get a warning sign – the chest pain of angina. But you may not and you could precipitate a heart attack. **Exercise can make your heart physically fit enough to enrich your life in more ways than one.**

When you exercise, you increase the ability of your heart and lungs to adapt to any sudden increase in the work they have to do. This in itself goes a long way to compensate for the decline in heart function that occurs with age. Exercise opens up spare arteries to your heart muscle, ensuring that blood will reach the hard-working tissues, even if one of the arteries gets blocked. In these two ways **exercise can lower the risk of a heart attack**. It also lowers your blood pressure, thereby reducing the risk of stroke.

exercise controls your appetite

We all have something called the **appestat**, which is a switch in the brain telling us we're full and should stop eating. All day long the appestat is bombarded with messages (chemical, electrical, hormonal, psychological) that turn it off and turn it on.

Exercise turns it on (STOP EATING!), and turns it on for as long as you exercise every day. The effects of this turn-on are both subtle and unsubtle. First of all **you don't feel hungry for an hour or so after exercising** because exercise saps your blood sugar and your insulin levels are really flat (high insulin levels make you eat, low insulin levels do the opposite).

Because of this stabilization of blood sugar, but especially of insulin, the appestat (which is blunted by high blood sugar and insulin levels) becomes sensitive again. It starts to give you really early signals that you're reaching satiety. That's the time to stop eating.

But the most subtle effect of exercise is on **what it makes you choose to eat.** When I was doing a cycle challenge through Israel, Jordan, and Egypt, I found that I automatically reached for oranges, tomatoes (both vitamin C), and bread (complex carbohydrates) every time we stopped. I didn't want protein, I didn't want fat, I didn't want sugar. **My muscles were telling my brain what they needed**. And my appestat was guiding my hand toward the fresh fruit and vegetables.

Exercise makes you listen to your appestat. On the training program for the cycle challenge, I would open the fridge door and take out fresh, healthy food. If I reached for sweet food my brain made me withdraw my hand. It made me choose the kind of food that would keep me strong and healthy and, incidentally, keep me from putting on weight – another reason, other than burning off calories, that exercise controls your weight.

exercise keeps the brain young and happy

Only five years ago it was thought that the brain couldn't grow new brain cells. Thanks to new research, the pessimists have been proven wrong. The discovery of neurogenesis – the creation of new nerve cells (neurons) – at the Salk Institute in California has opened many doors, including how to repair damaged brains by stimulating cell growth, bringing nearer a cure for diseases such as stroke, Parkinsonism, and even depression.

In animal experiments it's been found that **neurogenesis doubles** when a mouse has a running wheel in its cage. It's possible that the increased blood flow carries more growth factors into the brain, stimulating the growth of new brain cells. Another possibility is that running triggers a brain rhythm called theta rhythm, which in turn increases serotonin production – a known trigger for the **growth of new brain cells**, especially in the womb and in newborns.

...and not just in lab mice

Whatever the explanation of neurogenesis in mice, scientists believe that **exercise is good for the human brain** too. Indeed, some of the scientists at the Salk Institute started running regularly when they saw the results of putting treadmills in the cages of their laboratory mice. It would seem that the prescription for a long, healthy life is to **keep mind and body as active as possible**.

A well-known theory of clinical depression is that it arises from the brain's failure to grow enough fresh neurons. New brain cells form mainly in a part of the brain called the hippocampus, which plays a role in emotion, learning, and memory. They don't seem to form anywhere else.

Several recent studies have shown that patients with long-term depression have a consistently smaller hippocampus than people who aren't depressed, and it could be because new brain cells aren't being generated fast enough to replace the ones that are dying off. Stress combined with genetic factors is probably responsible for suppressing neurogenesis in the hippocampus. The rate at which neurogenesis proceeds is closely related to the level of stress hormones in the blood.

Some of the newer antidepressants such as Prozac and Seroxat **may stimulate the growth of neurons**, probably because they increase the amount of serotonin in the hippocampus.

I'm convinced that exercise is *the key* to a longer life and if you want some idea of the benefits of exercise, even in moderate amounts, just take a look at this picture of me on my exercise bicycle

KEY BENEFITS OF EXERCISE

"growth" hormones make **new brain cells grow**, so cognitive thinking and memory improve

endorphins released give you an eight-hour high

increased adrenaline controls appetite and stops cravings

exercise hormones treat anxiety and depression lessening need for antidepressants

reshapes your body

changes your eating habits …

cures jet lag

it's a treatment for irritable bowel syndrome

ankles don't swell any more

combats stress and lowers blood pressure

makes you get more exercise

good for migraines, cures headaches

vision gets brighter, can wear contact lenses longer

better sleep

increases heart/lung efficiency so you can be more active

lowers cholesterol

… into healthy ones

so fewer heart attacks and strokes

good for bones so less osteoporosis

skin gets pink because of **increased oxygen** in every cell in the body

increases suppleness, mobility, and stamina

better balance so fewer falls

TIPS FOR STARTING AN EXERCISE REGIMEN

◆ Always find out how *physically fit* you are before you start any exercise and if you're in any doubt about your fitness, **check with your doctor.**

◆ Always choose activities and exercises that you **enjoy** or you'll never stick to an exercise program.

◆ Exercises **shouldn't be a chore** – if they are, you're doing the wrong ones.

◆ Exercises should never be physically punishing – if they are, you're pushing yourself too hard.

◆ If you can't carry on a **conversation** while exercising, the activity is too strenuous.

◆ The best form of exercise is one that fits in with your **daily life,** like taking the dog for a walk, bicycling to work or to stores, climbing stairs rather than taking the elevator, and doing a few exercises while you're working in the kitchen.

◆ There's no need for you to spend a lot of money on exercise equipment. You can do all your exercises effectively without buying anything – except maybe a few gardening tools.

◆ **Never exercise on a full stomach** – always wait at least an hour and spend a few minutes loosening up before beginning any kind of strenuous exercise.

◆ Never be overzealous about increasing the amount of time you spend exercising. **Slowly and surely** should be your motto. Always check your pulse rate so that over a period of not less than six weeks you can reach the level of fitness appropriate for your age.

◆ Once you've reached your desired level of fitness try to exercise **at least three or four times a week** to maintain it.

◆ Simply increasing the amount of *walking* you do will increase your fitness.

◆ The aim isn't to exercise strenuously three times a week, it's to exercise *gently* every day.

how fit are you?

Remembering that mice never race around their treadmills and the Okinawans never hurry, starting on a gently active life is quite painless, but first of all you have to make sure that you're physically fit enough.

• To see how fit you are, run in place for 30 seconds, then take your pulse (count beats for 15 seconds and multiply by four). This is your pulse rate for mild exertion.

• During any exercise you should take your pulse rate and it shouldn't go any higher than the rate you have just calculated.

• The aim of heart-lung exercise is to keep up this pulse rate for about 15–20 minutes.

• Try for the appropriate exercising pulse rate as shown in the table on the right.

age	exercising pulse rate
50-54	117
55-59	113
60-64	109

the step test

Another simple test of how fit you are. Find a stool 8in (20cm) high and step up and down twice within five seconds. Now do 24 complete step-ups each minute, continuing for three minutes. At the end of three minutes, stop and find your pulse. Exactly 30 seconds after stopping, measure your pulse for 30 seconds – this is your aerobic fitness score. Check with the table opposite to find out how fit you are for your age and sex.

STEP TEST 30-second recovery heart rate

Age	20-29	30-39	40-49	50+
Men	Number of heartbeats in 30 seconds			
Outstanding	34-36	35-38	37-39	37-40
Very good	37-40	39-41	40-42	41-43
Good	41-42	42-43	43-44	44-45
Fair	43-47	44-47	45-49	46-49
Low	48-51	48-51	50-53	50-53
Poor	52-59	52-59	54-60	54-62
Women				
Outstanding	39-42	39-42	41-43	41-44
Very good	43-44	43-45	44-45	45-47
Good	45-46	46-47	46-47	48-49
Fair	47-52	48-53	48-54	50-55
Low	53-56	54-56	55-57	56-58
Poor	57-66	57-66	58-67	59-66

GETTING STARTED

I'm going to describe for you a model called "stages of change" that's been used in clinics to help smokers and alcoholics overcome their addiction. It's effective for making any life change, such as trying to incorporate exercise into your life when you've never exercised before. These are the seven stages.

STAGE 1
Disbelief – you're still unconvinced of the need for change
What you can do:
1 Read as much as you can about *inactivity* and *obesity*
2 Read *inspirational* stories of those people who've changed their lives
3 Speak to people who've *changed their lives* and ask how they did it
4 Go to your doctor for a *checkup* and talk about how inactivity is affecting your health and how you'd *benefit from exercise.*

STAGE 2
You believe you should be a bit more active but can't get started
What you can do:
1 Think of yourself as a *new person*, how you'd look, how much you'd weigh, the new clothes you could buy, how energetic you'd feel, how much younger you would look
2 Write down the *health benefits* like how exercise will reduce your chances of heart disease, diabetes, osteoporosis, depression, and so on
3 Think about the new *social possibilities*
4 Think about the *alternative* – being a couch potato, being tired after work, watching life pass you by, getting fatter, losing your sex drive.

STAGE 3
You get down to actively planning the new you
What you can do:
1 You set a *start date*
2 You set small *achievable goals*
3 You make a *detailed plan* of how you would schedule exercise into your day
4 You become *specific* about your goals – when, how long, and where you would exercise
5 You decide to *tell people* so that you enlist support
6 You *set your goal*
7 You start *believing in yourself* and will let nothing stand in your way – you are going to take charge of your life.

STAGE 4
You've started exercising
What you can do:
1 Keep a *journal* of how your training goes
2 *Reward yourself* from time to time for sticking to your exercise
3 *Congratulate* yourself on your progress
4 *Be consistent*, do less rather than none at all
5 Don't worry if you *miss a session*, it isn't a competition.

STAGE 5
You start to think of yourself in a new way – you have a new image – you see yourself as someone who gets regular exercise, you're proud of yourself
What you can do:
1 *Be proud* of yourself for the changes you have made
2 Buy magazines that *reinforce your new image*
3 Try and find *somebody else* who's involved in the same sort of activities – the local gym is a good place.

STAGE 6
You're determined to keep your new self-image forever
What you can do:
1 Make a *backup plan* for setbacks
2 Keep *refining your goals* – do you want to exercise simply to be fit or do you want to set up another goal?

STAGE 7
You're a new person
What you can do:
1 *Help someone else* to become like you by telling them about what you do
2 Consider *writing* about your experiences
3 Keep up your *training journal*
4 *Buy books* so that you can read more about how your fitness is benefiting you
5 Think about splitting your exercise session into three parts – each part builds on the previous one to optimize your fitness. The three parts are warmup exercises, mobility exercises, and strengthening exercises.

GOOD *posture*

COMPARE PEOPLE IN THEIR 20S WITH PEOPLE IN THEIR 60S. THE MAIN DIFFERENCE YOU'LL SEE IS IN HOW THEY CARRY THEMSELVES. IN YOUR 20S YOU'RE ERECT, IN YOUR 60S YOU'RE SLUMPED. STRAIGHTENING SHOULDERS AND HOLDING YOUR HEAD UP TAKES TEN YEARS OFF YOUR AGE.

You can only do that if your back, neck, abdominal, and pelvic muscles are **toned and strong**. There's hardly one aspect of body function that isn't affected by exercise but one of the most important is **posture**, particularly as we get older. We cannot hold our bodies erect without **strong back and neck muscles**. In this respect posture isn't only important if we are to look better as we grow older, it's also a protection against developing backache, digestive problems, and heart disease. The bones in the spine tend to soften as we get older, particularly in women. As a result of osteoporosis after menopause, women may lose height because the vertebral bones become thinner and collapse, sometimes forming a dowager's hump.

keep back muscles strong

However, with good strong back muscles even slight softening in the spine can be mitigated, preventing rounded shoulders and an aging hump from developing. Just as important, an **erect spine** holds the chest at maximum capacity so that our lungs can **work efficiently**. Not only are our chests helped by an erect spine but also our hearts and our digestion. Strength and mobility exercises help to prevent a hesitant, shuffling walk so we're **steadier on our feet** and have fewer accidents. Joints remain supple, tendons don't tighten and weaken, and **this strength gives us confidence** so that

there's less likelihood of stumbling, falling, and fracturing bones.

Bad posture exacts a high price. Not least are neck and back pain, both due to the fact that the head and back fall out of the line of gravity so that the back muscles have to work extra hard to prevent the spine becoming crooked and to keep the body upright. Tired muscles ache.

For people with a tendency to slump forward, the back and neck muscles have to pull the weight of the head (the heaviest part of the body) back into the line of gravity. The muscles may even become distorted, causing more pain because the strain on the spinal ligaments damages them and may damage the disks between the spinal bones and, in time, the spinal bones themselves.

the importance of your abs to your back

The best protection for your back is to have really **strong, firm abdominal muscles**. They act like a front splint for the spine, holding it in place and taking a lot of the strain. Next time your back aches just **pull in your abs**. The relief will astonish you. Practice walking and sitting with tense abs for a few moments every half hour. Learn to separate your lower from your upper abs and exercise them independently as well as in unison. A few stomach crunches every day will keep your abs solid.

tips for protecting your back

The spine is one of the most overworked areas of the body. It's subjected to stress and strain 24/7, even in bed if your mattress and pillows aren't back friendly. Try to be on the lookout for ways of resting your back whenever you can. Start by thinking about and correcting the way you sit, drive, and sleep.

SITTING: well-designed chairs are a good start. A chair that is good for posture is one that keeps the angle of the spine to the hip at about 120 degrees, ensuring maximum comfort and minimum strain on spinal joints and spinal muscles. In addition, a chair should be convex where the back joins the seat so that the lower part of the spine is well supported. Look out for this feature when you're buying a new chair or choosing a car.

Sit back on the seat of the chair and make sure that you're comfortable and upright, with your **shoulders and head balanced over your hips**. Whenever you reach forward from this position, don't reach forward from the arms but **bend from the hips**. You can practice sitting correctly and stretching forward in the proper way so that it feels natural and comfortable.

DRIVING: examine your car seat. It should be designed to support the lower part of your spine. If you have a car in which the seats don't provide enough support, look for a cushion that can fit into the lower part of your seat to provide you with support. Most car accessory stores supply these.

TIPS FOR GOOD POSTURE

◆ Practice **walking along a straight line** so that you correct any tendency to walk with your feet too far apart or with your toes pointing out.

◆ When you walk, try to **balance** your head and keep your upper and lower torso in line.

◆ Try to **center your body** over the balls of your feet.

◆ Lead with your **thigh** not your foot.

◆ Every time you remember, bring your pelvis in under your spine, **tighten your abdominal muscles,** and bring your head back over your neck. Now your head's in line with your spine and your pelvis. The more evenly the weight of your body is carried around this line of gravity, the less work your muscles have to do.

◆ When sitting, become aware of slumping. **Sit up and lower the position of your head**. Learn to do that chin forward and backward motion that hens do so well – it does wonders for an aching neck.

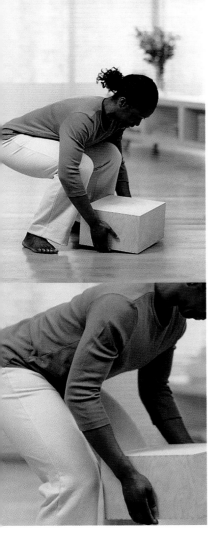

LIFTING AND CARRYING: it's important to maintain good posture when lifting or carrying heavy weights or bending. Not only does it make life easier, it also saves unnecessary wear and tear on muscles and joints. Here are some tips to remember.

• **Kneel right down** when doing a job at floor level, such as cutting a dress or weeding.

• Stooping is very tiring and a strain on the back.

• To shift a big weight, such as a dresser, **push with your back**, not your hands. It's always best to ask for help.

• To lift a large or heavy object, **bend down from your knees**, not your waist. Carry a heavy package close to your body, not out in front. Again, bend when putting it down.

SLEEPING: we spend about one-third of our lives asleep so it's worth paying attention to your mattress and the position you sleep in. As children we may love fluffy, soft mattresses, but they're bad for our backs as we get older, since they allow our spines to curve outward. A firm mattress is much better than a soft one. Old-fashioned beds with a box that provide an inflexible base are better than those without. Most of us know someone who, having injured their back, has been told by a doctor that the best way of curing back pain is to put an old door underneath the mattress to support the back during the night. This is good when we're in pain and even better when we're not. It prevents an overworked spine from being strained more than is absolutely necessary.

HOW WE MISUSE THE MUSCLES OF THE NECK AND BACK

Bending the head forward to work, instead of bending from the hips and keeping the spine straight, is a common fault. The rib cage and lower back tend to slump downward and a hump forms where the neck joins the back. This encourages misuse of the neck muscles, so that when the head is lifted to look straight ahead, the forward curve of the neck is exaggerated, resulting in neck ache and backache. This forward curve of the neck and backward curve of the upper back may become so ingrained that the distortion remains when standing, forcing the lower back to curve forward to compensate. Preventing back and neck ache involves a minimal backward curve of the upper back and forward curve of the lower back.

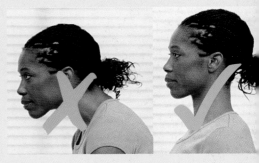

the Alexander Principle

The Alexander Principle is best learned from a specialist teacher. A coordinated approach to the health of both body and mind, it's based on the premise that most of us function inefficiently, both physically and mentally, because we develop **tension habits** in our muscles. This manifests itself in the form of back problems, fibromyalgia and a whole range of tension and stress problems. Asthma, hypertension, tension headaches, anxiety states, and general fatigue can all be worsened by this misuse. It's apparent, too, in the majority of people who cope well in normal circumstances but find that their bodies let them down when they want to be at their best, whether it be in a major crisis, competitive sport, making love or music. The Alexander Principle teaches an intimate **awareness** of body use. If we know what our bodies are doing and why, we can use them to better advantage.

According to the Alexander Principle, the area around the **head, neck, and upper back**, through which the most important blood vessels and nerves pass, is where the misuse of the body shows itself most clearly. Faulty breathing patterns, for instance, throw the muscles of the lower neck and upper ribs into excessive spasm, while eating and speaking require good posture. Misuse often produces a hump on the back, created by wrongly distributed muscle tension.

An Alexander teacher starts by helping you develop an awareness of these abuses and at the most subtle level teaches the release of faulty tension patterns all over the body, which leads to a **better postural balance**.

The head and neck area must be gradually brought into correct **alignment** by gentle manipulation on the part of the teacher as well as by verbal direction. These directions are not instructions to be carried out by conscious effort, but are intended as a guide that the mind absorbs, so that the **body slowly reprograms itself** into a more efficient use. Eventually a balance should be achieved so that no part of the body has to work harder than any other.

balanced rest

The Alexander Principle is as much a **mental exercise** as a physical one and doesn't require a vigorous, exhausting routine. It can be helpful at a simple level, showing how to use muscles as they were designed to be used, or it can be developed into a comprehensive awareness of body use in every situation, including **rest**. Many people resort to alcohol, tranquilizers, or even self-induced hypnosis to relax. Alexander maintains that all these methods offer only temporary respite. **Balanced rest** is an important part of the approach and offers as much relief as correct use during activity.

body awareness

THE IMPORTANCE OF **YOUR QUADS**

From the point of view of youthfulness and fitness, the most important muscles in your body are your quadriceps, on the front of your thighs.

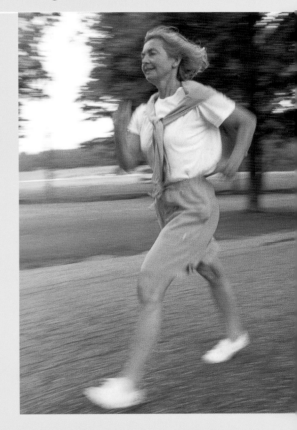

The quadriceps are the large group of muscles on the front of your thighs, the **biggest muscle group** in the whole body. The reason the quads are so crucial for defying age is that you can't get out of a chair if they're weak. If you want to resist that classic picture of an older person sitting in an armchair, *keep your quads well toned and strong*.

There are many ways of exercising your quads, like cycling, jogging, running, and walking to keep up muscle mass. Exercising your quads also improves the **fitness of your heart and lungs** – when the quads work hard they require a lot of oxygen and your heart and lungs have to provide it.

But the best way of strengthening your quads is to raise yourself out of any chair relying only on your **thigh muscles** and without using your arms to raise your lower body. The deeper the chair the harder it is, but persist in putting your quads through their paces as often as you can every day. That way you'll never let yourself become a prisoner of your armchair and on the sidelines of life.

keep your quads strong Don't find yourself at 70 or 80 operating at the limit of your physical powers – even when doing something as simple as trying to raise yourself from an armchair. If your quads aren't exercised they soon become flabby, weak, and easily tired. Along with your quads, the muscles in your back and those that control your balance become weaker too. You become unsure on your feet, you lose mobility, agility, and flexibility and you're more likely to fall and fracture a bone. A fractured bone in a young person will knit within six weeks. A fracture in an older person – particularly if they have osteoporosis – may never quite knit. A proportion of all women who go into the hospital with a fractured hip bone never come out – they die in the hospital, usually of pneumonia. And all because they didn't exercise and keep their quads strong. **So keeping your quads fit is one of the most important ways in which you can defy age**.

INACTIVITY *stress*

A DECREASE IN PHYSICAL ACTIVITY IS DIRECTLY RELATED TO AGING – THE OLDER YOU GET, THE LESS ACTIVE YOU FEEL LIKE BEING AND IT'S MAINLY BECAUSE YOU START TO DECLINE IN VIGOR.

If for any reason your vigor decreases, your desire and ability to take part in physical activities is blunted. Mental stress from depression and anxiety can further dampen your desire to get up and go, and you tend to withdraw from the world.

It's possible then to find yourself getting into a **downward spiral of less and less physical activity**. More stress, withdrawal, and deeper depression may follow, with results that should concern us all.

As we lose our vigor and withdraw, the **inactivity-stress syndrome** drains our energy and motivation, no matter what we try to do. It's insidious, it pervades all aspects of our lives and it follows that we get less out of life. We're less able to participate and enjoy ourselves – we become less and less happy. To my mind, no other argument is needed in favor of retaining our physical fitness.

As we get older, however, we can no longer rely on having mobile joints, fit muscles, and

ALL YOU HAVE TO DO IS WALK

Here are a few things to remember when you're going to take up walking:
◆ You're not in a hurry.
◆ You won't progress in days but in weeks.
◆ At the end of four weeks I guarantee you'll notice *changes* in your body and your mental well-being.
◆ Since you're going to take it easy, don't worry about measuring your heart rate, just get up and go.
◆ All you have to attempt is **half an hour** at a pace slightly above a stroll.
◆ If you've never exercised before, go and **get checked out by your doctor**.
◆ Always do your **flexibility** exercises before you go out to walk.
◆ To start with, **walk on level ground** and avoid hills.
◆ Always walk "**within your breath.**" This will mean that your heart is beating at about 60 percent of its maximum rate.

◆ The level of **intensity** of exercise that you should be aiming for is one that allows you to have a conversation while you're moderately out of breath.
◆ Never push yourself further than you feel you want to go and **never strain yourself**. As soon as you feel strain, stop.
◆ Don't try to increase the speed at which you walk, but try to **increase the distance or the time** you spend walking.
◆ At the beginning, never walk into the wind. This will increase your workload quite a lot.
◆ If you suffer from heart disease you can walk along quite comfortably for a while when the wind is behind you, but you can get severe angina if you turn and face the wind.
◆ Work at your walking until you are able to walk about **3 miles (5km) without stopping** in 45–55 minutes.

strong bones. Our insurance policy is exercise. **Exercise promotes an agile, healthy body that will respond quickly and safely in most situations.** We need to have strong muscles that give us endurance and stamina and allow us to live life to the fullest.

a healthy mind means a healthy body

Just as important, we need to have **healthy minds** that are eager to encourage our bodies. None of this will happen if we let them slide into neglect. They have to be put regularly through their paces to bring them up to a level of physical fitness that enables us to live the lives we want to. In this respect **exercise undoubtedly keeps us young**.

MAXIMIZE your performance while you're walking

◆ Add a **weight belt** or weighted wrist bands.
◆ **Lengthen** your stride, smoothly and slowly, but make sure it's comfortable.
◆ Think about your **posture** and correct it. Don't lean from your waist or you'll put undue stress on your back.
◆ Always keep your **arms swinging**. The forward swing should end with your fists at about shoulder height and your backward swing with the upper arms at a 90-degree angle to the trunk.
◆ Stop halfway and do some **stretching** exercises, see pages 128–30 for some examples.

◆ **Good walking shoes are key**, so make sure your feet are comfortable and wear good walking socks
◆ **Wear layers** that you can peel off if necessary or put on when it gets a bit colder. Make sure they're loose fitting.
◆ Plan your route, measure out 2 miles (3km).
◆ Keep tabs on yourself. Time how long it takes you to walk for 1 mile (1.6km) on level ground without getting short of breath. Most of us should be able to do this in about 20 minutes. Keep track of your increasing fitness when measured from this base line.
◆ If you possibly can, keep to your plan of regular exercise. Walk a minimum of three times a week.
◆ Enjoy yourself – this is leisure not work.
◆ A good tip is to walk a useful trip that you might otherwise do by car – for example, shopping or to the train station. This builds the walking into your daily pattern rather than making it an optional extra.

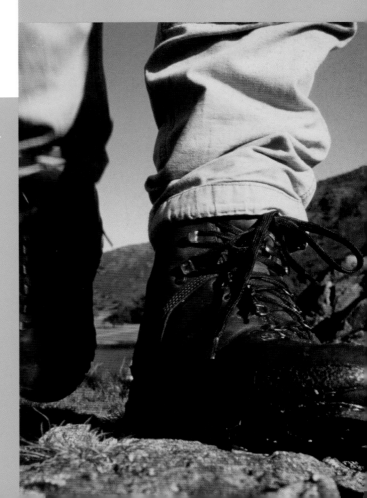

KEEP*active*

EXERCISE IS THE BEST WAY I KNOW OF DEFYING AGE. TRY THESE SIMPLE EXERCISES AND KEEP YOUR BODY SUPPLE.

Warm-up exercises improve the mobility and flexibility of our bodies, ensuring that they stay as **supple as possible** and help promote agility and good posture. After warm-up exercises come **mobility** exercises. Then we should go on to **strengthening** exercises, which help to increase our muscle power so that we can go through our daily tasks easily and prevent undue wear and tear, and most of all injury. Lastly come the **heart and lung exercises**, which give us the stamina to make a sustained effort and give us endurance – these are sometimes called aerobic exercises because our breathing rate increases.

WARM-UP EXERCISES

The older we get, the more time we should spend on warm-up exercises. The following promote circulation and "oil" the major joints:
• **Arm circling** – stand with your feet hip-width apart and arms hanging loose. Begin by slowly circling one shoulder backward,

then the other. Increase to circling your arm bent at the elbow, and then to circling your whole arm.
• **Hip circles** – stand with your feet hip-width apart, knees slightly bent, and hands on your waist. Slowly circle your hips clockwise, then reverse. Repeat several times.
• **Walk in place** – stand with your feet hip-width apart and gently walk in place. Imagine there's gum under your feet so you have to "peel" them off the floor.
• **Forward curl** – stand with your feet hip-width apart, knees slightly bent and stretch both arms above your head. Slowly curl forward, bringing your elbows down toward your waist, around your shoulders, and tuck in your bottom and head. Don't bend too low.

MOBILITY EXERCISES

These are designed to take all **major muscles and joints** through a complete range of movement. Once you've achieved mobility fitness you'll be able to move, stretch, twist, and turn in all directions with freedom and without feeling

any discomfort or pain in your muscles or joints.

Arm swings and shoulder rolls (repeat 5 times)

Stand with your feet slightly apart and swing forward with your right arm, then backward. Repeat with your left arm. Now slowly roll each shoulder forward and then backward in a full circle.

Body bends (see right) (repeat 3–5 times)

Stand with your feet slightly apart and place your hands on your hips [1]. Bend slowly forward as far as you can manage and then backward [2]. Do this exercise gently at first.

Body turns and side stretches (repeat 5 times)

Stand with your feet apart. Now turn your body to the right and back, and then to the left and back. Next, place your left hand on your left hip and extend your right arm over your head. Now change hands, placing your right hand on your right hip and stretching up with your left arm.

BODY BENDS

1

2

ARM LIFTS

1

2

NECK, SHOULDER, AND ARM EXERCISES

Arm circling (repeat 3 times)
Stand erect with your feet slightly apart and your arms by your sides. Bring one arm forward, upward, and backward to make a large circle. Next, reverse the direction of the swing.

Shoulder swing
(repeat 10 times)
With your feet apart, lean forward as far as you can comfortably manage. Swing each arm from side to side across your body. Next, swing both arms together.

Neck rolls (repeat 3–5 times)
Let your head fall forward, then slowly pull it up. Let it fall to the side, then pull it up again.

Arm lifts (see left)
(repeat 3–5 times)
This is quite vigorous so take it easy at first. Hold weights if you want but you'll still gain strength and mobility without them. Stand with your feet apart and knuckles facing away from your body [1]. Now, raise your arms, turning your hands so that your palms face the ceiling. Finally, raise your arms above your head [2]. Slowly return to your starting position.

BACK, HIP, AND LEG EXERCISES

Single knee pull

(repeat 5 times)
Lie with your back on the floor. Grasp one leg with both arms so you can pull it back onto your chest. Hold for a count of five, then repeat with the other leg.

Ankle circling

Sit down and cross your legs. Slowly trace a circle with your toes. Repeat this motion with your other foot.

Leg raising (repeat 5–10 times)

Lie on your side and raise your leg as close to 45 degrees as you can manage. Hold for a count of two, then lower. Try to keep your leg straight.

Reaching and bending

(see below, repeat 3–5 times)
Stand erect with your feet slightly apart and one hand in the air. Breathe in and stretch upward as far as possible, still keeping your feet flat on the ground [1]. Now, breathe out slowly, bend over, and touch the ground between your feet [2]. Bend your knees if you need to – this is quite a difficult exercise to master. Repeat the exercise, this time stretching up with your other arm.

Groin stretch (repeat 3 times)

Stand with your feet wide apart and your back straight. Bend your knee forward and count to 5. Rise onto your toes on 3.

Thigh stretch

(see below, repeat 3 times)
Stand at a right angle to the wall for support or hold on to a chair. With your free hand pull your ankle up toward your bottom and hold for a count of five.

Calf stretch (repeat 3 times)

Stand facing a wall. Lean against it and let your hips hang forward for a count of five Then rise onto your legs for a count of three.

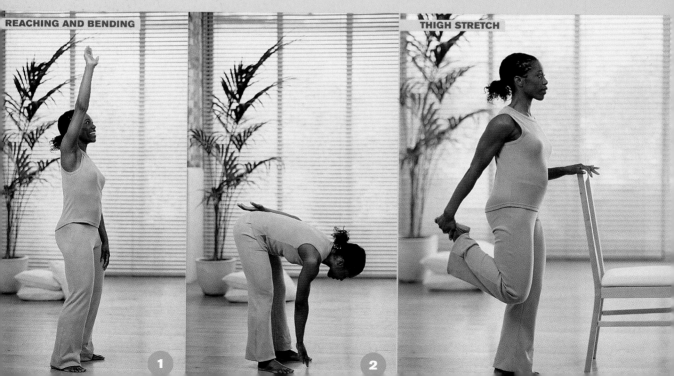

REACHING AND BENDING

THIGH STRETCH

1

2

strengthening exercises

These are designed to enable our bodies to cope with the **extra effort** we're sometimes called upon to make in special circumstances – so that we build in a safety margin of extra strength over and above the normal requirements. It's important that we have this reserve because when it isn't there, making a sudden and extreme effort can result in damaged muscles, ligaments, and tendons, even a slipped disk. To build up those extra resources we need to increase the **duration and force** of our exercise a little at a time. Strength won't suddenly appear; it will develop as we start exercising on a **regular** basis.

heart and lung exercises

Any exercise that increases your breathing rate (aerobic exercise) will keep your heart and lungs healthy if you repeat it frequently and keep it up over the weeks and months. In order to look forward to exercise and do it consistently, you should find an activity you really **enjoy** or something that has to be done (walking the dog) or **fits neatly into a corner of your life**. My daily 30 minutes on my exercise bike covers the television news, but there's a lot to choose from.

SWIMMING This is for almost all of us **the perfect activity** and one of the few all-body sports. Once you're immersed, the water takes the weight off your body, so that your limbs become weightless and your **joints are relieved of strain**. Just floating in water is a treatment in itself for your muscles, joints, and bones. The water supports all your movements through the full excursions of your joints and limbs, so that

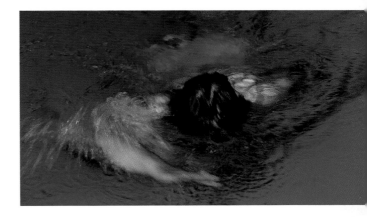

you can exercise with very little discomfort. As a result, your joints can gain in flexibility and your muscles can **gain in movement and elasticity** with you hardly being aware of it.

Swimming is good for the whole body, exercising all your muscles. If you do it for pleasure, even once a week, you can do an awful lot to keep your body **flexible and strong**. It's extremely good for relaxation and rehabilitation after an illness, especially for your back and legs. Swimming can also be used as a method for keeping fit, though it would involve swimming fairly hard for 20 to 30 minutes, at least four times a week.

GOLF will keep you as fit as you need to be because of all the walking. It's very good for improving your **strength, flexibility, and muscular coordination**. Because golf is mainly walking, and slow walking at that, the calorie expenditure is quite low – about 1,000 calories for 18 holes. So it really can't be used as a means of shedding weight. The amount of energy that you expend during golf depends very much on whether or not you carry your golf clubs yourself or drive around in a golf cart. Obviously you'll be fitter if you do the former, but as you get older it's very nice to take things more easily and slowly, with less strain and fuss. Carrying your clubs will certainly exercise your body and your heart more than traveling around in a cart. It's been shown that the heart rate will rise to an average of about 113 beats per minute if you carry your clubs, whereas it stays at a fairly steady 80 if you drive around in a cart. Thus, you're asking your heart and lungs to work about 50 percent faster if you opt for carrying your clubs.

CYCLING An excellent way to exercise since it involves the whole body, and again it's one of those sports that you can adapt according to how much you want to work your body. If you cycle steadily and energetically for 20 minutes or more, it's an extremely good way of increasing the strength and endurance of the whole body, including the heart and lungs.

It's one of those sports that can make you physically fit and in tip-top condition if you want since it's very good for strengthening the large muscles in your body. It's also efficient at strengthening your knees, ankles, and hip joints, and the quads on the front of the thighs.

TENNIS This is an enjoyable, sociable sport that you can play at any age. It is particularly good for keeping your shoulders, arms, and legs **supple and strong**, and for helping your **coordination**. Tennis is also very good for your posture and for keeping your youthful stride, and it can be played at any pace.

It's a sport that enables you to socialize before and after playing. It's important to play tennis at a **steady pace at first**, with partners of similar ability.

KEGEL EXERCISES

Keeping your **pelvic floor firm** really does confer benefits until the day you die. Kegel exercises alleviate incontinence and prolapse and improve sexual enjoyment. Here's how to do them:
◆ First, find the correct group of muscles by stopping the flow several times while you're urinating.
◆ **Tighten** the muscles for five seconds, **relax** them for five seconds, then **tense** them again. Make sure you're not just tightening your buttocks and try not to tighten your stomach muscles at the same time. You may not be able to hold the tension for the full five seconds at first, but you are likely to develop this ability once your pelvic floor muscles grow stronger.
◆ Next, **tighten** and **relax** the muscles ten times, as quickly as you can so that they seem to "**flutter.**" You will probably need to practice for a while to control the muscles in this way.
◆ Next, **contract** the muscles steadily. Hold the contraction for five seconds.
◆ The final step is to **bear down**, as if emptying the bowels, but pushing more at the front than at the back. Hold the tension for five seconds.
Gradually build up to ten contractions, ten times daily or more, spaced over several hours. Check your progress once or twice a week by stopping the flow when you urinate. After about six weeks of these exercises you should find stopping the flow is much easier than it was in the beginning. And once you've mastered the technique, you can do your Kegel exercises anywhere, any time.

TAKE *a seat* AND STRETCH

THESE EXERCISES FROM THE KFA (KEEP FIT ASSOCIATION) CAN BE DONE SITTING DOWN, AS ALTERNATIVES TO STANDING STRETCHES.

These exercises can all be done in a chair. Regular stretching will keep you **moving, mobile, and independent**. There are many benefits gained from including stretching in your daily routine. It will help maintain and improve your joint flexibility, encourage **good posture,** and assist breathing and **digestion**. These stretches can be performed on their own at home. They can also form part of a class exercise program, either as part of the warm-up process or at the end of a session.

WARMING UP

To avoid injury, warm your muscles thoroughly before stretching, with toe taps, knee bends, and arm swinging, which you can do sitting down. Read the following sections on safety, good posture and how to stretch effectively.

CHAIR SAFETY

It's important to check that the chair you are using is suitable (there should be no arms) and that the seat height is correct (your feet should rest flat on the floor). The chair should be stable, have a supportive backrest, and be placed on a nonslip surface.

SITTING POSITIONS

Ensure you're in the correct position on the chair before stretching. See Sitting Positions 1, 2, and 3 below.
1 Sit at the **back** of the chair.
2 Sit at the **center** of the chair seat, away from the back of the chair with an upright position.
3 Sit toward the **front** of the chair seat, ensuring you feel balanced and safe.

STRETCHING EFFECTIVELY

Always **warm up before stretching**. Be careful stretching muscles where the joints may already be lax or unstable due to a medical condition, such as rheumatoid arthritis or multiple sclerosis. **Always move slowly into a stretch**, easing into the correct alignment. You should be able to feel a gentle stretch in the "belly" of the muscle. Relax and hold the position for 10–30 seconds. Do not bounce, and breathe evenly. Release the stretch slowly and repeat up to three times.

SITTING POSITIONS

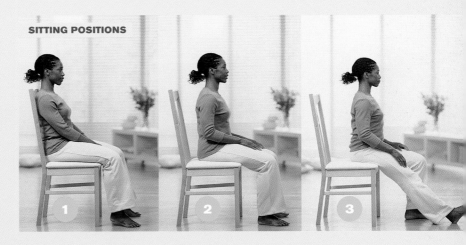

Fingers and wrists

Helps maintain hand function, reaching, and gripping.

Sitting position 1

With hands close to the body, place palms together as if saying prayers. Spread fingers and thumbs.

Upper arm (see below)

Strengthens triceps muscle, essential for shoulder flexibility and reaching upward.

Sitting position 2

Place the palm of your hand on the back of your neck. Using your other hand, gently ease the arm upward. Repeat on the other side.

Upper back (see below)

This stretch relieves tension in the neck and shoulders.

Sitting position 2

Clasp hands as if holding them around a beach ball. Curl spine by tightening stomach muscles. Relax and ease out between shoulder blades. Look at the floor in front of the knees.

Chest

Stretches the pectoral muscles, important for good posture and breathing.

Sitting position 2

Hold the back of the chair at both sides. Ease the elbows inward. Progress to placing palms on buttocks. Ease elbows together.

Waist

This stretch helps posture awareness and aches and pains around the lumbar area.

Sitting position 2

Hold the edge of the chair. With the other arm, reach upward, aiming for the ceiling. Bend gently to the side to increase the stretch, keeping the weight equal on both buttocks. Repeat on the other side.

Calf (see below)

Suppleness of this muscle is necessary for ankle flexibility and walking with a heel strike (not shuffling). The muscle gets tight if high heels are always worn.

Sitting position 3

With one leg stretched forward, and the heel on the floor, pull the toes toward the face and hold. Loop a scarf under the ball of the foot to assist the stretch. Repeat the stretch with the other leg.

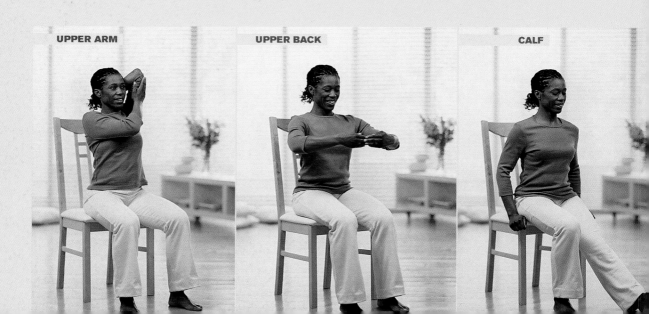

UPPER ARM UPPER BACK CALF

Back of thigh

This stretch is good for arthritic knees to prevent tightening at the back of the knee and increasing stride length.

Sitting position 3

Stretch one leg forward, heel on the floor. Support with one hand on the bent knee. Sit tall with head up. Slowly lean forward from the hip, keeping the spine upright. The stretch is felt at the back of the thigh. Pull the toes up toward the face, if necessary, to feel the stretch. Repeat with the other leg.

Front of thigh and hip

(see above)

This stretch is useful for helping you achieve a good upright posture.

Sitting position 3

Keep the body upright throughout and hold the chair for support.

Take one foot backward, under the chair until you feel a gentle stretch on the front of the thigh and hip.

Or, sit at one side of the chair and lower the outer leg toward the floor.

Or, sit sideways on the chair and lower the front leg toward the floor.

Repeat with the other leg.

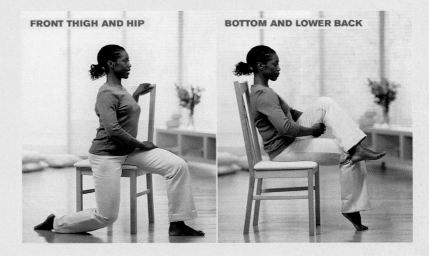

FRONT THIGH AND HIP

BOTTOM AND LOWER BACK

Inner thigh

This stretch is helpful for arthritic hips.

Sitting position 2 or 3 depending on the depth and shape of the chair seat

Place knees as far apart as possible, turning the toes outward. Place one hand on each thigh, with fingers toward each other. Slide the hands to the inner thigh and gently ease the knees apart.

Bottom and lower back

(see above)

This stretch helps maintain your hip flexibility.

Sitting position 2, then lean back against the chair

Place both hands underneath one thigh. Gently ease the leg toward the body.

Trunk

This stretch helps you stay flexible and turn easily. Ensure the twist occurs along the whole spine – not just the neck.

Sitting position 2

Keep an upright posture. Put both hands on one hip and turn the shoulders.

Or, with legs crossed, put both hands on the outer side of the knee and turn the shoulders.

Cooling down

At the end of an exercise program do some cool-down stretches to ease out the muscles that have worked hard during activity. This will increase flexibility and prevent muscle soreness.

FOR *mature* MOVERS

THESE STRETCHES FROM THE KFA (KEEP FIT ASSOCIATION) HAVE BEEN DESIGNED SPECIFICALLY FOR PEOPLE OVER THE AGE OF 65.

It's important to stretch all major muscle groups regularly, especially those that become tight due to the effects of gravity. Make these stretches part of your daily routine and keep yourself moving, mobile, and independent.

Start by warming up with a combination of walking in place, knee-bends and toe taps. Begin gently and gradually increase your movements. When you feel warmer and freer, stretch your muscles using the exercises described on these pages.

Remember to "cool-down" in the reverse way at the end of your stretching routine. Hold each stretch for 6–8 seconds. Breathe naturally throughout and intersperse the stretches with some activity to keep yourself warm.

Calf (see below)
Take a step back with one foot, keeping both feet facing forward. Bend the front knee, keeping your knee over your ankle, not toes. Lengthen/extend your back leg and gently ease your heel down. Repeat with your other leg.

Hip flexor
From the calf stretch position, raise your back heel. Tilt your pelvis under. Relax both knees. Align your shoulders over your hips and knees.

Upper back (see below)
Stand with your feet slightly apart and your knees slightly bent. Keep your pelvis tucked under and your stomach drawn in. Hold your arms as though you're encircling a large ball and look forward and down. Try to separate your shoulder blades as you stretch.

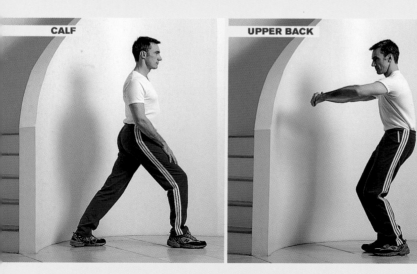

CALF

UPPER BACK

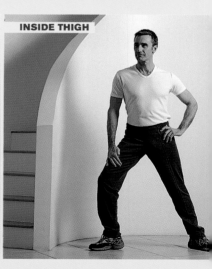

INSIDE THIGH

Inside thigh (see below)
Stand with your feet apart. Lunge to the side with the bent knee facing the same direction as your foot. Keep your knee over your ankle. The foot of your straight leg and your hips face forward.

Side stretch
Stand with your feet apart. Lunge to the side, supporting your weight on your bent leg. Keeping your hips and shoulder square to the front, reach toward the ceiling and slightly over.

Front thigh (see below)
Stand with your feet hip-width apart. Use a support if you need to. Bending your knee, slowly raise one foot into position. Do not pull it. Keep your supporting knee relaxed. Push your foot into your hand on the same side. Push your hip forward on the working leg and your knee down toward the floor. Repeat with the other leg.

Achilles tendon
Place one foot slightly in front of the other, keeping both feet facing forward. With your pelvis tilted under, bend your knees.

Hamstring (back of thigh)
Stand with both feet facing forward. Lengthen and extend your front leg, keeping your back leg bent. Support your weight on the thigh of your bent leg and then push your bottom up toward the ceiling. Repeat on the other leg.

Chest (see below)
Stand with feet hip-width apart and knees relaxed. Keep your pelvis tucked under and your stomach in. Place your palms on each buttock and ease your elbows toward each other.

Back of upper arm (see below)
Stand with your feet hip-width apart and knees relaxed. Raise one arm and place your hand at the back of your neck. Use your other hand gently to push the arm back so you feel a stretch. Repeat with the other arm.

Shoulder
Place your right arm across your chest. Use your left arm gently to draw the right arm close to your body. Repeat on the other side.

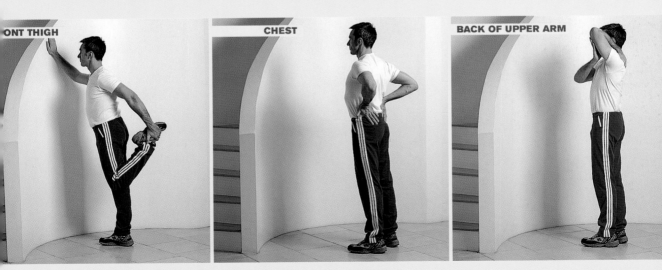

FRONT THIGH CHEST BACK OF UPPER ARM

DEFY AGE by adapting EXERCISES to your NEEDS

Age	Safeguarding bone density and developing stamina	Muscle tone
35+	Use large whole body movements to a quick tempo. Repeat each movement 4 times on alternate legs and repeat the whole sequence for a workout of 10–15 minutes. Make this part of 30 minutes of physical activity 5 times a week. **1** Do 4 runs in place. Step and hop on one leg and then the other, while raising one arm, then both above your head. **2** Hop on your right leg and raise the left leg out to the side like a pendulum. At the same time swing the arms in the same direction. Repeat by hopping on to your left leg. **3** Take a step to the side, bring feet together, then step and hop on one leg while raising your arms.	Try to do two sets of the exercises, 12–15 reps of each one. Moderate tempo. **4** Take a big step forward and bend both knees, ensuring your front knee is over your ankle. Raise the heel of the back foot. At the same time, raise both arms forward to shoulder level. Repeat on both legs. **5** Stand with your feet hip-width apart. Bending the supporting knee, lift one leg to the side. Repeat with the other leg. Repeat the previous exercise but lift your leg back behind you. **6** Kneel on all fours, with your hands below your shoulders and your knees slightly further back from your hips. Keeping the elbows slightly bent, lower yourself down toward the floor. Push to recover by doing a half press up. **7** Stand, sit, or lie – breathe in and as you breathe out pull your belly button toward your spine as though "zipping up" your pelvic muscles. Breathe normally but keep contracting for a slow count of 5 and then release.
55+	Repeat the exercises as for 35+ with the following adjustments if necessary. You may need to reduce the size of the movements and to reduce tempo to moderate. Build your reps gradually. **1** You may need to reduce the level of impact – how high you hop. You may need to lower your arms from high to shoulder level. **2** and **3** You may need to practice the leg movement first, then the arm movement before trying both together.	Repeat the exercises as for 35+ with the following adjustments if necessary. Try to do 1–2 sets of the exercises, 8–12 reps of each one. **4** Reduce depth of lunge – take a smaller step forward. Gradually try and increase the depth of the lunge. **6** Keep knees under hips – that is, box press up. Work to a slower tempo – 2 counts down and 2 up.
75+	Repeat the exercises as for 55+ with the following adjustments if necessary. You may need to reduce the size of the movements and to reduce the tempo. Build your reps gradually. **1** Simply rise onto the ball of the foot instead of hopping. **2** and **3** You may need to practice the leg movement first, then the arm movement before trying both together.	Repeat the exercises as for 55+ with the following adjustments if necessary. Try to do 1–2 sets of the exercises, 6-10 reps of each one. **4** Hold on to a chair for support while doing lunges. OR Stand with feet hip-width apart and bend knees slowly. **5** As for 35+ but hold on to a chair for support. **6** Stand facing a wall, a little way away. Place your palms against the wall and slowly bend your elbows to lower yourself toward the wall. Press against the wall to push yourself back to the starting position.

Balance and coordination	Flexibility and posture	Age
Try to do several sets of these exercises. **8** Take 3 steps to the side. Lean over to one side, taking your body weight on to one leg (you will get a feeling of being off balance). Sway and lift the other leg off the floor. Repeat several times. **9** Moving sideways to the right, step right left right, completing a full turn and finish with your feet hip-width apart. Then rise up on to the balls of your feet while lifting the arms as high above the head as feels comfortable. Avoid letting your ankles roll outward.	*Use large joint movements as you do these stretches.* **10** Stand with your feet hip-width apart. Bend forward, keep your knees relaxed and curl the shoulders forward, pulling in the stomach and rounding the spine. Return to standing, pulling your shoulder blades gently together. **11** Bend your knees and twist slowly to your right and then left. **12** Try the standing stretches on page 136.	35+
Repeat the exercises as for 35+ with the following adjustments if necessary. **8** Don't lean too far. If necessary, use your arms to help you balance. **9** Remove the turn or adjust into quarter turns. If necessary, reduce the speed.	*Repeat the exercises as for 35+. No adjustments necessary, but you may need to reduce size of the joint movements.*	55+
Repeat the exercises as for 35+ with the following adjustments if necessary. **8** Hold on to a chair and lean to the side. OR Keep your foot in contact with the floor. **9** Remove the turn or adjust to quarter turns. Keep your arms low.	*Repeat the exercises as for 35+ with the following adjustments if necessary.* **10** and **11** Reduce the size of the joint movements. **12** Try the seated stretches on pages 133–135.	75+

NOTES

• **Warm up** (see page 128) before starting the exercises. Progress gently and *build up* rather than throwing yourself into them full-tilt.

• **The age categories** are only a guide – an active 70-year-old may well be able to follow the advice for 55+.

• **Try to be active every day** as well as doing the exercises – take the stairs, walk instead of driving, and so on. Sitting in a chair causes body rust!

• The **coordination** required and remembering of sequences **gives the brain a work out too.** And increase in blood flow helps to offset the risk of Alzheimer's and stroke.

• If you prefer, try doing *several sessions* of five or ten minutes in a day instead of all in one shot – aim for a **cumulative effect**. Many find this easier to achieve and they are less likely to give up.

• Figure out your **maximum heart rate** – subtract your age from 220. Aim for a *moderate* rather than a vigorous workout at 55 percent of maximum heart rate.

• **Check** with your doctor before starting exercise.

• **Enjoy** your exercise.

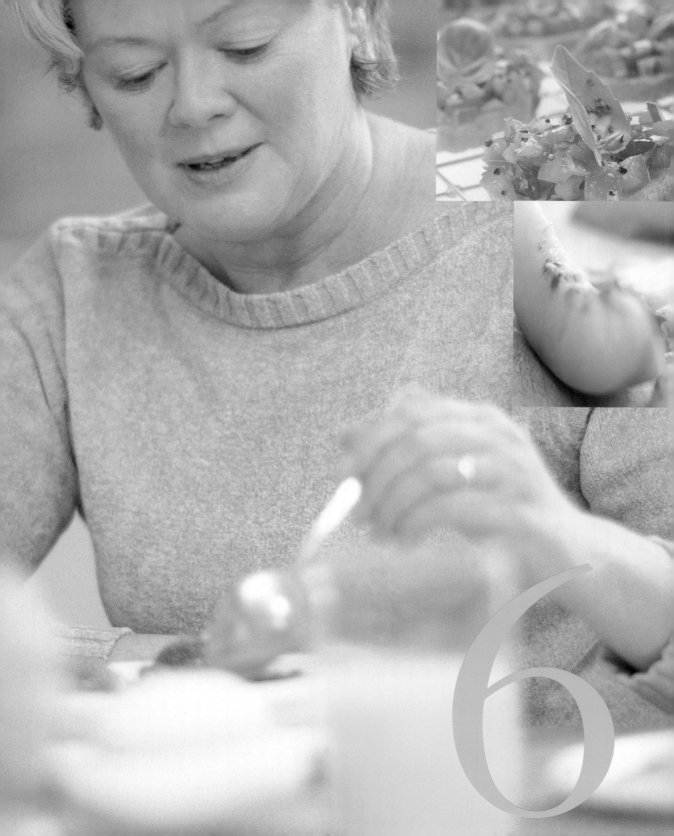

EATING
FOR A LONG LIFE

All fruit and vegetables *contain vast quantities* of known and unknown antioxidants, so having the minimum of five helpings a day is crucial. As we get older it may be that we need **as many as ten portions of fruit and vegetables**, indeed the Okinawan diet includes somewhat more than this. We know *antioxidants work better together* than alone, which is why popping pills isn't the answer, so if you can find foods containing beta-carotene, vitamin E, and vitamin C, *they really pack a punch*. Even after cancer is diagnosed, eating a lot of vegetables and fruits **can hinder its spread** and it's even possible that eating fruits rich in beta-carotene such as carrots, sweet potatoes, spinach, and leafy green vegetables could *cut cancer risk*.

EAT RIGHT, *stay well*

IN THIS BOOK YOU'LL COME UPON CERTAIN "RULES" TIME AND TIME AGAIN. THE REASON FOR THIS IS THAT THEY'RE GOLDEN RULES, RULES THAT RESEARCH HAS CONFIRMED AS HAVING MANY BENEFITS FOR GOOD HEALTH AND LONG LIFE. HERE ARE SOME OF MY FAVORITES.

GOLDEN RULE 1

Eat to stay young like the Okinawans

- **Eat a variety of foods, mainly from plant sources.** Each Okinawan centenarian eats an average of 18 different foods a day and 78 percent of these are plant foods.
- **Eat at least five servings of vegetables and fruits daily.** With the Okinawans this is at least nine, often ten and frequently 17 if you count two servings of peas and beans. Vegetables, potatoes, peas, and beans are the most common foods in the Okinawan diet.
- **Eat six or more servings every day of food made with grains.** In Okinawa they eat at least three servings of rice supplemented with whole grains such as buckwheat noodles and wheat noodles. Rice is the most commonly eaten single food in Okinawa. Brown rice, however, would contain more nutrients and more fiber.
- **Make complex, unrefined, unprocessed carbohydrates the basis of your diet.** More than half of your total calories should come from fruit, vegetables, rice, and whole grains.
- **Limit fat intake to a third or less of total calories.** Monounsaturates should comprise about 15 percent of total calories and polyunsaturates about 10 percent.
- **Limit total salt intake** to less than 3 teaspoons (6 grams) a day. Okinawans eat a little too much salt at 7 grams a day but much less than the mainland Japanese who eat more than ½ oz (12 grams).

GOLDEN RULE 2

Cut your calorie intake
No, this isn't just to control your weight, it's to prolong your life. Calorie restriction extends the life of every animal it's been tried on, sometimes by 50 percent. How might this work? A protein called SIR2 may hold the key. Yeast organisms given an extra copy of SIR2 **live twice as long as usual.** Now SIR2 can only exert an effect in the presence of another protein, NAD+, which is used up when we digest food. So eating less would make more NAD+ available to activate SIR2 and might help us to live longer. It's worth making a bit of an effort to lower your calorie intake. Here's how:

- **Drink water** before you eat. It decreases your appetite, stops you from eating too much, helps mix the digestive juices, and makes your stomach produce more acid, which stops flatulence.
- **Eat slowly** If you're ravenous, count to ten before taking a bite, then eat slowly. Before swallowing, hold food in your mouth for ten seconds.
- **Cut your calories** in an instant and satisfy your cravings by chewing sugarless gum or eating a low-calorie menthol mint.

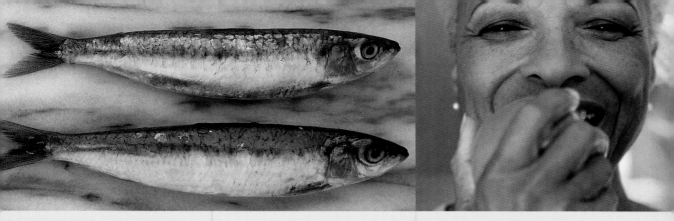

• **Put a motto** on the fridge door, on your mirror, or on your computer to remind you that you don't want to eat high-calorie snacks.

• **Chunky soup** with large pieces of vegetable makes you feel fuller and you eat a fifth less than you do of puréed soup.

• **Add chili to your food** We tend to eat less when food is spicy and hot.

• **A lunch box** may save you as many as 300 calories a day if you prepare your own meals.

• **Have a cup of tea** (black, green, or jasmine) before you walk. Fatty acids are liberated from your muscles so you burn fat faster.

• **Add interest to your salads** with celery, carrots, broccoli, onions, and other vegetables. Don't cut them up too small, and take more time so you'll be chewing more and eating less.

• **Instead of whole juice,** try a juice spritzer. Mix half your favorite juice with water and you'll cut up to 100 calories per glass. Over a year you'll weigh 7lb (3kg) less!

• **Get into the habit of reading labels** Always look for the number of calories per portion.

• **Don't pour oil** Spray it as the Japanese do for stir-frying. You'll use about a teaspoon of oil if you spray it, about six times less than if you pour it.

• **Don't cook too much food** or overeat.

• **Think small portions** Use smaller plates so that the portion looks larger.

• **Start to earn your calories** through exercise, even if it's just climbing up the stairs instead of taking the escalator or walking instead of taking a cab, then you won't overindulge.

• **Be inspired by a role model** to help you realize your goal and don't beat yourself up for not instantly achieving it.

GOLDEN RULE 3

Learn by heart which foods are high in which vitamins and minerals. For instance:

• **Good sources of folic acid** are spinach, curly kale, beet greens, vegetables, and nuts.

• **Good sources of B6** are seafood, whole grains, bananas, nuts, and poultry.

• **Vitamin E** is concentrated in vegetable foods containing fats such as soy beans, sunflower and corn oils, nuts and seeds, whole grains, and wheat germ.

• **You get selenium** (see page 146) in grains, sunflower seeds, meat, garlic, and seafood – especially tuna, swordfish, and oysters.

• **But for a major injection of selenium** nothing beats brazil nuts from the forests of the Amazon, where the soil is particularly selenium rich.

• **Chromium** is found in brewer's yeast, broccoli, barley, liver, shrimp, whole grains, mushrooms, and some beers.

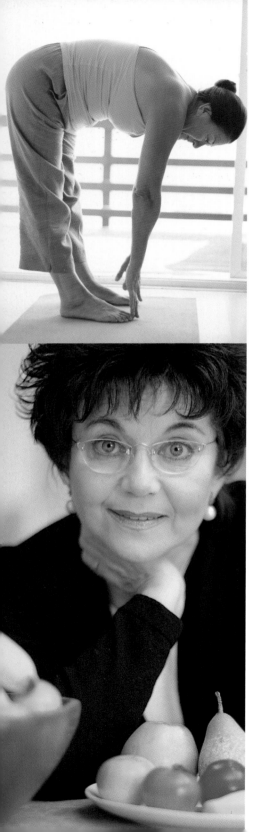

POWER*nutrients*

EATING HEALTHILY CAN CERTAINLY
INCREASE YOUR HEALTH SPAN AND MAY
CONTRIBUTE TO YOUR LIFE SPAN, GIVING YOU
THE CHANCE OF STAYING ACTIVE AND HEALTHY
FOR AS LONG AS YOU LIVE.

As Jean Carper says in *Stop Aging Now!*, we can all eat for a
longer life, especially since there are many **power foods**
containing anti-aging nutrients to help you achieve that goal.
First here's a rundown of some of the **power nutrients** for
which **life-prolonging properties** are claimed.

antioxidants

Antioxidants are the moppers-up of those damaging chemicals
known as free radicals (see page 13), which our cells turn out
every second of the day and night as the result of our metabolism.
However, compared to the potent antioxidants our own cells
can manufacture, the antioxidants that we might take on a spoon
or in a pill add little, even supposing that they could reach our
cells in an active form. **Nothing, for instance, comes close
to our own antioxidant enzyme, superoxide dismutase**.

The emphasis has to be on **food** as a source of antioxidants,
not supplements. The simple fact is that foods contain thousands
of micronutrients that help our bodies use antioxidants and
get them to the places they're needed – supplements don't. **Eat
as much antioxidant-containing food as you can**, but
popping supplements won't bring you added benefit. The most
powerful antioxidants supplied by foods (and supplements) are
vitamins C and E, selenium, and beta-carotene.

vitamin C

Because it's so short-lived in the body, this water-soluble vitamin
is needed daily in order to prevent a deficiency. These days vitamin
C from foods is better known for its role as an antioxidant, but it's
very doubtful that supplements help. Vitamin C does help make

collagen, the body's natural cement and scaffolding, found all over the body in tendons, cartilage, bones, and skin. It aids wound healing, increases iron absorption, and protects vitamin E from oxidation. It's important for the health of blood vessels and protects the tissues of the eyes against the free radical damage that can cause cataracts, macular degeneration (see page 105), and the irreversible loss of vision found in many old people. Lastly it has a role as a water-soluble antioxidant which **helps prevent free radical damage to cells** and cuts down on the production of cancer-causing nitrosamines in the stomach. What makes vitamin C so special is that **it's recyclable – our bodies can reuse it**. After mopping up free radicals, it's converted by an enzyme back into its original form and can do its job all over again.

vitamin E

In contrast to vitamin C, vitamin E is **oil soluble** and one helluva vitamin! It's famous as a free radical destroyer and appears to be **one of the main dietary guardians against free radical damage.** Vitamin C and vitamin E work in tandem: vitamin C protects vitamin E from oxidation by free radicals and leaves it free to do its job.

The membranes surrounding cells are made up of fats and are very rich in vitamin E, specifically to defend against free radical onslaught. If a free radical comes near a cell wall rich in vitamin E it's 1,000 times more likely to be snuffed out by vitamin E than it is to damage the cell wall. In this way **vitamin E lessens damage to the walls of the coronary arteries,** thereby lowering heart attack risk. Vitamin E also improves immunity by minimizing damage to immune cells. **It decreases cancer risk by lessening damage to cell DNA**, plus – because it's oil soluble and the brain is made up of fat – **vitamin E reduces the risk of dementia.**

The latest research points out that **vitamin E may help to inhibit the development of prostate cancer**. In prostate cancer, the body produces increasing levels of **prostate-specific antigen**, which helps the cancer develop and is used as a marker in the diagnosis and monitoring of the condition. But vitamin E

Top food sources of VITAMIN C

black currants
broccoli
brussels sprouts
cauliflower
strawberries
lemons
cabbage
oranges
spinach (fresh and frozen)
grapefruit
pineapple
turnips
potatoes
tomatoes
peaches
beans
bananas
peas

Top food sources of VITAMIN E

almonds
canola oil
hazelnuts
margarine
mayonnaise
olive oil
peanut butter
rice bran
sunflower oil
shrimp
sweet potatoes
sunflower seeds
wheat-germ oil
whole grains
cereals

suppresses the expression of prostate-specific antigen. There's also evidence that vitamin E helps to **prevent the growth of cancer cells in the prostate**. Vitamin E reduces the amount of androgen receptor, a key factor for the progression of prostate cancer. This finding could help to find new therapies for the prevention and treatment of prostate cancer.

selenium

The mineral selenium is a powerful antioxidant with diverse "anti-aging" properties. It's essential for a healthy immune system to **help us combat infections and cancer**. Selenium acts as an antioxidant, not only on its own but also as an essential building block for the creation of *glutathione peroxidase*, one of the body's most powerful antioxidant enzymes which neutralizes free radicals far more powerfully than any antioxidant you can take by mouth in food or supplement.

It's believed that **selenium's anti-aging power** is due to the way it can step up the production of the free radical busting glutathione enzyme. Selenium is a potent cancer fighting agent and may be particularly important in preventing lung cancer. **It appears to fight cancer** by preventing mutations and repairing damage to cells and, by stimulating lymphocytes to neutralize carcinogens, it boosts our cancer-killing immune cells. That it can **protect against heart disease** was shown in a large Finnish study where people with the lowest blood levels of selenium were three times more likely to die of heart disease than those with the highest levels. For people with HIV, it seems that as long as there's selenium in their cells, the HIV virus remains confined and doesn't invade the rest of the body. But when selenium is depleted, the virus switches to a high rate of replication that may go on to full-blown AIDS. Selenium also seems to have a **positive** effect on mood and mental functioning and increases blood flow to the brain.

beta-carotene

Beta-carotene, the orange-yellow pigment first isolated from carrots more than 150 years ago, has antioxidant powers that are thought to help **prevent and reverse** cancer, heart disease,

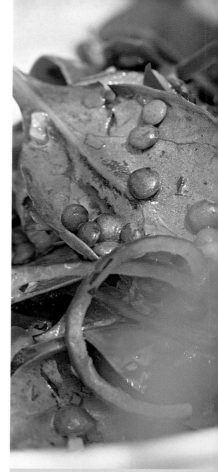

Top food sources of **SELENIUM**

whole grains
sunflower seeds
meat
seafood, especially tuna, swordfish, oysters
garlic
brazil nuts (these have the highest content of selenium of any food)

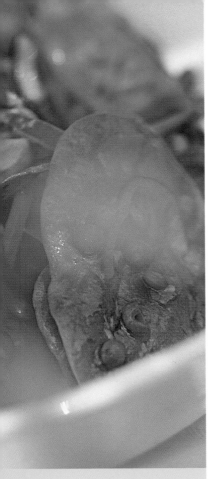

cataracts, and compromised immunity. It protects the integrity of cells by neutralizing free radicals that corrupt genes, turn fat rancid, and destroy cell structures. Beta-carotene converts in the body to vitamin A, which also boosts immunity. **Beta-carotene seems to block cancer**, particularly cancer of the cervix and the spreading of cancer cells. It may play a part in stopping heart attacks by preventing arteries from clogging with fat; it may even protect against strokes.

The wonderful thing about beta-carotene is that it comes in concentrated packages of single carrots. Women who eat at least five carrots a week are **nearly two-thirds less likely to have a stroke** compared with women who eat carrots once a month or less. Eating a lot of beta-carotene-packed spinach can cut the risk of stroke by 40 percent. Research suggests that high intakes of beta-carotene can reduce cardiovascular risk after two years but it takes at least 12 years for it to cut lung cancer risk. The simple carrot can also boost your immune system by activating T-lymphocytes, which help protect the body from cancer and infections, both viral and bacterial.

Top food sources of BETA-CAROTENE

carrot juice
sweet potatoes
apricots
chicory
raw carrots
spinach
cantaloupe
pumpkin
squash
tomato juice
pink or red grapefruit
mangos

flavonoids

Flavonoids — a current buzzword — are powerful antioxidants belonging to the **phytoestrogen group**, a weak plant estrogen. There are several — *flavonols, flavones, isoflavones,* and *bioflavonoids.* All seem to protect our health. Okinawans eat more flavonoids than anyone else in the world, largely in the form of soy and soy-based foods. The Japanese have blood flavonoid levels up to 50 times those of people in the West and the **lowest rate of hormone-dependent cancers** (such as breast and prostate) next to the Okinawans. This shows that the flavonoids they eat get into the bloodstream where they exert anticancer effects.

For us in the West who don't choose to eat much soy, **our best sources of flavonoids are tea, onions, apples, broccoli, and cranberry juice**. It's worth trying to get more flavonoid foods into your daily diet. After a high flavonoid meal you'll have measurable levels of flavonoid in your blood for up to 36 hours and **one such meal a day is adequate for protection**.

10 QUICK AND HEALTHY SNACKS

◆ Baked potato with chives and fat-free sour cream
◆ Veggie burger with lettuce and tomato
◆ Tablespoon of hummus on one piece of whole-grain bread
◆ Celery sticks with hummus or peanut butter
◆ Piece of fruit
◆ Tablespoon of fat-free cream cheese on a whole-grain roll
◆ Handful of soy nuts (roasted soy beans), unsalted
◆ Half a melon or papaya filled with low-fat yogurt
◆ Ricecake with low-fat cottage cheese and a slice of tomato
◆ Low-fat oatmeal cookie

TIPS FOR LOW-CALORIE EATING OUT

◆ **Order pasta or a baked potato.** If it comes with a high-fat creamy sauce or sour cream, ask for it on the side and eat very little.
◆ **Order fish or chicken** rather than red meat and have it baked or grilled, not fried.
◆ **Avoid margarine,** butter, and fried foods.
◆ **Eat a few crackers** or bread sticks rather than hunks of white bread.
◆ **Always** get a sandwich without mayonnaise.
◆ **Split dessert** with your partner or better still, have a sugarless mint tea.
◆ **Fill up first** with a salad, little or no dressing.
◆ **Eat vegetables** and resist ordering french fries. Steal a few from your partner instead.
◆ **Drink water** instead of high-calorie soft drinks.

Tips for increasing your flavonoid intake.
• **Find out as much as you can about soy products** like tofu, silken tofu, tempeh, miso, soy milk, soy flour, textured soy protein, defatted soy flakes.
• **Eat soy beans** – whenever you're in a Japanese restaurant snack on edamame (fresh soy beans) or buy them frozen in supermarkets and in health food stores. Roasted dried soy beans make another tasty snack.
• **For a healthy breakfast** make a smoothie by blending silken tofu with some fresh fruit.
• **Try soy alternatives** – soy milk, ice cream, and yogurt, soy hot dogs, bacon, and cheese, soy burgers, even soy turkey.
• **Add a scoop of flaxseed** (linseed) to your breakfast cereal and salads. It has a delicious nutty flavor, especially if you grind it into a powder.
• **Drink tea – green or black**, there's hardly any difference. Tea is the major source of flavonoids for Europeans. All forms of tea supply 12–16mg per cup.
• **Green vegetables contain flavonoids** so include broccoli, kale, celery, onions, snowpeas, turnip greens, alfalfa sprouts. All of them are terrific sources of flavonoids, so eat them often.
• **Many fruits contain flavonoids** – apples, cranberries, strawberries, grapes, and apricots all score high. Mix them into fruit salads and eat them fresh or dried.
• **Flavonoids are not lost** in freezing or cooking.
• **Flavonoids and phytoestrogens** – bump up your own estrogens with the phytoestrogen contained in flaxseed, carrot leaves, textured vegetable protein, red clover, cranberry juice, kale, celery, snowpeas, broccoli, black tea, soy milk, and chickpeas.

Top food sources of **CHROMIUM**

brewer's yeast	shrimp
broccoli	whole grains
barley	mushrooms
liver	beer
lobster	

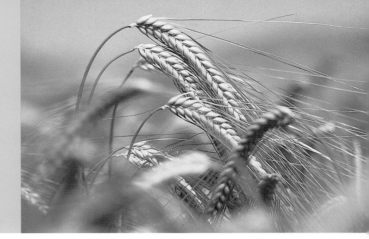

fiber

Fiber is the indigestible part of fruit, vegetables, and whole grains – complex carbohydrates – and it's useful to us because it steadies the absorption of the sugars, which provide most of our calories. Fiber therefore is a **slow-release food** and as such **keeps your blood sugar steady** and prevents the high spikes of insulin that cause cravings and binges.

If you eat 1oz (30g) of fiber a day, your blood sugar will remain absolutely **rock steady**. One can of beans will give you 30 grams of fiber and fiber supplements such as psyllium are excellent. If you add too much fiber too suddenly to your diet, watch out for intestinal cramps and gas. They're common but temporary side effects of adding fiber to your diet, and can be avoided by upping your fiber intake slowly.

Fiber helps to **keep your weight steady**: over a period of ten years, men and women who ate at least 20 grams of fiber a day gained 8lb (3.5kg) less than people who ate the same number of calories but 40 percent less fiber.

How to increase fiber in your diet

• **Buy breakfast cereals** with at least 7 grams of fiber in one serving.

• **Eat high-fiber vegetables** such as celery, cabbage, radish, fennel, and sweet potato whenever you can.

• **Eat whole grains**, brown rice, and oats as often as you can. They contain soluble fiber which keeps your cholesterol down.

• **Eat oatmeal** several times a week to increase your intake of soluble fiber.

CHROMIUM

Chromium is a heavy metal which is crucial to the body in two major respects: first, it's a main constituent of red blood cells and they cannot develop properly in its absence. Second, it's part of an enzyme system that generates most of our energy. Recently we discovered a third way it contributes to our long-term health – it assists insulin in regulating our blood sugar levels (see page 32). There are even some authorities that claim it has anti-aging properties.

FOODS *that* BLOCK AGE

SO FAR YOU HAVE SEEN THAT PRACTICALLY ALL THE NUTRIENTS THAT ERASE AGE ARE PLENTIFUL IN FRUITS AND VEGETABLES. AS IT HAPPENS VEGETARIANS ARE VERY GOOD ADVERTISEMENTS FOR A DIET BASED ON FRUITS AND VEGETABLES.

THE VEGETARIAN LIFESTYLE

Forgoing meat and eating only plant foods seems to give you a good chance of aging slowly and lengthening your life. You'll benefit from:
◆ lower weight
◆ lower cholesterol
◆ lower blood pressure
◆ fewer heart attacks
◆ less cancer
◆ a strong immune system

Vegetarians **simply outlive** meat eaters. Even vegetarians who smoke and are fat are less likely to die than fat, meat-eating smokers. Women vegetarians seem to be **spared cancers of the breast and ovary**; they also have less type 2 diabetes, gallstones, kidney stones, osteoporosis, and arthritis. Vegetarians have a **more vigorous immune system** with white cells that are twice as lethal to tumor cells as those of meat eaters. In fact, vegetarians need only half as many white cells to do the same job.

It's thought that vegetarians age more slowly because they have higher levels of plant antioxidants in their bloodstreams to ward off cancers and chronic diseases. They have **more robust immune systems** to resist infections and other immune-related diseases including cancer. They eat fewer calories and fewer dangerous fats, both of which we know to be life-prolonging.

the magic of fruits and vegetables

Most of us in the West are fruit and vegetable deficient. We all know that eating five fruits and vegetables a day will make us healthier, but if you want to eat sufficient **to stay young**, you have to eat much more than that, like the Okinawans, the longest-living people on the planet. Here's how eating more fruit and vegetables will help reduce your cancer risk.
• **Even smokers** can partially reverse cancer damage by eating fruits and vegetables rich in beta-carotene like carrots, sweet potatoes, spinach, and green leafy vegetables – **eating one carrot a day may cut cancer risk by 50 percent.**
• **Cabbage, broccoli,** cauliflower, and other cruciferous vegetables contain chemicals that **protect against breast cancer.**
• **Tomato eaters** are five times **less likely to develop pancreatic cancer.**
• **Women eating fruit and vegetables,** particularly the deep orange and green varieties,

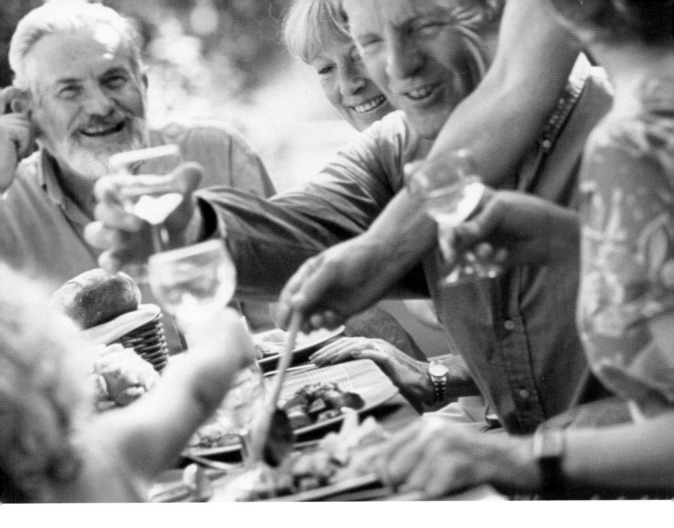

have about **half the risk** of cancer of the uterus.
• **Even after cancer is diagnosed** eating a
lot of fruit and vegetables can **hinder its
progression**. Among men, tomatoes, oranges,
and broccoli appear to improve survival chances.

more benefits of fruits and vegetables

**Fruits and vegetables prevent heart disease and
high blood pressure**. A recent study found that
women who ate an additional carrot a day slashed
their risk of a heart attack by a fifth and of a stroke
by more than two-thirds. A diet high in fruits and
vegetables also curbs high blood pressure.

**Fruits and vegetables keep your mental and
physical faculties in good shape**. It may be that
a deficiency of a chemical contained in tomatoes
impairs your ability to cope in old age. This is a
red pigment called lycopene. It's an antioxidant
and virtually the only way to get it is to eat
tomatoes. In women over the age of 75, those
with low blood lycopene levels were less able to
perform self-care tasks such as walking, bathing,
dressing, feeding, and toileting than women who
ate tomatoes! The deep pigment is a pure give-
away for antioxidants so go for the darkest

AGE-DEFYING FRUITS AND VEGETABLES

broccoli contains a lot of calcium but also a great selection of antioxidants, particularly one called *sulphoraphane*, as well as vitamin C, beta-carotene, *quercetin*, *glutathione,* and *lutein*. It's also one of the richest food sources of the trace metal chromium, which attacks insulin resistance and helps normalize blood sugar. Broccoli eaters also have less colon and lung cancer and heart disease.

carrots A must every day and legendary in fighting off the effects of aging. Eat five carrots a week and you'll reduce your risk of a stroke by almost two-thirds. A couple of carrots a day will lower your cholesterol by 10 percent and cut your lung cancer risk by half, even in smokers.

grapes Red are best. Grapes contain 20 known antioxidants mainly in the skin and seeds – the more colorful the skin the greater the antioxidant effect. Grape antioxidants lower LDL cholesterol and relax blood vessels. Three glasses of purple grape juice and one glass of red wine have equal anticlotting effect in the arteries. Raisins are even more potent than fresh grapes.

berries The darker the berry the more antioxidants it has, so go for blueberries which have an antioxidant called *anthocyanin*. Both blueberries and cranberries help ward off urinary tract infections. Strawberries may ward off cancer and all berries are rich in the antioxidant vitamin C.

citrus fruits The orange contains a vast array of antioxidants, including carotenoids, terpenes, flavonoids, and vitamin C. Grapefruit has a unique type of fiber, especially in the membranes and the juice sacs, that reduces cholesterol and may even reverse atherosclerosis.

tomatoes Never go a day without them. They're practically the only reliable source of the antioxidant *lycopene*, which preserves mental and physical functioning as we age and lowers the risk of pancreatic and cervical cancer. Cooking and canning tomatoes doesn't destroy lycopene. Cooked tomatoes may even be more cancer-protective than fresh and may lower the risk for prostate cancer.

cabbage Like broccoli, cabbage is high in antioxidant activity and cabbage eaters have a lower risk of colon, stomach, and breast cancer. Savoy cabbage is the most potent.

onions Red and yellow onions are richest in *quercetin*. Quercetin helps keep bad LDL cholesterol from attacking the arteries and helps prevent blood clots.

avocado One of the most potent antioxidants. Though avocados contain a lot of fat, it's healthy fat in that it lowers cholesterol; it also delivers potassium to protect blood vessels.

spinach may protect against cancer, heart disease, high blood pressure, strokes, cataracts, and even psychiatric problems because of its powerful antioxidant lutein. Eating large amounts of spinach may cut the risk of the vision-destroying disease macular degeneration (see page 105).

oranges and carrots, the deepest-green leafy vegetables, the reddest grapes, the reddest onions, and the deepest-color berries. Blueberries contain an exceptionally high concentration of antioxidants.

Fruits and vegetables may save your eyesight. People who eat less than three servings of fruits and vegetables a day are four times more likely to get cataracts. In particular carotenoids, vitamin C, and folic acid, found in fruits and vegetables, seem to **oppose the free radical damage** that causes opacity of the lens. Spinach seems to have particular eye-protecting powers.

the magic of soy

That most uninteresting vegetable, the soy bean, turns out to be a **virtual magic bullet** of antioxidant and other anti-aging agents, including *genistein, daidzein, phytates, saponins, phytosterols, phenolic acids,* and *lecithin.*

Genistein may be an inhibitor of breast and prostate cancer and interferes with fundamental cancer changes at virtually every stage.

• **It blocks an enzyme** that turns on cancer genes.

• **It inhibits** *angiogenesis*, the growth of new blood vessels needed to feed growing cancers.

• In the laboratory it **curbs the growth** of all types of cancer cells, breast, lung, colon, prostate, skin, and leukemia.

• As far as the heart is concerned genistein helps **prevent fatty plaque** buildup and clogged arteries and, in damping down the activity of thrombin, which promotes blood clotting, it

HOW TO DEFY AGE WITH FRUITS AND VEGETABLES

◆ Eat at least five servings of fruits and vegetables a day but try for ten.

◆ Eat a lot of different fruits and vegetables.

◆ Choose fresh and frozen fruits and vegetables over canned ones where possible.

◆ Eat both whole fruits and vegetables and juices or blend your own.

◆ Eat vegetables both raw and lightly cooked. Both have advantages.

◆ To get the most antioxidants, choose deeply colored fruits and vegetables.

◆ Cook vegetables in a microwave oven to retain as many antioxidants as possible.

helps prevent heart attacks and strokes.

• **Daidzein** is a second-class type of genistein but still blocks cancer in animal experiments.

Soy is rich is two amino acids, *glycine* and *arginine*, which reduce blood insulin levels and so it may help ward off type 2 diabetes. It may also help build strong bones because eating soy protein conserves calcium, whereas eating animal protein tends to wash calcium out of the body. Soy also prevents unhealthy LDL cholesterol from harming the arteries.

how to get soy into your diet

• Drink a cup of soy milk every day.

• In baking recipes, replace one third of wheat flour with soy flour.

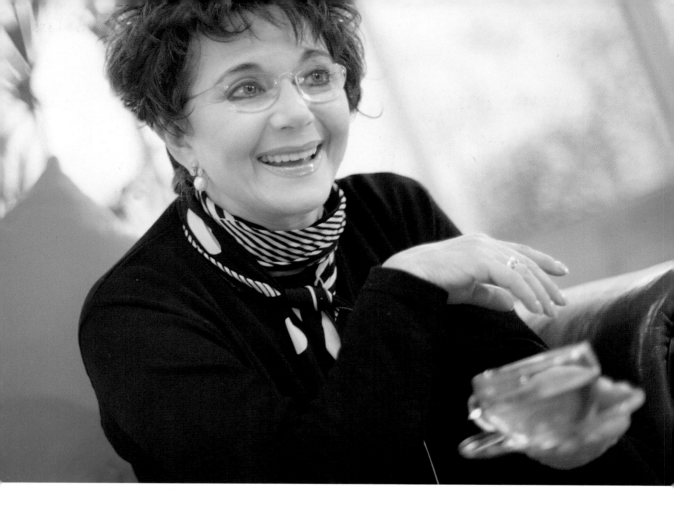

• Put **nonfat soy milk** on your cereal and use soy milk when making cakes and desserts.

• Use **soy protein powders** to make beverages: one-third cup fruit juice, one-half cup water and 8oz (225g) of soy protein powder. Stir until powder is dissolved.

• Use **roasted soy nut**s as a snack. They are readily available in most grocery stores.

• Make fruit shakes with **tofu** or soy milk.

• Add chunks of **tofu or tempeh** (fermented soy bean cake) or both to stir-fried vegetables.

• Cook fresh green soy beans as a vegetable.

• Eat imitation meat products – "hot dogs" and "hamburgers" made primarily with **soy**.

• Use dried soy beans as you would other dried beans, such as navy beans.

• Substitute **textured vegetable protein** for part or all of the meat in recipes.

tea

Tea contains many antioxidants, indeed five cups of tea a day delivers **as much antioxidant as two fruits or vegetables**. The antioxidants are polyphenols such as catechin and quercetin. After you drink tea your antioxidant blood levels soar by as much as 50 percent in 30–50 minutes. Tea works by revving up the liver's detoxification system that rids the body of

After drinking tea, your *antioxidant blood levels soar* by as much as *50 percent* within 30–50 minutes. Tea also *revs up* the liver's detoxification system.

free radicals and other cell-damaging chemicals. **Tea fights aging for the following reasons.**

• **It cuts the rate of fatal heart disease.** Even drinking two cups of tea will give you a cardio-protective dose of flavonoids.

• **It reduces cholesterol** and if you drink five cups of tea a day you'll halve your risk of stroke.

• People who drink tea **reduce their risk of cancer.** Tea works in at least five different ways to block both the formation and the growth of malignant tumors.

• **If you want healthy gums, drink tea** because it combats the bacterial activity that causes gum disease, a lot of tea being as powerful as the antibiotic, tetracycline.

• **Tea seems to prevent tooth cavities** by attacking *Streptococcus mutatis*, the main bacterium that causes tooth decay.

• Tea isn't the only drink that contains catechins; red wine and red grape juice do too, but you have to drink three times as much grape juice to get the same antioxidant effect as wine. **And here's the evidence:**

• In a Japanese study involving around 500 patients with breast cancer, researchers found that premenopausal women who drank green tea **had fewer lymph nodes affected by cancer.** Five or more cups of green tea daily seemed to offer the best cancer defense.

• **Scientists in America report that drinking tea could reduce the risks of dying from heart disease** after having a heart attack. Doctors at the Beth Israel Deaconess Medical Center in Boston studied 1,900 patients who had all suffered a heart attack between 1989 and 1994. The lowest mortality rate was among those who had been moderate or heavy tea drinkers in the year before their heart attack – a 44 percent lower death rate among heavy tea drinkers and 28 percent less chance of death among moderate consumers compared to non-tea drinkers.

• People who drink tea every day were shown in trials at the University of Minnesota to suffer **fewer clogged arteries and blood clots.**

• **Ordinary tea is a useful source of vitamin E and K as well as small amounts of B vitamins.** Drink it regularly and it will contribute to your intake of manganese, a mineral that is essential for bone growth and hormone production.

alcohol

A glass of wine or a portion of grapes a day is cardio-protective and it's possible that the redder the wine and the redder the grapes, the greater the benefits for your heart.

the age-defying effects of chocolate – yes chocolate

Good news for all chocoholics – you've been right all along. **Chocolate is the new health food** – one might almost say a magic bullet. Not only does it contain the same chemicals that make you feel good after sex, but it can also protect your heart, thin the blood, and **lower your cholesterol and blood pressure** – the list is endless. A study by researchers at Harvard University suggests that if you eat chocolate three times a month you'll live almost a year longer than those who don't.

The unique combination of aroma, texture, and taste stimulates the emotional feel-good centers of the brain. **In short, chocolate tastes good, so we feel good.** This has been proved by scans tracking changes in the brain activity of the frontal cortex, which analyze the reward value of incoming information to the brain. Scans on a group of volunteers showed that the frontal cortex really glowed when they were munching a bar of chocolate, more than when they were listening to pleasant music.

It turns out that both smelling and eating chocolate activate areas of the brain that are known to be involved in creating feelings of pleasure. It seems chocolate has a unique blend of **sensory qualities** which make us feel good, activating pleasure centers in the brain. Some researchers believe one ingredient in chocolate can produce a real high. *Tryptophan* is a natural chemical that the brain uses to make serotonin. High levels of serotonin can produce **feelings of elation**, and it's thought to be no coincidence that the drug ecstasy and some antidepressants work by increasing serotonin.

Another ingredient, *phenylethylamine*, stimulates the brain's **pleasure centers**, reaching peak levels during orgasm. It's the chemical that makes you feel so good after sex. This could explain why it was used as an aphrodisiac in the 16th century and why some women claim that chocolate is better than sex.

Most recently *anandamide* has been found responsible for chocolate's most universal appeal. It's said to target the same brain structures as the active ingredient in marijuana. These structures could be described as **reward center**s – after chocolate you feel rewarded.

Another of the magical ingredients in chocolate is **cocoa flavonoids – potent antioxidants**. Here are just a few of the health benefits they confer – but beware the fat and sugar in most forms of chocolate!

• **Lower cholesterol.** Eating chocolate rich in flavonols may counteract LDL (bad) cholesterol, and that helps protect blood vessels against oxidative damage by free radicals. Both free radical damage and poor blood vessel health are recognized factors in the development of heart and vascular disease.

"chocolate – the

• **Blood clotting.** Blood platelets contribute to clotting of the blood and make a heart attack or stroke more likely in susceptible people. Cocoa flavonols may reduce platelet stickiness and increase the time it takes for blood to clot. These blood-thinning effects are similar to those seen with aspirin. Aspirin is widely used to reduce platelet activity in people at risk of coronary heart disease or deep vein thrombosis, and to treat patients who have had a heart attack or stroke. Eating a bar of chocolate might have the same effect.

• **Blood pressure.** Certain cocoa flavonols may increase levels of nitric oxide in the bloodstream. This is good because nitric oxide opens up arteries to increase blood flow so is important in keeping your blood pressure healthy and, in turn, your heart. This may explain why there's so little high blood pressure among the Kuna Indians – a tribe living on islands off the coast of Panama in Central America, who have a diet rich in cocoa.

• **Immune system.** In addition to enhancing antioxidant defenses, compounds in cocoa may have a positive impact on the immune system. The mechanism by which certain flavonoids modulate the production of cytokines (inflammation-causing proteins) remains unclear but the suggestion is that cocoa flavonoids are potential immune modulators and may have therapeutic advantages in humans by activating the immune system against cardiovascular disease, eczema, cancer, and arthritis.

But it's not all good news. Don't think of bingeing on chocolate – the research suggests that people who eat too much chocolate have a lower life expectancy. Chocolate's high fat content means excess indulgence can contribute to obesity, leading to an increased risk of heart disease. Moderation is the key.

If you think you're eating too much chocolate here are a few things you can do.

• Look for **low-fat chocolate** products such as mousses and drinks, but don't kid yourself into thinking you can now consume more.

• **Crave control patches** have been developed for the true chocoholic and are modeled on nicotine patches for smokers. But instead of releasing the addictive chemical into your body through your skin, it emits a powerful smell that is supposed to remind you of sweet food like chocolate. The idea is that, as you're exposed to the smell all day, you will lose your appetite for such things. A clinical study at St. George's Hospital, London, has shown that those wearing the patches lost more than twice the weight of those who did not use them

• There's a brand of tiny long-lasting **chocolate drops** on the market that give you all the pleasure of the taste and smell of chocolate without the fat and calories. Try them for damage limitation.

new health food?

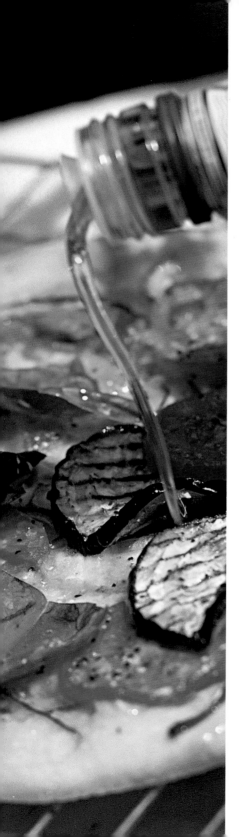

GOOD FATS, *bad fats*

FATS IN FOODS CAN AGE YOU – SO AVOID
THE NASTY ONES. ONE OF THE REASONS WHY
CORONARY HEART DISEASE IS SO COMMON IN
THE U.S. IS OUR UNHEALTHY DIET. FAT INTAKE –
ESPECIALLY SATURATED FAT IN THE FORM OF ANIMAL
FAT – IS MUCH TOO HIGH.

We should **get no more than a third of our calories from fat**,
but many people get way in excess of that. The Japanese, on the
other hand, get only 15 percent and that may account for their
healthy hearts. Fats are made from fatty acids and provide the
body with energy in its most concentrated form. They are known
as **saturated** or **unsaturated** depending on how saturated
they are with hydrogen. Saturated fatty acids tend to be harder,
becoming solid at room temperature, whereas polyunsaturates
remain liquid at room temperature. With the exception of coconut
and palm oils, **almost all plant oils are unsaturated**. Most of the
saturated fat we eat comes from animal sources – milk, cheese,
butter, and meat.

   You can keep your fat intake down by eating these foods rarely,
or only if they have a low fat content. Better still, **avoid most
red meat** and eat poultry, fish, and legumes instead.

   BUT – just as some amino acids can't be made by the body,
so certain fatty acids, all polyunsaturates, are impossible to
manufacture ourselves, we have to eat them. So they're essential
to our diet and are therefore called **essential fatty acids or
EFAs**. Everyone's diet should include foods containing these
essential fatty acids, such as **oily fish, vegetable oils, and nuts**.

fats and your cholesterol

In recent years everyone has started to worry about the role
of saturated fat in the development of coronary heart disease.
The concern revolves around the different ways saturated and
unsaturated fats are transported in the bloodstream. Because
fats (lipids) are insoluble in water, to get around the body they

have to be combined with protein, so making a **lipoprotein**. The third component in this transport system is **cholesterol**.

When lipids are traveling to and from fat reserves or muscle they have a very low density. These lipoproteins are called *very low-density lipoproteins*. After the fatty part has been delivered, its place is taken by cholesterol and it becomes a *low-density lipoprotein* or *LDL*. Finally, the transport system can load up with extra protein for some journeys making *high-density lipoprotein* or *HDL*. Dangerous cholesterol deposits in the coronary arteries are derived from cholesterol-carrying low-density lipoproteins (LDLs). If your LDL level is high, your risk of a heart attack is raised. HDLs on the other hand, protect you because they're the healthy form of lipoprotein. So, biochemically speaking, it's good to have a lot of HDL in your blood.

the age-defying fats

Oleic acid is our main **monounsaturated fat** and is found in olive oil, which can protect the heart by reducing the amount of artery-clogging LDL cholesterol in the blood and make blood platelets less sticky and so less likely to form blood clots. This may be the reason why people in Mediterranean countries, who consume large amounts of olive oil, have **lower death rates** from heart disease.

For monounsaturated fats, eat olive oil, canola oil, peanut oil, nuts, and margarine. There are now cholesterol-lowering margarines that are very effective — if more expensive.

Polyunsaturated fats tend to have a liquid consistency, whether at room temperature or refrigerator temperature — most of our EFAs are polyunsaturated fats. There are two families of essential fatty acids (EFAs) in our diet: omega-6 (derived from linoleic acid) and omega-3 (derived from alpha-linoleic acid).

Omega-6 fatty acids are found in vegetable sources such as sunflower, corn, safflower, soy oils and margarines, grapeseed oil, and sesame seeds. **Omega-3 fatty acids** are found in oily fish, such as mackerel, trout, salmon, and herring, as well as in canola, linseed, soy and walnut oil, pumpkin seeds, and green leafy vegetables. Both are needed for growth and the repair of cells and

Healing FOODS and HERBS

apples
cranberries
lemons
papayas
rhubarb
garlic
ginger
hot peppers
onions
parsley
peppermint
tomatoes
chamomile
echinacea

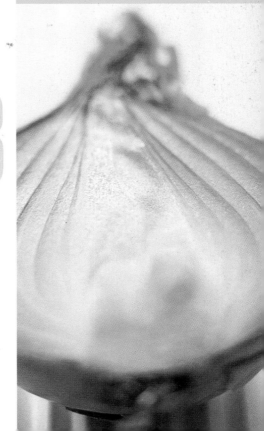

NOT ALL FATS are bad

Good	Better	Best	Bad
Monounsaturated fats	*Polyunsaturated fats*	*Omega-3 fats*	*Saturated fats*
flaxseed oil	corn oil	fish oil	coconut oil
walnut oil	sunflower oil	herring	palm oil
olive oil	soy oil	mackerel	meat (beef, lamb,
peanut oil	some margarines	sardines	pork, suet, lard,
canola oil	white fish	herring	drippings)
avocado oil	cod	salmon	dairy fats (butter,
some margarines	nuts	tuna	cheese, milk)
		trout	processed fats
		anchovies	(cakes, cookies,
		linseed	pies, sausages,
		soy	snacks)
		pumpkin seeds	
		green vegetables	
		walnut oil	
		olive oil	
		Omega-6 fats	
		sunflower oil	
		corn oil	
		safflower oil	
		margarine	
		grapeseed oil	
		sesame oil and seeds	

tissues in the body, but the **balance between them** is more important than the amounts in the diet. The way we in the West eat now has ruined that balance.

the fatal omega-3/omega-6 imbalance

To start, our modern intake of fats is very different from what our ancestors were eating when the human brain evolved. We used to have a taste for fish and seafood, all of which are high in omega-3s. With settled agriculture, which began about 10,000 years ago, people started to rely more on cultivated foods and the consumption of fish and wild game declined. The result was a **decrease** in omega-3 intake and an **increase** in the alternative type of polyunsaturated fatty acid, omega-6.

But the most dramatic change in what we eat has happened in the past century with industrialization and the development of the food industry. Manufacturers favor foods with long shelf lives, so they mostly use soy, corn, palm, and cottonseed oil. All contain high amounts of omega-6 fatty acids and very little omega-3. In fact, there's been **a thousandfold increase in our omega-6 intake** in less than 100 years. It accounts for 83 percent of all fats we eat.

This is not what our bodies want at all. A century ago we were eating **equal quantities of omega-3 fats and omega-6 fats**. These days, unless we make a conscious effort, few of us eat the foods high in omega-3 like fatty fish, walnuts, linseed, and olive oil.

It could be that we're eating ourselves into a collective depression by consuming the wrong kind of fats. Globally, more working days are lost through depression than any other illness and it is one of the most serious health threats worldwide. One in ten people are depressed. For one in 20, it's a chronic lifelong condition. The age at which it first strikes is falling.

Omega-3 might be all-important in the brain and essential to keeping you happy. Brain cell membranes are 20 percent fat and the more omega-3 they contain, **the more efficient they are at producing serotonin**, the mood-enhancing neurotransmitter.

People with little omega-3 in their spinal fluid also have low levels of serotonin and a tendency to depression. Early in a baby's development, serotonin acts as a signal to guide migrating neurons to their correct locations. Serotonin also assists to correct growth of brain connections. So lack of omega-3 fatty acids early in life may forever alter the way the brain develops and operates. This much has been widely recognized with the move to add omega-3s to infant formula milk.

fatty acids and depression – is there a link?

More important to us looking for ways to stay active as we go through life is the strong relationship, demonstrated by cross-cultural studies, between **a nation's consumption of fatty acids and its level of depression.** In countries where people eat the least fish the rate of depression is highest, and vice versa.

The average New Zealander, for example, eats only 40lb (18kg) of fish a year and 6 percent of the population suffers from depression. In Japan, where they eat 140lb (64kg) of fish a year, depression strikes fewer than 1 percent of people. This correlation seems to hold true across the world. The case for a real correlation between depression and low omega-3/high omega-6 consumption is convincing. What's more, the imbalance leads to other mental disorders.

So countries where people eat a lot of fish have lower rates of homicide, bipolar disorder, and suicide. And there's varying omega-3 fatty acid levels in breast milk across countries, with low levels in women from non-fish eating cultures. Those same women have the most postpartum depression.

So could foods rich in omega-3s be a treatment for depression? In one study patients showed significant progress within two weeks of starting to take fish oil high in omega-3 fatty acid.

And in a 2002 Israeli study, depressed patients who weren't responding to drugs showed significant progress within two weeks of taking fish oil high in omega-3 fatty acid.

By week four, six of the ten taking fish oil had a **50 percent drop in symptoms such as low mood, insomnia, and feeling worthless.** Only one of the ten patients on placebo improved similarly.

After all, eating more fish, flaxseed, and walnuts while using olive oil and cutting down on processed food can only make you healthier, if not happier.

why we need more omega-3s

It's the omega-3s found in oily fish and fish oils that the body needs because **they're protective against:**

- heart disease
- stroke
- certain cancers (breast, colon, prostate)

and they're therapeutic for:

- mildly high blood pressure
- arthritis
- autoimmune diseases (lupus, certain kidney disorders)
- Crohn's disease
- inflammatory skin diseases (eczema, psoriasis)
- depression, schizophrenia.

So, for general good health, try to make sure that you eat a minimum of two fish meals a week. Alternatively, take 150–200mg daily of omega-3 in cod liver oil supplements.

And for heart disease prevention, eat three meals rich in fish oils weekly, or take 400mg of omega-3 in fish oil supplements.

lessons in healthy eating from around the world

The **Japanese diet**, rich in soy protein, oily fish, and vegetables, may hold the key to improved health in the West.

- The key could be **high levels of omega-3 fatty acids** in the Japanese diet which tend to lower blood pressure, lower the level of triglycerides in the blood, and reduce the risk of clots forming.
- Also linked to tumor suppression, omega-3s may explain the **lower incidence of many forms of cancer** in Japan.
- Japanese women **develop three times fewer cases of breast cancer** than women in the UK
- The Japanese consume **much less fat** than those in the West: Europeans, for example, take in 33 percent of their calories through fat, while in Japan it's around 15 percent.
- Inuit people in the frozen north are thought to owe **their freedom from heart disease** to omega-3 fats from the oily fish that's a staple part of their diet.
- Those who enjoy a Mediterranean diet **may owe their longevity partly to olive oil**, which contains omega-3 essential fatty acids, and partly to the amount of omega-6 and omega-3 in the rest of the Mediterranean diet.

No, you don't have to eat sushi every day. Simply by **eating more fish and fresh vegetables** to boost your intake of omega-3 fatty acids and antioxidants, and **reducing the amount of meat and dairy products you eat** to lower your saturated intake, you can enjoy the health advantages of the Japanese diet without dramatically changing the way you eat.

FOOD*worries*

WE HEAR SO MUCH NOW ABOUT WHAT IS AND ISN'T GOOD FOR US THAT IT'S EASY TO GET CONFUSED. HERE ARE MY THOUGHTS ON SOME COMMON QUESTIONS.

Is coffee bad for you?

Coffee is neither good nor bad for you. Some people need the caffeine in coffee to jump-start the day; others can't stand it and claim it makes them jittery. It's hard to believe this effect is universal, given the toffee-like coffee drunk throughout Greece, Turkey, the Middle East, Eastern Europe, and countries like Austria, France, and Italy.

Some people seem especially susceptible to the stimulatory powers of caffeine found in many drinks. They may feel unpleasant but they do you no harm, nor do they shorten your life.

Look out for caffeine in over-the-counter medicines too – read the labels if you want to avoid caffeine.

Is breakfast the most important meal of the day?

No. There is research showing that the efficiency of our blood sugar regulating mechanisms involving insulin are vulnerable and fragile in the morning, so we should refuse the traditional eggs and bacon breakfast and lightly snack on fruit, cornflakes, oatmeal, or toast.

Does it help to eat certain foods at different times of day?

No. Our bodies evolved to digest food no matter what it is, no matter what time of day we eat it. To suggest anything else runs counter to evolutionary theory.

Are high-protein and high-fat diets safe?

No. Worse, they're dangerous, encouraging heart disease, stroke, and cancer.

ORGANIC PLANT FOODS

Are they better for you?

No. Organic foods are mostly a mind-set. A mind-set that believes organically produced fruit and vegetables taste better,

CAFFEINE counter

	Serving	Caffeine (mg)
Coffee	5fl oz (150ml) cup	
Drip		115
Percolated		80
Instant		70–100
Tea	5fl oz (150ml) cup	33–64
Soft drinks	12fl oz (325ml) can	
Cola drinks		38–46
Diet cola drinks		36–46
Dark chocolate	1oz (30g)	24

are healthier, fresher, free of fertilizers and pesticides, and more ecologically friendly than foods grown by traditional farming methods.

But these perceived benefits aren't necessarily real. In fact, many plants produce their own pesticides, many of which are more toxic to human beings than synthetic ones. **Everything that's natural plainly isn't good for us.**

In addition, organic food isn't free of chemicals. Many tests have shown that organically grown foods do indeed contain pesticides and are prone to contamination with toxic bacteria, molds, and viruses.

The certification agency for organic foods actually does allow the use of pesticides under certain conditions. **And the pesticides used by organic farmers are no less harmful than those used conventionally.**

There is convincing evidence that organically grown food is not superior in quality to conventionally grown produce, even though the organic growers, suppliers, and retailers claim that it is. A carrot is a carrot is a carrot no matter where or how it's grown.

A CARROT IS A CARROT IS A CARROT

In its report *Organic Farming, Food Quality and Human Health*, published in 2002, the Soil Association, a cheerleader for organic farmers, states that organic fruits and vegetables contain more vitamin C and may also have higher levels of minerals and natural plant chemicals that are good for us.

However, Professor Robert Pickard, director general for the British Nutrition Foundation, thinks that the Soil Association's claims are unlikely. "Green crop plants such as fruits, vegetables, and grains absorb their nutrients from the soil as inorganic molecules," he says. "This means that crops grown in organic soil cannot use the nutrients until bacteria converts them into the sort of chemicals that conventional farmers use in bags."

"Essentially, it doesn't matter how their food is delivered to vegetables, be it in top-quality manure or nitrogen fertilizers, they're still going to make the same molecules and **therefore have no biological or nutritional difference.**"

MORE ABOUT CARROTS

In a particular study, while the nonorganic carrots tested were free of pesticides, the organic carrots were found to contain 0.08mg/kg of the insecticide – four times over the government's maximum recommended limit.

The tests also found 0.01mg/kg of an insecticide called methamidophos – an amount equal to the MRL – in the organic batch. Both these pesticides belong to a group of chemicals called organophosphates, which are thought to have nerve-poisoning qualities and aren't permitted in organic farming.

... MEAT MAY BE DIFFERENT

Animals, however, are different because, like us and unlike most plants, they cannot form all of their own nutrients and need to take them from food. "Meat and products from animals raised organically will be nutritionally better because what they eat affects their makeup. For example, the beef from cows fed on grass and not on feed usually has a higher level of the healthy polyunsaturated fats," says Professor Pickard.

THE DOWNSIDE TO ORGANIC FOOD

Last year, a report was published by Dennis Avery, director of the Center for Global Food Issues. Using figures released by the US Centers for Disease Control, he claimed that people who eat organic foods are **eight times more likely to be attacked by the deadly new strain of E. coli** and also have a higher risk of contracting salmonella.

Dennis Avery's view is that organic food is more dangerous than conventionally grown produce because organic farmers use animal manure as the major source of fertilizer for their food crops. "Animal manure is the biggest reservoir of these nasty bacteria that are afflicting so many people. Organic farmers compound the contamination problem through their reluctance to use antimicrobial preservatives, chemical washes, pasteurization, or even chlorinated water to rid their products of dangerous bacteria."

Over the past few years, organic lettuces, apple juice, and even baby food have been linked with outbreaks of these pathogens – bacteria or viruses that can cause disease. And in the recent scandal involving the high level of the food-poisoning bug *campylobacter* found in supermarket chickens, a small sample of 70 organic chickens was included in the research. The findings suggest the bacteria was more common in these than in conventionally farmed chickens, with 60 percent of the organic poultry having the bug.

It seems to me that the organic food story is one which serves producers and retailers very well (organic food is between 20–30 percent more expensive than non-organic) and those who feel driven for themselves and their children to eat pure food.

GM FOODS
Can they do us any harm?

I don't think so. Here's why. In a series of studies for Britain's Food Standards Agency, a research team at Newcastle fed burgers and milkshakes containing genetically modified soy to 12

healthy volunteers and to seven volunteers who'd had their colons surgically removed. By examining stools from healthy subjects and material from the others' ileostomy bags, the researchers could see how different parts of the digestive system affected DNA in the GM soy.

THE FINDINGS

The team found no trace of DNA from the soy in the stools of the volunteers with intact digestive systems. But they found that up to 3.7 percent of the soy DNA remained in the contents of the bags. When they grew bacteria from these samples, they were able to detect trace amount of GM DNA.

That suggests a very few bacteria had taken up a foreign gene or transgene from the soy food. However, the Newcastle team wasn't able to isolate any bacteria containing the soy transgene. Nor was there any evidence that the gene had actually started to function in the bacteria.

THE CONCLUSION

The researchers concluded that while some DNA might survive as far as the small intestine in people with normal digestive tracts, it's broken down on the way through the colon. Even if some bacteria take in some of the DNA, they don't make it out the other end. This led the team to confirm that we have no evidence the foods could have any adverse effects on human beings.

These results don't surprise me at all. "GM foods" are all around us. Genes in plants are changing all the time and have been since time began.

Evolution sees to it that genes mutate to protect plants from their environment, be it extremes of temperature, changes of climate, or a new insect predator. It would be odd if, after millions of years, we hadn't found a defense against those mutant genes. And we have – the large intestine has evolved so that it can destroy them.

Another team at the Rowett Research Institute in Aberdeen has tried and failed to get human gut bacteria to take in

genes for resistance to the antibiotic ampicillin, present in some GM food crops.

What's more, such resistant genes are already widespread in the gut bacteria of many animals. This is probably because of the misuse of antibiotics in agriculture and medicine.

So even if gut bacteria did manage to acquire and turn on antibiotic resistance genes from GM food crops, they would be a drop in the ocean of *existing* resistant bacteria.

DRUGS of a lifetime

Statins
HRT
Selegiline (for Alzheimer's)
Retinoic acid (for the skin)
Aspirin

FOODS of a lifetime

Oily fish
Fresh food
All fruits and vegetables
Eat vegetables rather than meat
Oatmeal every morning
Carrots, tomatoes, and a few nuts and seeds every day
Dark-coloured fruits and vegetables – dark red or black fruit and dark green leaves

SUPPLEMENTS of a lifetime

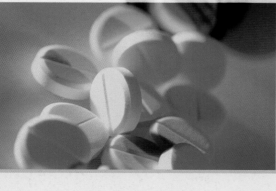

HABITS of a lifetime

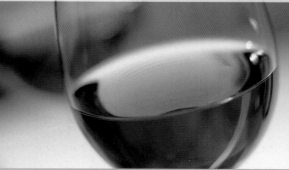

WATER

As we get older, does water get any more important to us?

I really don't think so. I can only think of one example where it does. As we age the stomach becomes worse at secreting acid, which purifies our food and prevents gas being produced in the large intestine. Drinking a glass of water before a meal stimulates acid production and cuts down on gas. Still, mild to moderate dehydration is a widespread problem in older people. The body becomes worse at signaling its need for water via the thirst-awareness messages.

Is water important to our long-term health?

Not as important as is often represented. Yes, we need 2.6–4.2 quarts (2.5–4 liters) of fluid a day depending on how active we are and how hot it is, but the body doesn't care where that fluid comes from.

Your body can't distinguish between the purest water, a cup of tea, or a glass of lemonade. All it wants is fluid. As it happens, the body can get a great deal from what you eat. Think of a juicy pear, an orange dripping with juice, a stick of celery stiff with water, a tomato – which is 99 percent water. In fact most fruits and vegetables are more than 90 percent water.

Water is a waste product of the body – the body must get rid of it because it's the waste from cellular metabolism. We excrete water with every breath we take (as water vapor) and as urine.

GET USED TO CHOOSING
HEALTHY FOODS

- ◆ Substitute **seafood** for red meat whenever you can – eat dark-fleshed fish like salmon, tuna, and shellfish.
- ◆ Try **grilled salmon** instead of beef.
- ◆ Try a **tofu burger** instead of a hamburger.
- ◆ Try **crushed and seasoned tofu**, tuna, vegetarian sausages, or soy bacon bits for your pizza topping.
- ◆ Try a **tuna sandwich** instead of beef or chicken.
- ◆ Next time you barbecue, try **trout, salmon, or tuna** seasoned with herbs – barbecued fish is delicious.
- ◆ Eat **eggs** for breakfast no more than three times a week.
- ◆ Don't have more than one or two servings of dairy products a day – and make them **low-fat**.
- ◆ **Vegetables** should be the centerpiece of most meals.
- ◆ Don't give yourself any more meat than can cover the palm of your hand.
- ◆ **Wean yourself off red meat** slowly – the less red meat you eat, the less you'll miss it, and soon a couple of bites will be enough.

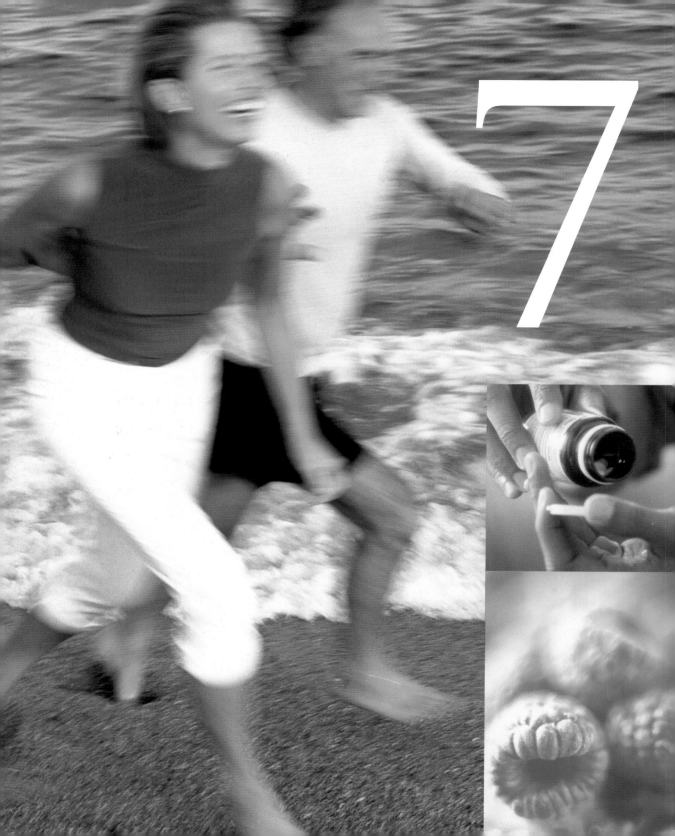

7

IN SEARCH OF
THE ELIXIR
OF YOUTH

We've all read or heard of claims to have found the **formula for long life and eternal youth**. The fact that there are so many means *none of them works*. Each claim represents the sound of an axe being ground. Worse, it may simply be the current fashion or fad. But after exhaustively researching the possibility of there being a single magic pill or potion that will prolong your life, and carefully examining the science behind the various claims of supplements, vitamins, herbs, and alternative therapies, *I believe all but a handful are false*. I'll get to those later in this chapter, but first I'd like to touch on a few areas where the claims can't be supported and to explode **a few common myths**.

DO *supplements* WORK?

I'M AGNOSTIC ON THIS POINT. THERE'S NO QUESTION THAT WE ALL NEED AND BENEFIT FROM VITAMINS, MINERALS, AND HERBS, BUT I'M NOT CONVINCED THAT TAKING SUPPLEMENTS IS THE WAY TO ENSURE THAT OUR BODIES GET ENOUGH OF THEM.

The simple reason is that the human body isn't equipped to use vitamins and minerals parceled into capsules. **It's equipped to use vitamins and minerals parceled into food.** There's little good science to prove that supplements are beneficial, except in specific situations like folic acid in pregnancy.

One of my main objections to self-administered supplements and vitamin pills is that they're marketed as "foods" not drugs. **Because of this they don't have to undergo the rigorous testing that prescription medicines must.** It also means that there is virtually no research to monitor them or find possible side effects. Furthermore, because supplements aren't controlled, many don't contain ANY active ingredient at all.

high doses can be harmful

Research confirms that high doses of vitamin supplements **may do you more harm than good**. Some can cause toxic reactions or other severe side effects like peripheral neuropathy – damage to the nerves in the fingers and toes. But today's enthusiasm for natural remedies is encouraging many people to overdose on supplements. The one in three people who swallows vitamins in an attempt to ward off illness could in fact be **damaging their health** instead of protecting it.

Despite the fact that a **diet including a lot of vitamin-rich fruit and vegetables** can help prevent heart disease and cancer, it doesn't follow that taking supplements has the same effect. The US National Academy of Sciences panel spent two years studying supplements of beta-carotene, selenium, and the antioxidant vitamins C and E.

All of these are said to mop up the body's free radicals – which are a consequence of normal cell metabolism, disease, smoking, and possibly pollution – and neutralize their effect, thereby, theoretically at least, helping the body stay healthy. The supplements are taken by millions in North America to ward off illness and act as an insurance policy against possible deficiency – **although, in fact, none of us eating a good, balanced diet should be deficient in anything**.

But the US report says that although not getting enough of a particular vitamin or nutrient can have a damaging effect, there's no convincing evidence that taking excessive supplements is necessary or good for you. **Neither is there proof that either selenium or beta-carotene supplements cut your chances of getting cancer, heart disease, diabetes, or Alzheimer's disease.**

Myths about vitamins and supplements abound. Here are the facts.

dispelling myths about vitamin supplements

Q If a vitamin is good for us, can the body use it if we swallow it in any form? Are pills, capsules, jelly, or powders just as good for us as food?

A NO, this is a MYTH. The body simply can't use a vitamin or mineral unless it's surrounded with the thousands of micronutrients in a natural food. Once you take a nutrient out of a food and digest it on its own it loses its effectiveness.

Taken alone as a pill, the body can't use most of the nutrient and you literally flush it down the toilet. In the table below I outline what some essential nutrients need (and they're by no means all) to be assimilated by us. These additional nutrients aren't found in the capsules you take, only in foods.

Q If a little of a vitamin does you good, is a lot better?

A NO, this is a MYTH. Most vitamins and minerals are poisons – they'll stop the body working properly or injure it if taken in excess. And that can mean megadoses taken in a single dose or moderate doses over a long period. Here are some examples.

• **DON'T** take megadoses of vitamin C for a cold – or moderate doses over a long period.

WHAT VITAMINS NEED to make them work

Vitamin C appears to protect against heart disease and speed up wound healing	**but not without** bioflavonoids, calcium, and magnesium at the same time
Vitamin B complex contains the so-called antistress B vitamins	**but you also need** calcium, plus vitamins C and E for it to work
Vitamin B6 can sometimes help to relieve PMS	**but it needs** potassium, all the B vitamins, and vitamin C to be effective
Vitamin A can help to treat acne and possibly protect against cancer	**but it needs** essential fatty acids, zinc, and vitamins C, D, and E to do its job
Vitamin D is important for strong bones	**but it needs** calcium, essential fatty acids, and phosphorus as well as vitamins A and C before it increases bone health
Calcium is crucial for strong bones	**but it's no good without** vitamins A, C, D, and F, essential fatty acids, magnesium, manganese, and phosphorus
Magnesium, essential for the health of nerves and muscles, is wiped out by stress and is the second most common deficiency in women	**but you can't** raise levels without calcium, potassium, vitamins B6, C, and D
Essential fatty acids are important for energy and brain health	**but they need** vitamins A, C, E, and D to work effectively

• **DON'T** take vitamin B6 every month for premenstrual syndrome.

The way overdosing on a vitamin or supplement harms you is that taking an excess of one vitamin can lower levels of another. **In addition, falling short of one mineral can prevent absorption of another seemingly unrelated one.**

Put another way, **too high a dose of one vitamin or mineral can produce the same symptoms as a deficiency of another.** So:

• **TOO** much calcium can cause a deficiency in iron, zinc, magnesium, and phosphorous by preventing their absorption. All these minerals are vital for bone health and prolonged deficiency can lead to osteoporosis – the condition you were trying to prevent in the first place by taking calcium supplements.

• **TOO** much vitamin D, which enhances the absorption of calcium, can cause a potassium deficiency.

• **TOO** much vitamin A, the antioxidant loosely claimed to help prevent premature aging, increases the body's need for another antioxidant, vitamin E, which is said to protect against heart disease.

HOW vitamins and minerals are depleted

Depleter	Vitamin or mineral
Alcohol	Vitamins A, B, and C; magnesium, zinc
Cigarettes	Vitamins A, C, and E; calcium, selenium
Caffeine	Vitamins C and B, especially thiamine (B1); calcium, potassium, and zinc
Nitrites (found in processed and smoked meats)	Vitamins A, C, and E
Aspirin	Vitamins C and B, especially pyridoxine (B6) and folic acid
Antibiotics	Vitamins B, C, and K; potassium
Antacids	Vitamin B, especially thiamine (B1); phosphorus
Antihistamines	Vitamin C
Barbiturates (sedative drug)	Vitamins A, C, and D; folic acid
Cortisone	Vitamins A, C, D, and B, especially pyridoxine (B6); potassium, zinc
Indocin (antirheumatic drug)	Vitamins C and B, especially thiamine (B1)
Laxatives and diuretics	Vitamins A, D, E, and K; potassium

• **TOO much vitamin E** is now thought to cause strokes.

• **TOO much selenium**, the popular antioxidant, can lead to brittle nails and hair loss. If you take a multivitamin containing iron at the same time as a calcium supplement, iron may interfere with calcium's absorption. Likewise, caffeine will cause you to lose calcium.

Q Can you rely on supplements to boost an unhealthy lifestyle?

A NO, this is a MYTH. It's no good thinking that you can be careless with your body and then pop a handful of vitamins and expect them to make you fireproof. Far from it.

If you smoke, for instance, you need **an additional 35mg of vitamin C every day** to combat the depleting effects of tobacco. **So cigarettes can be thought of as vitamin depleters.** There are many other vitamin and mineral depleters that we come in contact with every day (see left).

Q Does a supplement always contain exactly what's printed on the label?

A NO, this isn't always true. Top of the list is **ginseng**. In a laboratory analysis published recently in the US, 8 of the 21 brands tested were found to contain high levels of pesticides, and some also contained significant amounts of lead. Neither were stated ingredients.

Nearly a quarter of the **gingko** brands tested did not contain the advertised amounts of the active ingredient.

In the case of **glucosamine-chondroitin**, nearly half the brands tested had lower than claimed chonodroitin levels.

Q How can manufacturers get away with this?

A The US Food and Drug Administration doesn't regulate the supplement industry the way it does prescription drugs and over-the-counter drugs. **In Britain, supplements don't get the rigorous premarket testing that drugs get, nor are labels scrutinized for accuracy and honesty.** This is because they're classified as foods not drugs, even though many supplements are as powerful as drugs.

Q Can I always believe a supplement's claims? For example, if a vitamin or mineral is shown in the laboratory to "boost the immune system," "protect from cancer," or "prevent heart disease," will taking it regularly confer these benefits in real life?

A NO, not strictly true. None of these much-touted laboratory cause and effect relationships of supplements has been proven in human beings. The claims are empirical and as such can't be relied upon. **They're only theories based on laboratory studies,** and the fact that they've been taken up as proof by alternative practitioners doesn't make them any truer.

An example of fallacious thinking on supplements goes like this.

• Some men with low sperm counts have low levels of zinc – true.

• Normal zinc levels are essential for normal sperm production – unproven.

• Giving zinc supplements will improve sperm counts – unproven.

• All men trying for a baby should take zinc supplements – false and unnecessary.

the downside to supplements

Vitamin E Taking more than 1,000mg of vitamin E a day could thin the blood by interfering with the action of vitamin K, which promotes blood clotting, and consequently increase the risk of a hemorrhagic stroke.

It's worth saying again because it's counter-intuitive – unlike drugs, **vitamin and mineral pills don't have to be rigorously tested to establish their benefits** or their safety, or to define harmful interactions with prescription medicines.

Vitamin C The American study warns that taking megadoses of vitamins C or E can cause **severe side effects** and may stop other essential substances being absorbed by the body. Although it isn't possible to maintain high levels of vitamin C as the kidneys excrete any excess in urine, intakes of more than 2,000mg a day can lead to gastric irritation with diarrhea and make urine acidic, which may negatively affect people prone to kidney stones and bladder infections. It may also, if taken in large doses, reduce the effect of the contraceptive mini-pill.

Excess beta-carotene, which is converted to vitamin A in the body, is known to increase the risk of **lung cancer** in some people, especially smokers. And it can turn the skin yellow.

Beta-carotene supplement should never be taken unless proven vitamin A deficiency is present. It should only ever be ingested in foods.

Selenium can cause a toxic reaction, leading to hair loss if more than 400 micrograms are taken daily. **The UK Government's Committee on the Medical Aspects of Food Policy says everyone should avoid taking high doses of selenium and beta-carotene supplements.**

The US government has already announced it is revising its recommended maximum limits for all supplements. **The panel's new recommended daily intakes are:**
Vitamin C: men 90, women 75 milligrams
Vitamin E: men and women 15 milligrams
Selenium: men and women 55 micrograms
Beta-carotene: no recommendation since it shouldn't be taken at all except by people with a vitamin A deficiency.

vitamins work best in teams

So what's the truth about vitamins and supplements? There's so much inaccurate information about that it's difficult to pick your way to the truth.

The general rule has to be that you take your vitamins and minerals in the form of foods – and it will come as no surprise to find

"natural doesn't

that all fruits and vegetables are perfectly designed natural packages of the most valuable and protective minerals, vitamins, and chemicals – the so-called phytochemicals.

The truth is all vitamins and minerals work best in **unison**, like the instruments of an orchestra. If one instrument is missing or too loud, the orchestra sounds out of tune. Our bodies fall below par.

The best examples are the **B vitamins**, which all help each other. They're more potent when used together, and neatly they often come **packed together** in foods. Known as nature's stress-busters, they're all water-soluble, which means that any excess can't be stored by the body. They're excreted quickly by the kidneys – thus we should eat them every day, but in food not pills.

Vitamin B1 is widely known as a **morale-booster** because it can affect mood. But it can't work alone. It always works best in balance with other members of the B-vitamin family, including B2, B6, and B12, plus folic acid and pantothenic acid. That's where a salad of dark green leaves comes in – it contains nearly all the B family in one tidy parcel.

natural isn't harmless

Unfortunately many people think that because something is natural it can't do them any harm.

THE WINNING VITAMIN TEAMS ARE FOODS

◆ Foods are a convenient, efficient, and tasty way to get all the vitamins and supplements you need.
◆ When eaten in a food, each essential nutrient comes in a neat little package with all the other micronutrients your body needs to use it.
◆ You can't overdose on a mineral or vitamin if you take it in food.

The assumption is that if a remedy is natural, it has to be better and safer than anything doctors prescribe.

Yet, as with most substances, it's the amount consumed that's the key. **Many natural substances are toxic if they're consumed in excess.**

The British Nutrition Foundation doesn't recommend huge doses of vitamins or minerals since they can prevent other nutrients from being absorbed by the body.

mean *harmless*"

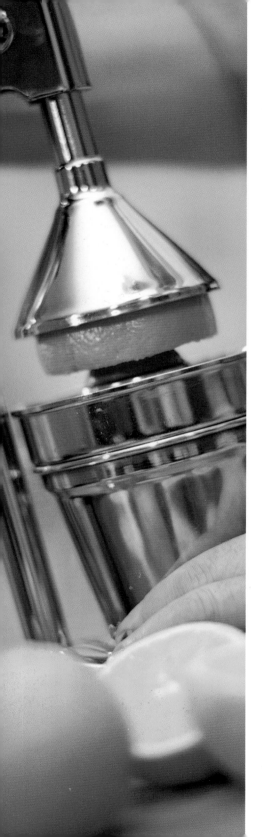

phytochemicals – foods are "supplements"

Phytochemical is a current buzzword but it's not fancy or particularly significant. A phytochemical is simply a chemical (for example, a vitamin or mineral) that's found in a plant. We eat phytochemicals every day. In fact, I've covered most of them in the chapter on foods and eating (see pages 140–167). However, some people believe a few have anti-aging effects.

bioflavonoids

If you ask an alternative practitioner which nutrients are anti-aging they'll specify **bioflavonoids**, one of the supplements of the moment. Though not vitamins, they're a group of biologically active substances found in plants and one of the phytochemicals. They're sometimes called vitamin P.

As well as theoretical cancer-fighting properties, they're said by some to have an antibacterial effect in the body, where they're supposed to promote **healthy circulation, stimulate bile production, lower cholesterol levels, and keep you young**. Quite a list of claims. If they're only half true we will benefit from eating them – the Okinawans seem to, but in the form of food, not pills.

So, if you want to start popping flavonoids, which foods do you eat? You'd be surprised: apples, beets, blackberries, blueberries, cabbage, carrots, cauliflower, cherries, dandelions, lemons, lentils, lettuce, oranges, parsley, plums, peas, potatoes, rhubarb, rosehips, spinach, tomatoes, walnuts, and watercress. **Flavonoids are more efficient when taken with vitamin C. And would you believe it, all the above foods come with vitamin C as part of the package.**

what about phytoestrogens?

Phytoestrogens, mainly in the form of soy-based foods, are postulated as being one of the major contributors to the low prevalence of menopausal complaints in women from Asia and the Pacific Rim. And it was an attractive theory that encouraging Western women to eat soy-based products might help with the

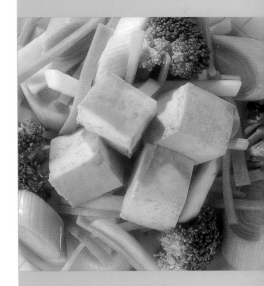

treatment of menopausal symptoms. **Again foods are better than supplements. Several studies examining commercial products extracted from soy revealed disappointing results in relieving menopausal symptoms.** An explanation for this could be that Asian women eat soy foods throughout their lives and popping a daily soy supplement isn't an effective alternative.

There's no evidence to support the belief that even very high intake of soy products is powerful enough to alleviate hot flashes, night sweats, and other symptoms such as vaginal dryness, mood changes, and osteoporosis.

Nor have phytoestrogens, including extract of red clover, been shown to improve other symptoms of menopause such as anxiety, joint pains, muscle aches, bone loss, and headaches. Phytoestrogens should never be taken with Tamoxifen, which protects against breast cancer, because isoflavones may antagonize the desired antiestrogen effects of Tamoxifen.

Many commercially available soy products contain very little actual soy. This is because the manufacturing processes result in destruction of the active substances in the natural product. Let me give you an example: when two commercial "textured vegetable protein" soy products were compared with soy flour, the concentration of the active ingredients daidzein and genistein were 25 times less in the textured vegetable protein than in soy flour. Many products recommended for menopausal symptoms contain virtually no active soy. You, the purchaser, may not be able to discern this because the labeling of such supplements is inadequate, so buying natural soy products to relieve menopausal symptoms may be a waste of money.

Soy concentrate is another matter – indeed, one study from Israel has shown that a significant number of women may get relief from menopausal symptoms while taking soy concentrate each day and it **might turn out to be an alternative for women** who do not, or cannot, take hormone replacement therapy.

Most other phytochemicals that have anti-aging properties are covered in depth in Chapter 6 – chemicals such as lycopene (tomatoes), carotenoids (carrots), and anthocyanodins (grapes, red wine, garlic, and tea).

> "taking soy concentrate every day may help to relieve menopausal symptoms"

ARE *herbs* ANTI-AGING?

THE MAJORITY ARE NOT – A FEW MAY HAVE SOME ANTI-AGING EFFECT BUT SOME MAY INFLICT GREAT HARM.

The most authoritative work on this subject is by Professor Edzard Ernst, the eminent Professor of Complementary Medicine at the University of Surrey in Britain. He dismisses most herbs because there is no trustworthy research to confirm any useful effects. In 2001 one of the oldest – 5,000 years old – of the complementary therapies, traditional Chinese herbalism, was found to be actually **KILLING** its patients.

Two British women suffered kidney damage after taking a herbal preparation to treat eczema.

A toxic herb was implicated as the main cause of an outbreak of kidney disease in Belgium in 1993 when it was an ingredient in some Chinese sleeping pills. Seventy people were affected and some had died of kidney failure.

While there are many places to buy Chinese herbs in North America, few provide guidance.

One of the problems is deciding, on insufficient evidence, whether the benefits of herbal remedies outweigh their risks because most are sold as food supplements and therefore escape regulation of quality and safety. They're unlicensed and so the public doesn't have systematic protection against low quality and unsafe, unlicensed remedies. Furthermore, because of their lack of control on herbal preparations, toxic, even disallowed ingredients may be included. In Britain, for example, a recent study of Chinese herbal creams showed that 8 of the 11 preparations tested contained undeclared **dexamethasone – a very powerful topical steroid** – in the cream, which accounted for its effectiveness in treating eczema and psoriasis, rather than the herbal components. **This practice is illegal and dishonest.** In hoodwinking the public it brings alternative medicine into disrepute.

In 2001 Professor Ernst issued a warning to pregnant women about a widely taken herbal

BLACKLISTED HERBS

TThe US Food and Drug Administration wants warning labels on certain herbs and has banned others, such as ephedra, from being sold in stores and being used by herbalists. This is because there is clear evidence some traditional Chinese medicines in the US are at best unreliable. Some have been found to contain potentially dangerous and often illegal ingredients, including

◆ arsenic
◆ mercury
◆ prescription-only steroids
◆ a herb that may cause cancer or liver damage
◆ gingko biloba seeds that can cause convulsions.

The act of faith, the suspension of belief, is part of the deal with alternative therapies and it has to be if, like Chinese herbalism, it employs such outlandish ingredients as singed human hair, ground tiger bones, seahorses, seal testicles, and bear's gall bladder, several of which are very cruelly collected.

supplement, **gingko biloba. It was discovered to contain** *colchicine*, **a toxin dangerous to the newborn.** He described it as a disaster waiting to happen, a catastrophe like thalidomide. **Just because something is natural or green doesn't mean it's safe.** Everything with a beneficial effect will have side effects.

so do ANY herbal medicines work?

Yes, there's a small body of good clinical evidence that would support for instance:
• **St. John's wort** for mild or moderate depression
• One specific formula of **gingko biloba** for improving memory in 59-year-olds
• **Saw palmetto** as a symptomatic treatment for benign enlargement of the prostate
• **Horse chestnut seed** extracts for varicose veins with swelling of the lower legs. There's very little else and all of the above **cause side effects and dangerous interactions** with prescribed medicines, which the manufacturers don't necessarily warn about.

Doctors have to face the fact that we haven't fully understood how herbal medicines work. Evidence is now accumulating that *hyperforin* and *hypericin* of St. John's wort are effective because they cause the same chemical reactions within the brain as mainstream antidepressant treatments.

the possibility of herb/drug interactions

Remember, manufacturers of herbal remedies rarely research how their products might interact with life-saving medicines. On its own, for

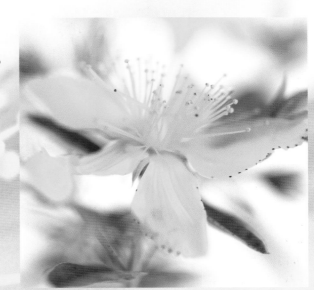

St. John's wort flower

instance, **ginseng** has few adverse effects but **when combined with warfarin its blood-thinning activity might cause bleeding.** Many other interactions between herbal remedies and prescription drugs have been uncovered.

Drugs can interact with substances such as vitamin supplements and herbal remedies in two main ways:
• Sometimes the overall effect of one or both of the substances may be **greater than desired** like ginseng and warfarin
• Sometimes, however, the opposite happens when two or more substances are taken and **make a drug less effective.** If this happens, the medicine may not work as well – or may not work at all.

And a third consideration is that not all plant-based medicines are cheap. The standard daily dose of St. John's wort costs more than the standard prescription antidepressant.

SETTING *the record* STRAIGHT

I'D LIKE TO TAKE A STRAIGHTFORWARD LOOK AT THE CLAIMS OF COMPLEMENTARY THERAPIES. IN MY VIEW, MOST HAVE LITTLE EFFECT.

Based on science, I'd have to say **very few alternative therapies can prolong life**, and we know what those few are. The rest are what I'd describe as weird and freaky but over the past 20 years have become alternative, complementary, and respectable. And while some therapies may indeed complement conventional medicine, this unquestioning attitude has given false respectability to many dubious practices, even charlatanism.

what research shows

Some alternative therapies like acupuncture and osteopathy have been shown to have more than **a placebo effect** in a very small number of conditions. But the most recent research with such a well-established complementary therapy as homeopathy showed that specific remedies for specific conditions have no convincing evidence of effectiveness. Herbal medicines that are well researched, and **thoroughly tested**, are helpful.

Then there are **harmless** therapies which have never been shown to do either good or harm such as Bach flower remedies and simple feel-good therapies like yoga. They won't cure a disease, but if we enjoy them why not indulge in them? But there's a third category **that's downright dangerous or simply silly**, such as crystal therapy, dousing, iridology, and kinesiology.

In the US, the National Institutes of Health (NIH) have begun studying the benefits and risks

THE PLACEBO EFFECT

Having seen the results of studies that verify that particular alternative therapies have no validity whatsoever yet still attract a faithful following, **I'm convinced that most alternative remedies are working in the placebo area.** Let me explain. It's well known in general medical practice that a third of all patients will get better with a dummy pill – a placebo. These patients are susceptible to the suggestion that the pill will do them good. I'm saying that many of the cures claimed by alternative practitioners work in this way. And if they do there is no basis for the claim of an authentic remedy – or of prolonging life.

The truth is that anyone can set themselves up as a therapist or expert in some obscure method of healing without any certificated training and offer "medical treatments" that have no scientific basis nor any evidence of proven usefulness, let alone effectiveness. **Nor is attention paid to side effects or interactions with prescription medicines.**

Millions of people in the US seek some form of unconventional treatment every year, usually with no reference to a qualified doctor. **For a few that delay seeing a doctor the time lost may be critical because important investigations, diagnosis, and conventional treatment is delayed.**

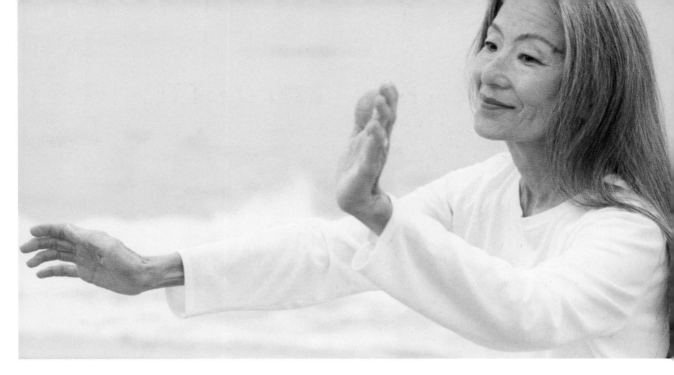

of complementary medicines such as Chinese herbalism and Ayurveda, a very fashionable and even older Indian system which is all about balancing the body's energy channels and the five elements: earth, water, fire, air, and the ether. The NIH hopes to provide scientific study, in place of the existing **anecdotal evidence,** to see if alternative therapies do us any good.

the appeal of complementary therapies

It could be that these medical practices appeal because they're **deliciously old-fashioned and ancient**. They thrive on personal and anecdotal evidence – case histories that of course are interesting but totally unreliable. They can't form the basis for treating large numbers of people, no matter how zealously they're preached.

With alternative and complementary therapies the story inevitably starts with the emotional,

first-person account of the illness, the failure of conventional medicine, despair, recourse to alternative therapy, the miracle cure. Hard facts, tested figures, and verifiable results are always thin.

Many people are susceptible to a miracle and we love stories about having to fight the medical profession. It's thrilling to take power into our own hands and away from the medical professionals, so robbing them of their superiority. However, that doesn't change the fact that therapies such as Chinese herbalism and Ayurveda use substances that are powerful drugs and poisons, sometimes without disclosure.

So **avoid the harmful and enjoy the harmless** but don't expect too much. As long as we only expect to be pampered rather than to be treated and healed we can come to little harm from taking alternative remedies. And we could even feel the warm, satisfying glow of the placebo effect.

NEW*ideas*

IS DHEA THE MUCH SOUGHT AFTER ELIXIR OF YOUTH? SOME CLAIM THAT IT IS, BUT AS YET TOO LITTLE IS KNOWN ABOUT IT.

DHEA, or dehydroepiandrosterone, has become the most fashionable supplement used by workers in the field of anti-aging. It's normally manufactured by the adrenal glands in both men and women. Indeed, in postmenopausal women it becomes crucial and fortunately our adrenals go on producing it long after our ovaries have failed. In women it is converted to a weak estrogen, estriol, but we need any estrogen, even a weak one. **The great news is that exercise converts DHEA to estriol faster than anything else,** which is why postmenopausal women must, for their own sakes, exercise.

Levels of DHEA in the blood, however, start to drop from the age of about 25 and get low in older age. **This is the logic behind DHEA supplementation and the results, according to its supporters, are spectacular:**
• a feeling of **mental well-being**
• **memory** much improved
• loss of fat, **improvement in shape,** and increased muscle mass
• new-found **physical energy**, stamina, and endurance
• renewal of **sexual pleasure** and performance.

Other claimed benefits are not enjoyed by all users but would include appetite control by counteracting the taste for fatty foods and encouraging a feeling of fullness by affecting

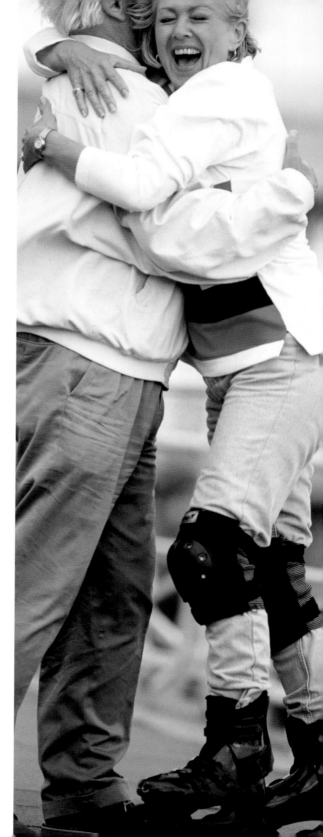

the appetite center in the brain and the way the liver uses glucose.

In laboratory mice DHEA is said to prolong life by 50 percent and in men over 50 it lowers the death rate from all causes, mostly probably because DHEA lowers cholesterol. Patients with certain cancers (breast, stomach, bladder) seem to have particularly low DHEA levels but that doesn't mean that deficiency of DHEA played a part in their cause or that supplements of DHEA would prevent them. Bearing this out is the fact that **high doses of DHEA increase the risk** of prostate cancer and ovarian cancer.

we're in the dark on DHEA

Furthermore, there seems to be no general agreement between doctors using DHEA about dose. Most start off with a low dose, say 5, 10, 20, or 50mg a day according to your age, but in one study with women that rose to 1,600mg a day, and some doctors go as high as 2,500mg a day. This extraordinary range of daily dosage means only one thing to me: **we don't know what we're doing, we're in the dark**. And that seems too dangerous a place for me to be an advocate of DHEA in our present state of knowledge. **And we can't forget the well-documented side effects:**

• excess hair in men and women
• reemergence of periods in postmenopausal women
• increased risk of prostate cancer in men
• increased risk of ovarian cancer in women
• sleeplessness and aggressiveness
• mood changes.

I find it difficult to persuade myself that DHEA is a safe medication that can

Stem cells could be *"grown"* into heart muscle cells that could then be transplanted

be widely advocated to stave off aging when there isn't even agreement about the reliability of tests to establish accurate levels of DHEA in the body. The effect of this ignorance is that DHEA dosage can't be tracked but nor can the effectiveness of treatment. We have a long way still to go.

stem cell treatment – the answer to defying age?

Stem cells are special cells, typically found in embryos and in the umbilical cord. Stem cells are found in adults too, though they are less able to transform themselves into many types of tissue, including bone, nerve, heart muscle, and liver, than embryonic stem cells. It's stem cells that explain many phenomena in animals, causing lizards to grow new tails, earthworms to regenerate half their bodies, and humans to grow new skin over wounds and cuts.

It's hoped that if scientists learn how to control stem cells they could be used to **regenerate parts of our bodies** that are failing or are worn out. Stem cells could be "grown" into heart muscle cells then transplanted into the muscular wall of the heart where they would repopulate unhealthy heart tissue with young, healthy heart tissue. Theoretically, this technique could be used to treat quite a number of serious ailments associated with aging, such as diabetes, Parkinson's, Alzheimer's, strokes, certain cancers, and osteoarthritis.

As a result of the Human Genome Project it may be possible to reseed the body with our own cells that are made more potent and younger so that the whole body can be repopulated. I say theoretically because having one rejuvenated organ ahead of the rest could itself be a cause of death. Keeping an overall steady pace of rejuvenation throughout the whole body is still a pipedream.

My own **PERSONAL RECIPE** for long life

I'm forced to the conclusion that there is no single elixir of life, no pill, no potion, no single food, no single rule. There is a LIFESTYLE, which includes most of the above, but it requires more effort than simply reaching for a bunch of supplements.

To live longer you have to invest, work, commit, and remain vigilant. Even if my recipes didn't result in a single extra day of life I can promise you you'll have more life in every day of your life.

- ◆ Have oatmeal for breakfast
- ◆ Don't eat fatty foods, except oily fish
- ◆ Eat fruit and vegetables at every meal if possible
- ◆ Eat fresh food whenever you can
- ◆ Eat fish, especially oily fish, whenever you can

DRUGS of a lifetime

Statins
HRT
Selegiline (for Alzheimer's)
Retinoic acid (for the skin)
Aspirin

FOODS of a lifetime

Oily fish
Fresh food
All fruits and vegetables
Eat vegetables rather than meat
Oatmeal every morning
Carrots, tomatoes, and a few nuts and seeds every day
Dark-colored fruits and vegetables – dark red or black fruit and dark green leaves

SUPPLEMENTS of a lifetime

Vitamin E
Cod liver oil
Selenium
Gingko biloba (but only this form: EG6761)
Folic acid

HABITS of a lifetime

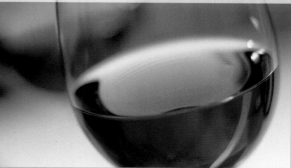

HERB/DRUG INTERACTIONS

Certain herbal medicinal products and food supplements can interact with prescription drugs. They may increase the action of the medication so that it is greater than desired, or they may make the medication less effective so that it does not work or works less well. If you are taking prescribed drugs, always check with your doctor before taking any more. Here are some examples:

Interaction with **ANTICOAGULANTS**

If you're taking anticoagulants to prevent blood clots from developing, certain herbal medicines or supplements may affect their action. The following herbal medicines and food supplements may **increase** the action of anticoagulants:

Alfalfa	Chondroitin	Garlic	Lugwort	Senega
Angelica	Cinchona	Ginger	Meadowsweet	Sweet clover
Aniseed	Clove	Ginkgo	Mugwort	Tonka bean
Asafetida	Coenzyme Q10	Ginseng, panax	Pau d'arco	Turmeric
Bilberry	Coryceps	Horse chestnut	Pill-bearing spurge	Vervain
Black haw	Danshen	Horseradish	Pineapple	Willow
Bogbean	Devil's claw	Irish moss	Poplar	Wintergreen
Buchu	Dong quai	Kelp	Prickly ash	Woodruff
Cat's claw	Fenugreek	Khella	Quassia	
Celery	Feverfew	Licorice	Red clover	
Chamomile	Fucus	Lovage	Reishi	

The following herbs may **decrease** the action of anticoagulants:

Agrimony	Arnica	Goldenseal	Mistletoe	St. John's wort
				Yarrow

Interaction with **ORAL CONTRACEPTIVES**

Certain herbal medicines and supplements can interact with oral contraceptives.
The following herbal medicines and supplements may cause an **increase** in plasma levels of oral contraceptives:

Chaste tree	Pokeweed	Siberian ginseng
Hop	Red clover	

The following herbal medicines and supplements may cause a **decrease** in plasma levels of oral contraceptives:

Guar gum	Herbal laxatives	St. John's wort
Licorice	(e.g. aloe vera, senna)	

Interactions with **HEART MEDICATIONS**

CARDIAC GLYCOSIDES

If you're taking cardiac glycosides for a heart disorder the following herbal medicines and food supplements may **increase** the action of the drug:

Adonis	Figwort	Night-blooming cereus	Sarsaparilla
Aloe vera	Fumitory	Oleander	Senna
Bearberry	Ginseng, panax	Psyllium	Shepherd's purse
Boldo	Hawthorn	Queen Anne's lace	Squaw vine
Buchu	Lily-of-the-valley	Red clover	Squill
Buckthorn	Lugwort	Rhubarb	St. John's wort
Cascara	Motherwort	Rue	Strophantus

ANTIHYPERTENSIVES

If you're taking antihypertensives for the treatment of high blood pressure, the following herbal medicines and food supplements may **increase** the action of the drug:

Agrimony	Cowslip	Ginseng, panax	Mistletoe	Shepherd's purse
Asafetida	Dandelion	Goldenseal	Motherwort	Squill
Avens	Devil's claw	Hawthorn	Nettle	St. John's wort
Betony	Elecampane	Horehound, white	Parsley	Vervain
Black cohosh	Fenugreek	Horseradish	Plantain	Wild carrot
Broom	Fucus	Indian snakeroot	Pokeroot	Yarrow
Calamus	Fumitory	Irish moss	Prickly ash	
Cat's claw	Garlic	Kelp	Queen Anne's lace	
Celery	Ginseng,	Khat	Rue	
Cornsilk	eleutherococcus	Khella	Sage	

The following herbal medicines and food supplements may **decrease** the action of hypertensives

Arnica	Capsicum	Ephedra	Licorice
Bayberry	Cola	Gentian	Maté
Blue cohosh	Coltsfoot	Ginger	Yohimbine

BETA-BLOCKERS

If you're taking beta-blockers for the treatment of a disorder of the heart or circulation, the following herbal medicines and food supplements may **increase** the action of the drug:

Broom	Khat	Shepherd's purse
Fumitory	Lily-of-the-valley	

Interactions with **HEART MEDICATIONS** continued

ANTIARRHYTHMIC DRUGS

If you're taking antiarrhythmic drugs for the treatment of abnormal heart rates and rhythms the following herbal medicines and food supplements may **increase** the action of the drug:

Aloe vera	Khat	Squill
Calamus	Night-blooming cereus	

ACE INHIBITORS AND CALCIUM CHANNEL BLOCKERS

If you're taking ACE inhibitors or calcium channel blockers for heart or circulation disorders, the following herbal medicines and food supplements may **increase** the action of the drug:

Coenzyme Q10	Lily-of-the-valley	Pill-bearing spurge	Squill
Fumitory	Night-blooming cereus	Shepherd's purse	

The following herbal medicines and food supplements may **decrease** action of calcium channel blockers:

Coltsfoot

Interactions with **ANTIDIABETIC MEDICATIONS**

If you're taking medication for diabetes, certain herbal medicines and food supplements may affect the action of the drug. The following herbal medicines and food supplements may **increase** the antidiabetic effect:

Alfalfa	Cornsilk	Ginseng, panax	Myrtle
Aloe vera	Damiana	Guar gum	Nettle
Basil	Dandelion	Horehound	Night-blooming cereus
Burdock	Eucalyptus	Juniper	Onion
Celandine	Fenugreek	Marshmallow	Sage
Celery	Garlic	Melatonin	Tansy
Coriander	Ginseng, eleutherococcus	Myrrh	

The following herbal medicines and food supplements may **decrease** the antidiabetic effect:

Bee pollen	Elecampane	Gotu kola	Licorice
Devil's claw	Figwort	Hydrocotyle	St. John's wort

PLANTS with ADVERSE AFFECTS

The *Complete German Commission E Monographs: Therapeutic Guide to Herbal Medicines* is the most comprehensive list of approved complementary products in Europe.
The following medicinal plants are not approved by the Commission because of safety concerns.

Plant	Possible adverse effect	Constituent responsible for effect
Angelica (seed and herb)	Photosensitivity (sensitivity to sunlight)	Coumarins
Bilberry (leaf)	Intoxication	Not known
Bishop's weed (fruit)	Allergic reactions; photosensitivity (sensitivity to sunlight)	Khellin
Bladderwrack	Hyperthyroidism (overactive thyroid)	Iodine
Borage	Liver damage	Pyrrolizidine alkaloids
Bryonia	Numerous risks	Not known
Chamomile (Roman)	Allergic reactions	Not known
Cinnamon (flower)	Allergic reactions	Not known
Cocoa	Allergic reactions, migraine	Not known
Colocynth	Gastrointestinal problems, kidney damage, cystitis	Cucurbitacin
Coltsfoot	Liver damage	Pyrrolizidine alkaloids
Delphinium (flower)	Bradycardia (low heart rate), hypotension (low blood pressure), heart attack, paralyzing effect on breathing	Alkaloids
Elecampane	Irritation of mucosa, allergic contact dermatitis	Alantolactone
Ergot	Wide spectrum of adverse effects	Alkaloids
Goat's rue	Hypoglycemia (low blood sugar)	Galegin
Hound's tongue	Liver damage	Pyrrolizidine alkaloids
Kelp	Hyperthyroidism (overactive thyroid)	Iodine
Lemongrass, citronella oil	Toxic alveolitis (lung inflammation)	Essential oil
Liverwort (herb)	Irritation of skin and mucous membranes	Protoanemonin
Madder (root)	Possibility of genetic mutations and cancer	Lucidin
Male fern	Wide spectrum of adverse effects	Not known
Marsh tea	Poisoning, can cause miscarriage	Not known
Monkshood	Varied spectrum of effects	Cardiotoxic component
Mugwort	Can cause miscarriage	Not known
Nutmeg	Affects mental activity, can cause miscarriage	Not known

Plant	Possible adverse effect	Constituent responsible for effect
Nux vomica	Possible damage to central nervous system	Strychnine
Oleander (leaf)	Poisoning, sometimes fatal	Oleandrin
Papain	Bleeding in patients with clotting disorders	Not known
Pasque (flower)	Severe irritation of skin and mucosa	Protoanemonin
Periwinkle	Suppression of immune system	Not known
Petasites (leaf)	Liver damage	Pyrrolizidine alkaloids
Rhododendron, rusty leaved	Poisoning	Grayanotoxin content
Rue	Possibility of causing genetic mutations and sensitivity to sunlight, liver, and kidney damage	Furanocoumarins
Saffron	Adverse effects noted in doses over 10g used for abortion	Not known
Sarsaparilla (root)	Gastric irritation and temporary kidney impairment suspected	Not known
Scotch broom (flower)	Contraindicated for patients on MAOI (monoamine oxidase inhibitors) for depression, and hypertension	Not known
Senecio (herb)	Liver damage	Pyrrolizidine alkaloids
Soapwort, red (herb)	Mucous membrane irritation	Saponins
Tansy (flower and herb)	Poisoning due to abuse	Thujone content of oil
Yohimbe (bark)	Nervousness, tremor, sleeplessness, anxiety, hypertension, and tachycardia (raised heart rate), nausea, vomiting associated with therapeutic administration of yohimbine; interaction with psychoactive herbs	Nerve stimulators

The following plants have also been listed as "potentially unsafe" in *Complementary and Alternative Medicine*, by C. W. Feltrow and J. R. Avila. Adverse effects are described in brackets.

American yew (cell damage), **Autumn crocus** (gastrointestinal toxicity, vomiting, neurologic toxicity, renal failure), **Betel palm** (malformations in fetus), **Bird's foot trefoil** (cyanide poisoning, seizures, paralysis, coma, death), **Black locust** (low heart rate, nausea, vomiting, dizziness), **Black nightshade** (cardiac toxicity), **Blue flag** (severe nausea, vomiting, diarrhea)

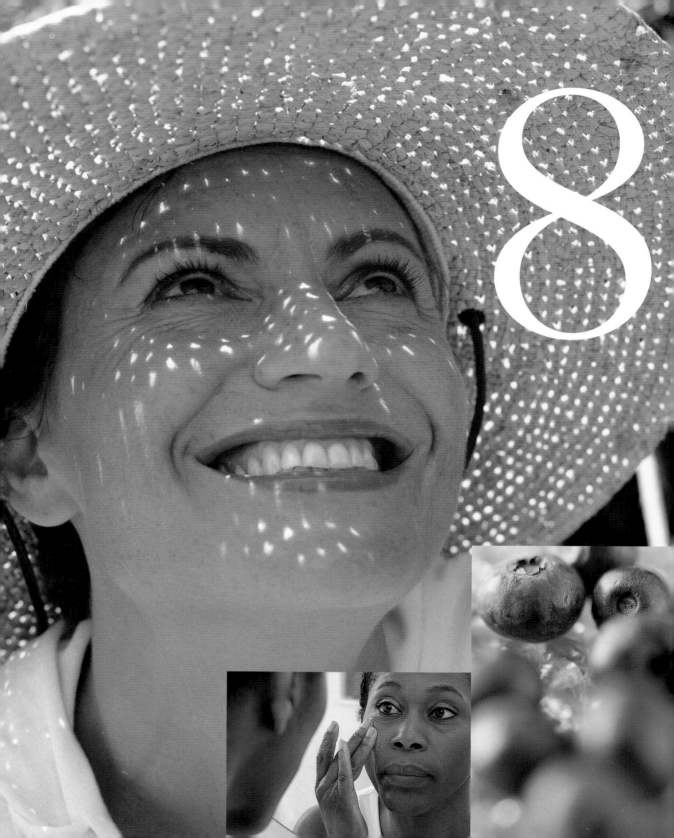

8

INSTANT REJUVENATION

Many people in their fifties are **not ready** to resign themselves to being thought of as getting old. Both men and women feel that middle age would be more comfortable if they could *avoid obvious signs* of wear and tear. Furthermore, they feel it is **unjust** that they should begin to show some superficial features of their age when they are at the **height** of their *intellectual and emotional* powers. So, when fine lines, wrinkles, and sags appear, many of us decide to *fight back* with creams, potions, and cosmetic surgery. But there are also **other ways of helping yourself**, with a more **spiritual** approach based on the belief that *inner calm and inner strength* reflects in the way we look.

KEEP *your skin* YOUNG

THE SUN, NOT TIME, IS YOUR SKIN'S GREATEST ENEMY. WHAT SHOWS IN YOUR FACE ARE NOT THE YEARS YOU'VE LIVED BUT THE TOTAL NUMBER OF HOURS YOU'VE SPENT IN THE SUN.

Besides the sun, there are other factors in your lifestyle and in the environment that age your skin. Here are some of the most important.
• **Cigarette smoke**, whether you're a smoker or you simply spend time with smokers
• Diet **short of vitamins** such as A, C, E, folic acid, and B12
• Diet that's **high in fat and salt**
• **More than moderate** alcohol consumption
• **Stressful** life or job
• The use of **soaps and water** on your skin
• Going without **sleep**.

stub it out

Smoking has long been associated with premature aging. The face of a 20-a-day smoker **ages by 14 years** for every 10 years of smoking.

Smokers look older than nonsmokers because tobacco triggers a protein that attacks the skin's elasticity. The protein breaks down collagen, the fibrous material that helps to prevent wrinkles.

Smokers who sunbathe **wrinkle even faster** because the sun's ultraviolet rays also encourage anticollagen protein in the skin. The protein, known as matrix metalloproteinase-1 (MMP-1), was found by accident during a study of ultraviolet light and aging on 33 volunteers. Researchers were at a loss to explain why background levels of MMP-1 were higher in some volunteers,

until they asked about their smoking habits. The concentration of MMP-1 was found to be **much higher in the smokers' skin**, while the nonsmokers had undetectable amounts.

Smoking exerts such a noticeable effect on the skin that it's often possible to know whether or not a person is a smoker **simply by looking at their face**. Smokers have more wrinkles and their skin tends to have a grayish pallor. The changes in collagen caused by smoking can't be restored by diet or other supplements. Collagen is the major structural chemical present in skin, but once it's gone, consider it gone for ever. For smokers, wrinkles around the mouth and eyes begin in their early thirties. Young female smokers are wasting money on anti-aging face creams.

DO ANTI-AGING CREAMS WORK?

Dr. Nicholas Perricone in his book, *The Wrinkle Cure*, certainly advocates a variety of creams for keeping wrinkles at bay. I'm a little less sure. From the point of view of putting right some of that accumulated damage to your skin, some creams might be helpful. The chart opposite shows what they can and cannot do.

ANTI-AGING creams – the verdict

Product or ingredient	Good	Bad	Overrated
Alpha-hydroxy acid (see page 194)	Fine at low concentrations of not more than 10 percent. On dark skin, test a small area to see if the product irritates.		
Cleansers	If they're formulated to remove oil and makeup without drying	If they contain harsh alkalis	
Elastin products (collagen)	No, useless	Not intrinsically bad	Yes, because the elastin molecule is too big to penetrate the skin
Eye creams and gels	Only if they contain nonirritant anti-inflammatories or antioxidants	Those containing grease or oils can migrate into the eye	Don't believe claims to remove dark circles, nothing can
Facial masks	If they moisturize	Can cause irritation and shouldn't be used more than once a week	Anything claiming facial rejuvenation is overrated
Hypoallergenic	In a limited way		Name means only that the ingredients are hypoallergenic; no guarantee that these products will not cause allergic reactions
Moisturizers, with petrolatum or mineral oil	OK for normal to dry skin	If used on oily skin	
Moisturizers, with Co-enzyme Q10	Because they have some antioxidant/anti-inflammatory effects		Possibly
Moisturizers, oil-free	For oily and/or acne-prone skin		For normal/dry skin (moisturizers with oil are better)
Moisturizers, with oil/non-comedogenic	Proper use does not cause acne	If overused because they can clog pores	
Sunscreens	If SPF (sun protection factor) is 15 or higher	If used instead of avoiding sun exposure	If used as protection from long sun exposure
Vitamin C Ester/Ascorbyl Palmitate	May act as an anti-inflammatory		Possibly

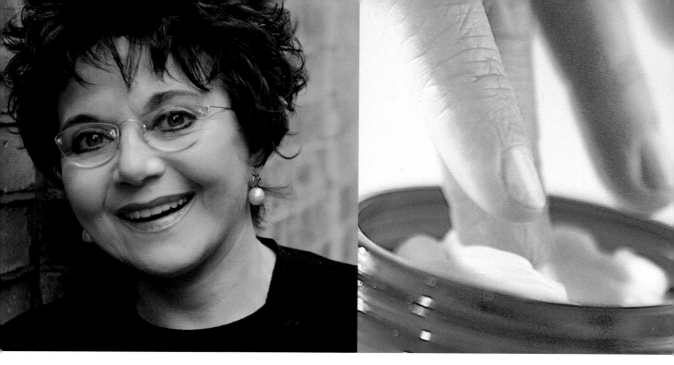

how antioxidants can help give you a youthful glow

I well remember in the 1980s the discovery of the alpha- and then the beta-hydroxy acids, AHAs and BHAs, and how cosmeticians looked on them as **miracle agents for making skin look more youthful**. Hardly a face cream exists without them these days, their secret being that they induce a very mild peel, removing dead skin cells and leaving the skin smooth and glowing, visibly different.

AHAs and BHAs used properly and in low concentration can have an **instant rejuvenating effect** on the appearance of the skin, although they don't lessen wrinkles. What they can do is dissolve **keratin** – the tough shells of dead skin cells that continually pile up on the surface of the skin and accumulate day and night.

Skin cells grow from the lower levels of the skin and migrate upward, dying as they do so and leaving only their skeletons on the surface.

These dead skin cells are dry, scaly, and give the skin a withered appearance. Daily removal of them gives the skin **a refreshing glow**, so from the age of 40 onward these creams should become part of everybody's early morning skin-care routine. They're certainly part of mine.

AHAs and BHAs have an antioxidant effect and can work synergistically with other antioxidants. The most famous antioxidant is the lactic acid in milk – Cleopatra knew this and had a daily bath in asses' milk to keep her skin smooth and youthful looking. Another is **aspirin, or acetylsalicylic acid,** as it's known among dermatologists. When I was a practicing dermatologist, we used acetylsalicylic acid cream on scaly skin conditions because it gently exfoliates the skin, getting rid of redundant scales, and it's standard therapy to get rid of the silvery scales in psoriasis. Acetylsalicylic acid is used in astringents, skin cleansers, and creams that are meant to dry and defat the skin and are useful for acne. This medicinal use could have benefits to the aging skin too, especially when used in conjunction with AHAs and BHAs.

... and slow down skin aging

Vitamin E is a powerful antioxidant, too. It's a constituent of many skin creams, especially for skin under the eyes because it's supposed to make **fine lines** disappear.

However, it's a particular type of vitamin E that holds the promise of rejuvenating aging skins. It's called high potency E or HPE.

Vitamin E is a complex substance made up of several different components. Those that could have a **possible anti-aging effect** on the skin are the tocopherols and the tocotrienols. The latter are the newer and more effective form that could be really helpful to the aging skin. In the late 1980s scientists found that tocotrienols had the ability to inhibit a particularly damaging enzyme implicated in cell aging by being able to mop up free radicals very quickly.

HELP FROM VITAMIN E

Preliminary research shows that preparations containing tocotrienol – a component of vitamin E – make hair glossier, heal redness and scaling, and prevent fingernails from splitting. Tocotrienol will also probably make sunscreens more effective while calming the redness and inflammation caused by sunburn. To give all-day protection to the skin, tocotrienol can be added to other skin-care products and to makeup.

the only antiwrinkle cream that works

Many promises are made to you at the cosmetic counters about creams to keep wrinkles at bay. Be skeptical about them all except those creams that contain a derivative of vitamin A called **tretinoin**, which comes as a cream, gel, or liquid.

Tretinoin is well known to dermatologists because it's been used for decades to treat many skin conditions, including acne and psoriasis. Quite incidentally it was discovered to have an **antiwrinkle effect** and since then quite detailed and reliable research has shown that tretinoin increases the blood flow to the skin, so improving the quality and quantity of collagen fibers in the lower level of the skin, the dermis. The result is a smoother, plumper, younger-looking skin. Even for use as an antiwrinkle cream, tretinoin is only available by prescription.

Tretinoin has many actions in the skin and is extremely good at **preventing scarring in acne and scaling in psoriasis**. Research shows it works as a true **rejuvenator**. Cells that have become damaged and inefficient with age are switched on again so they repair and renew themselves, making skin look more youthful.

how to use tretinoin

The use of tretinoin must be carefully supervised because it's not free of side effects and can cause severe inflammation if incorrectly used. Treatment usually starts with the lowest dose cream (0.25 percent) used every other night and then every night if there are no signs of inflammation. You rub it into the wrinkled parts of the skin, including the areas around the eyes which respond best – good news for crow's feet.

The effect of the cream takes several months to show. You'll notice some redness, peeling, and itching of the skin from the tretinoin, but this will be counteracted by the soothing and moisturizing ingredients in the cream. If you're applying tretinoin in the summer you have to be very careful because it makes your skin more sensitive to sunlight and more vulnerable to aging from the sun. You could burn badly if exposed to strong sun. So use a long-acting sunscreen on your skin several hours before you apply the tretinoin and before you go out.

what you'll see

During the first four weeks of application you'll notice your skin takes on a pinkish color and you'll feel that it's tightening up. After a couple of months the fine **wrinkles tend to flatten out** and after six months there's even some tightening of the sagging skin around your mouth. The greatest benefit happens in the first 12 months and thereafter you can apply the cream once or twice a week to keep up appearances. Tretinoin isn't free of side effects. It causes dryness, redness, tenderness, and swelling of the skin (which may account for its antiwrinkle effect), but these side effects lessen with time.

Precautions

• Don't smoke while applying tretinoin because the gel is flammable.

• If you plan to have hair removed by waxing, especially of the upper lip, stop the tretinoin three to four weeks prior to the treatment. Otherwise, you may be left with a sore area, which could heal and leave a brown patch.

• Don't apply tretinoin to broken skin or creases around your nose, lips, or eyes.

can foods stop wrinkles?

The research is no more than theoretical, but scientists from the Human Nutrition Research Center at Tufts University in Boston have discovered **which fruits and vegetables keep us looking youngest**. They have come up with a list of 25 top foods – and **prunes, raisins, and blueberries** are the leading three wrinkle-zapping snacks.

The key to these age-defying foods is the **high level of antioxidants** that they contain. Antioxidants are the defensive chemicals that our bodies make to protect us from free radicals, the harmful chemicals we produce when we burn up oxygen (see page 13).

They can also enter our system from the outside – smoking, environmental pollution, radiation, too much sunlight, and irritant chemicals will all produce free radicals. It's these free radicals that have the power to destroy our body's cells and cause sagging skin and wrinkles.

Dr. Ronald Prior and Dr. Guahau Cao, the scientists who conducted the research, devised a measurement that shows the strength of antioxidants in certain foods. This is called the ORAC value (Oxygen Radical Absorbance Capacity). The theory is that by eating foods with a high number of ORAC units you can **maximize the number of antioxidants in your body and help prevent aging**. Foods rich in ORACs will theoretically help **stop the development of wrinkles**, protect your joints from arthritis, reduce your risk of heart disease, and increase your chances of avoiding many forms of cancer. It's even claimed that they could **halt early dementia** and senility. Eating foods with a high ORAC value could be

ZAP THOSE WRINKLES
with the top 25 age-defying foods

Fruit/vegetable	ORAC units per 100g	Serving	ORAC units
Prunes	5,750	one pitted prune	462
Raisins	2,830	¼ cup	1,019
Blueberries	2,434	½ cup	1,620
Blackberries	2,036	½ cup	1,466
Garlic	1,939	one clove	58
Curly kale	1,770	½ cup (cooked)	1,150
Cranberries	1,750	½ cup	831
Strawberries	1,536	½ cup	831
Raspberries	1,227	½ cup	755
Spinach	1,210	one cup (raw)	678
Brussels sprouts	980	one sprout	206
Plums	949	one plum	626
Alfalfa sprouts	931	one cup	307
Broccoli	888	½ cup (cooked)	817
Beets	841	½ cup (cooked)	715
Avocado	782	½ pear	149
Oranges	750	one orange	982
Black grapes	739	10 grapes	177
Red peppers	731	one medium pepper	540
Cherries	670	10 cherries	455
Kiwi fruit	609	one fruit	458
Pink grapefruit	483	½ fruit	580
Onions	449	½ cup (chopped)	360
Corn	402	½ cup (cooked)	330
Eggplant	386	½ cup (cooked)	185

maximize the number of anti-oxidants in your body and help prevent aging

important as we get older, as the body tends to produce more free radicals and fewer of its own antioxidants. The research team figured out that we need between 3,000 and 5,000 ORAC units a day to slow down the aging process, though I'm highly skeptical of such a simplistic formula.

In the table of ORAC-rich foods, **prunes come out on top**. They contain 5,770 units per 3½oz (100g), which works out at around 462 units in just one pitted prune. So, if you were only getting your antioxidants from prunes, you would need to eat seven a day.

The reason these fruits are so full of antioxidants is because they contain enormously high levels of plant pigments called polyphenols. But there is a huge gap between finding polyphenols in prunes and seeing a measurable anti-aging effect when you eat them. The other reason prunes and raisins have such a high ORAC value is because they're dried. Drying plums and grapes **concentrates the antioxidants** by removing all the water that dilutes them.

All the foods that are high in antioxidants contain other vital nutrients too. Kale, spinach, brussels sprouts, and broccoli contain folic acid; blueberries, blackberries, strawberries, raspberries, red peppers, oranges, cherries, and kiwis are rich in vitamin C; blackberries, spinach, alfalfa sprouts, and avocado all include vitamin E; prunes, raisins, spinach, and beets also contain iron. **Onions and garlic are both natural antiseptics and antifungals** – and they also boast cholesterol-lowering properties.

MEDICAL*skin*TREATMENTS

ANY TECHNIQUE OR TREATMENT WHICH IS CAPABLE OF ALTERING THE SKIN'S APPEARANCE PERMANENTLY SHOULD BE UNDERTAKEN ONLY BY A MEDICALLY QUALIFIED PERSON, SUCH AS A DERMATOLOGIST OR A PLASTIC SURGEON.

I'm categorical in making this statement because treatments that have such radical effects have side effects as well and can damage the skin if the treatment isn't properly done. **Only a person who is medically qualified** has sufficient knowledge to make the keen judgement about how and when a treatment can be given safely. If one of the following treatments is being offered by a nonmedically qualified person, then **don't have it**. Treatments such as skin peeling and dermabrasion, if badly administered, **can seriously damage the skin and leave permanent scars**.

skin peeling

Chemical skin peeling can be done for medical or cosmetic reasons. The agent most commonly used by doctors is **phenol**, which causes coagulation, inflammation, swelling, and peeling when painted on the skin. Phenol may be absorbed through the skin and in large doses it may harm the kidneys. It must therefore be used **cautiously and infrequently** and never applied over a large area. It's usually used in small local areas for the treatment of acne scarring or small blemishes and cysts.

Skin peeling treatment for cosmetic purposes may involve larger areas in order to get rid of discolored areas of skin and freckles. It may soften the facial lines but doesn't stop aging and the rejuvenating effect usually wears off within a year. The skin peeling agent is often an acid such as trichloracetic acid, which produces a second-degree burn and turns the skin a whitish gray color. A brown crust forms within three to five days and then drops off. The skin becomes pink and tight with fewer lines and wrinkles.

Beauty clinics offer skin peeling using fruit and vegetable extracts, which have only a transitory effect.

dermabrasion

This is useful for improving **acne scars** on the face or to treat large birthmarks and it may also give fairly good results for **stretch marks and fine lines around the mouth**. First introduced in the 1930s, dermabrasion is now highly sophisticated. **Results on the face are generally good** because the skin is well supplied with hair follicles and sebaceous glands which allow the skin to regrow quickly. Scarring is rare. Dermabrasion is usually done with a high-speed rotary drill plus a cooling device. You're generally sedated or tranquilized beforehand and the area to be treated is cooled with cold packs

and cleansed with soap and water followed by rubbing alcohol. Ears, nostrils, and hair are carefully protected and the eyes are covered with an ointment and a lead shield held by an assistant. The skin is frozen with a stream of cold gas and then the drill abrades the skin to the required depth. Obviously, experience and great skill are required to perform this correctly without causing scarring.

The area may bleed for 15–30 minutes after treatment and nonadhesive surgical dressings are used for 12–24 hours. Crusts form over the treated area and drop off 7–10 days later. The wound should be left dry and open thereafter. If necessary, the treatment can be repeated after about four weeks.

electro-desiccation

This involves killing the cells of the skin with an electrical current either by a spark, which solidifies the cells, or by heat, which coagulates them. In either case the skin cells shrivel. It's usually used for the treatment of broken veins on the face and legs and sometimes for treating warts. **A valuable technique in the dermatologist's clinic**, it can treat small skin tags, several of which can be removed in one treatment session without any anesthesia.

Skin tags are coagulated by the application of the fine metal electric desiccator needle for only a few seconds, and because the blood vessels are coagulated, there's no bleeding. The surrounding skin may become inflamed by the burning and crusts may form which fall off in about two weeks. Scarring is rare. In a beauty clinic, electrocoagulation or diathermy is also used to remove unwanted facial hair.

BEAUTY TREATMENTS

Here are some quick fix treatments offered at many beauty salons – and my opinion on their effectiveness or otherwise.

facial microdermabrasion – a rejuvenating treatment – is a quick way of "resurfacing" the skin by blasting tiny salt crystals on to it to exfoliate the dead cells and then vacuuming them off again. This is done with a machine that both sprays on the crystals and sucks them up again. The experience is pleasant – it doesn't hurt at all, and a rich antioxidant cream is smothered over the face afterward. **Opinion:** The skin looks soft and pink for a few days.

light laser wrinkle treatment uses "intense pulsed light" which is supposed to stimulate the production of collagen, eventually making the skin plumper and filling out the lines. A nurse holds the laser – which looks like a pen – just above the skin, you see a red flashing light and hear the clicking of the laser. **Opinion:** Results are disappointing, so expect little.

cellulite-busting squeezes you into an unattractive white body suit to have the cellulite on your bottom pummeled with an Endermologie machine. This machine (whose name is a purely pseudoscientific confection) is guided by the nurse and feels like a toothless "bite." It also feels like a deep massage and is aggressive and intense. After around 30 minutes, you feel as though your muscles have been working overtime. **Opinion:** Standing after the treatment is difficult and cellulite looks much the same.

spider vein removal by sclerotherapy is an injection of sterile salt and local anesthetic into a small patch of spider veins. The intention is to shrink the veins and eventually make them disappear. The treatment feels like a pinprick, painful for only a few seconds. The veins disappear during the treatment, then later reappear in a red patch to fade gradually over the next two to three weeks. **Opinion:** Quick, but only worth it if the veins are very obvious.

nose-to-mouth lines filled – your cheeks are smeared in a thick layer of anesthetic cream. After 15 minutes you're injected with the hyaluronic acid "filler" several times down the lines, which will certainly make you wince but the pain is fleeting. At first you notice the area round your mouth looking a little "thick" and the pinpricks are visibly red. **Opinion:** You'll be able to see that the lines have plumped up nicely. Lasts a few months at most.

lip plumper with collagen can plump the top lip or reshape lips that have lost their shape. A local anesthetic is injected into the gum, the same as you'd have before a filling, then you won't feel the injections. The lip will swell but by the next day it will settle down. **Opinion:** There is a visible difference – but the effect lasts four months max, then you must re-do.

COSMETIC *surgery*

THESE DAYS YOU CAN CHOOSE TO CHANGE YOUR BODY IN VIRTUALLY ANY WAY YOU LIKE IF YOU CAN FIND A GOOD COSMETIC SURGEON TO COOPERATE. BUT, IF YOU DO FIND SUCH A COOPERATIVE SURGEON, HESITATE – HE MAY NOT BEST SERVE YOUR PURPOSE.

If you decide on plastic surgery, **choose your surgeon carefully**. It's better to select your surgeon on the recommendation of a friend, whose results you can see, or through your own family doctor than from an advertisement in the newspaper or a magazine. **Be suspicious** of a surgeon who says you can have exactly the operation you require without giving you a professional opinion of what you really need.

I'd also be skeptical about a surgeon who's overly optimistic about the results of the operation. **No good surgeon will give you a 100 percent guarantee of success**. A trustworthy surgeon will always give you some idea of their results by showing you before and after photographs of their patients.

Ask your surgeon to draw exactly what they're going to do and if you don't understand ask for further clarification. If you're in any way uncertain or don't feel that you have a rapport with your surgeon, **go elsewhere**. As a general rule you should never trust yourself to a surgeon with whom you cannot establish a good relationship at your initial consultation.

fat transfer surgery

A face that becomes somewhat haggard and drawn with age can be **instantly plumped out** with fat transfer surgery. Fat is harvested from somewhere where there's plenty of excess, say the thighs and buttocks. It's then injected by a skilled plastic surgeon into hollows and contours on the face to give it the **bloom of youth**. Laughter lines and crow's feet can vanish making the face smooth and, if overdone, almost doll-like. This technique can be used anywhere, the face is only one place. It's also used on the back of the hands to fill out signs of aging.

liposuction and liposculpture

It's worth seeking out an experienced surgeon of excellent reputation to perform liposuction because it can go seriously wrong. On the tops of the thighs, for instance, the results can be worse than the original condition since liposuction can scar and leave a pitted, uneven surface.

The best practitioners of liposuction are experienced surgeons with the most modern techniques who are able to extract fat from a

A *trustworthy* surgeon will always give you some idea of their results by showing you *before and after photographs* of their patients

deep level and leave a flat, even surface to the skin. Liposuction can be used anywhere and has made the tummy tuck virtually redundant.

An incision is made in the area from which the fat is to be extracted and a glass or metal tube is inserted. The tubes vary in thickness, the thicker the tube, the greater the unevenness of the scar that will be left. However, the finer the tube, the longer it takes to suck out the fatty fluid. Surgeons therefore tend to use thick tubes which reduce operation times but leave unsightly ridges in your skin.

The tube is attached to a surgical device which will suck up soft, fatty tissue, but before fat is sucked out, saline mixed with an enzyme that breaks down fat is injected into the site and then the mixture is removed. Liposuction requires a general anesthetic and there's often bruising and some considerable pain after surgery.

Quantities of fat in excess of half a liter – approximately one pint – should never be removed on a single occasion. Fat is liquid in circulation round the body. Losing more than half a liter of fat is similar to losing a half a liter of blood and can make you ill. When large quantities of fat are removed – a liter or more – you may even go into surgical shock with low blood pressure, and need transfusion in order to stabilize your blood pressure.

Fatty tissue can be removed from one part of the body and inserted at another site to change your shape. For example, fat from the abdomen can be used to augment breast size, to plump out the backs of aging hands, or even to increase the girth of a small penis.

facing up to defying age

Cosmetic surgeons say that typical patients are energetic, active people who are less interested in hiding their age than in **looking as youthful as they feel**. These patients find that an aging face erodes self-confidence and may even cause panic. A typical question such a patient should ask herself if, "Why should I go on looking like this when every other part of me feels young?"

"NATURAL" FACE-LIFTS

Before going into detail about the radical (surgical) approach to face-lifts, let me touch on the subject of so-called **natural** face-lifts, claimed to be achieved through exercising the facial muscles. The claims are entirely fake. You can never make your face look different from the way it is now with special exercises because your face gets all the exercise it can possibly need from talking, laughing, and chewing.

what can cosmetic surgery do for me?

No cosmetic surgeon will attempt to make a face conform to a current ideal or appear impossibly youthful. It is essential that each person's face **retains its own individuality** after surgery and a good surgeon strives to make changes that are almost imperceptible to others. He attempts to create an overall effect without pinpointing any single feature and is careful

PREPARATION FOR COSMETIC SURGERY

Most people who have cosmetic surgery are pleased with the results. But you'll need to prepare yourself for the immediate aftereffects of surgery, which can be quite a shock to the system. After the operation, the mind has to recover as well as the body and of course the results are not instant. When the dressings first come off, your face will be swollen, the skin bruised, and there may be stitches. It will be some time before you know if the operation has been a success. Confidence in your surgeon and the team as well as support from family and friends are a great help here.

to preserve the character of the face. The old saying that **beauty comes from within** has a great deal of truth in it. An indefinable quality of the spirit and disposition can combine to make quite nondescript or irregular features have their own charm and that must be maintained.

Most people who have a face-lift do not want friends and relatives to gasp with surprise at their first sight of them. They want **a natural look, an almost indefinable improvement** in their appearance so that people comment on **how well they look**. For this reason, a totally smooth skin is not the desired outcome. If the skin is overstretched a false look around the eyes may rob the face of much of its expressive qualities, taking the spontaneity from the smile and producing an impression of continual tension. The best advertisement for a good cosmetic surgeon is a patient who looks **naturally young**, not one whose smooth skin seems artificial.

how is a face-lift done?

This operation demands **great precision, accuracy, and attention to detail** on the part of the surgeon. An unsuccessful face-lift can leave the patient looking – and certainly feeling – far worse than before.

These days most surgeons don't touch the visible hairline – they make incisions in the scalp above the forehead, in front of (and just behind) the ears and underneath the earlobes and under the chin. These cuts allow your surgeon to loosen the skin and pull what is judged to be an appropriate amount of muscle upward and backward. After the skin has been trimmed, the surgeon uses stitches or metal clips to close the edges of the incisions with meticulous care.

The effect of pulling the muscle is to reposition sagging areas (around the cheeks and jawbone, for example). To some extent peels can smooth out frown lines on the forehead, crow's feet around the eyes and wrinkles generally. Botox injections can temporarily erase some skin creases. Scars left behind by the incisions are quick to blend with the surrounding skin and are normally hidden by hair and the natural fold in front of the ear.

A face-lift takes at least three hours to perform and is usually performed in the hospital under a general anesthetic. The usual length of stay in the hospital is one night. Because the surgeon generally treats the incised skin with a local anesthetic, it is rare for there to be a lot of pain immediately after the operation, though discomfort can last several weeks. The area of the operation is covered with a bulky dressing at this stage and when this is removed the following morning, your face will look red and swollen. Surgeons adopt different rules for timing the removal of stitches, but generally stitches come out between four days and ten weeks after the operation. The superficial swelling and bruising wear off gradually over two to three weeks. A headscarf and dark glasses will camouflage the worst of the swelling and discoloration.

The full effect of the face-lift will not be evident until at least three months after the operation and **may go on improving for a year**. During this period the swelling gradually subsides and healing of the deeper tissue takes place. People heal at different rates, so it may take a slightly longer or shorter time for the wounds to heal completely. It is even possible for the incisions on opposite sides of the face to heal at different rates.

The results of a good face-lift usually last about eight years. You go on aging all the time, thus after eight years your face is back to where you started but you yourself are eight years older.

eye-lift or blepharoplasty

This operation can be performed to remove sagging skin that makes the eyes look puffy, to raise a drooping eyelid, or to reshape an eyebrow, and is often combined with a face-lift. An incision is usually made in the natural fold of the upper lid, extending out into the smile lines around the eyes. For a lower lid, the incision comes just below the eyelashes and also extends into the smile lines. After excess fat and tissue have been removed, the incision is stitched up. The lower lid may also be corrected from the inside, thus leaving no scars.

The stitches come out three or four days after the operation and within ten days the scars should have blended sufficiently so that they can be hidden by makeup. Immediately after a blepharoplasty dark glasses can conceal the aftereffects (bruising and swelling). Blepharoplasty is often done as an outpatient procedure using general anesthesia or as an "office" procedure under local anesthesia and sedation.

FACIAL REJUVENATION

An approach advocated for older patients by some surgeons in the US is "total facial rejuvenation." This embraces a face-lift, eyelid repair, dermabrasion of the deep wrinkles around the top lip, and neck rejuvenation (removal of loose folds of neck skin). If there is a nasal deformity, rhinoplasty is thrown in. The nose is said to grow longer with advancing age and so shortening it is supposed to give a more youthful appearance. All the operations may be done at one session or staggered over several months. Some patients complain of a feeling of tightness round the neck or numbness around the ears for a few weeks or even months after this surgery, but the feeling disappears eventually.

BOTOX – THE FACTS

Thanks to Botox injections we can all have smoothed-out foreheads. The downside is that our faces, without laughter lines, can become unattractively expressionless. Before you rush off to be Botoxed, get informed.

botulinum toxin is a toxin produced by the bacterium *Clostridium botulinum*. Originally introduced for the safe and effective treatment of muscle spasms, it causes muscle paralysis and prevents sweating. In patients treated for facial spasm it was noted that wrinkling decreased over the treated muscle, leading to the use of Botox for the treatment of facial wrinkles. Botox works best on the upper third of the face, on frown lines between the eyes, crow's feet, and horizontal lines in the forehead. Botox can be combined with implantations such as collagen or hyaluronic acid injections to further improve the appearance.

how does Botox work? Tiny quantities of the toxin are injected directly into the affected muscles. It takes three small injections between the eyebrows to treat the frown line. The treated muscles weaken over the following week or so. Most people don't notice anything. They simply become aware that they are no longer able to contract the frown muscles. They can still lift their eyebrows normally and blink without problems. The injection is almost painless. It's important to remain upright for four hours after the injection. You can frown as often as you like in the first day or so, but the treated areas should not be touched. Don't have a facial massage!

how long does Botox last? The effect starts wearing off within a few weeks, but retreatment isn't usually needed for three to six months. Treatment can be repeated as required. Many people find after three or four treatments that they don't need another – the muscle has permanently weakened or they have broken the bad habit that led to the frowning or squinting.

are there side effects? Some people have a slight headache after treatment and it's safe to take acetaminophen to relieve it. There may also be some bruising at the site of the injection. The most common complication, which fortunately is rare, is "ptosis" – a drooping of the eyelid caused by the botulinum toxin tracking into the eyelid muscle. It generally lasts just a few days, but more prolonged weakness is possible. Iopidine eye drops can be prescribed to lessen this effect. Botox injections cannot be used in pregnancy or when breast-feeding.

is Botox always successful? Occasionally the injection fails to result in the desired muscle weakness. The treatment can be repeated safely. In 2001 Americans spent 310 million dollars on Botox and it's believed that this will rise to over a billion in a few years time. It would be wrong to use Botox all over your face – you'd find you had a freakish death mask that didn't permit your face to move properly and you'd be horribly bereft of expression.

BREAST*surgery*

THERE ARE SEVERAL DIFFERENT WAYS IN WHICH COSMETIC SURGERY CAN CHANGE THE SIZE, SHAPE, AND UPLIFT OF YOUR BREASTS. THESE INCLUDE BREAST-LIFT (MASTOPEXY), BREAST ENLARGEMENT (AUGMENTATION), AND BREAST REDUCTION.

BREAST-LIFT

The smaller the breast, the better the result. A lift can be combined with augmentation if your breasts are small or reduction if your breasts are very large. Without reduction, a breast-lift is not very effective on large breasts because gravity will pull them down again.

Be realistic. Mastopexy can't give you the pert breasts of a teenager and it will leave scars. Discuss the operation with your surgeon in some detail before proceeding.

You should keep in mind that your breast-lift, just like a face-lift, is by no means permanent. Your breasts will continue to age and eventually sag all over again.

THE OPERATION

A general anesthetic is usual. Your surgeon will remove excess skin and fat from under the breasts and move the nipple upward by pushing it through a hole in the skin higher up your chest. The operation takes two to two and a half hours.

AFTEREFFECTS AND FOLLOW-UP

Mastopexy is usually very successful and there are few side effects, although you may notice loss of sensation in your nipple and areola.

You can expect to have all the stitches removed after two weeks and, if you're an active person, you'll have full movement of your arms and shoulders and be able to play sports after about three weeks.

Although it may be slightly uncomfortable, **it's advisable to wear a good supporting bra after the operation** to support the inflamed breast and skin and help healing.

You should be prepared to wear your bra day and night for at least three months after having surgery.

BREAST REDUCTION

There are two groups of women who look for breast reduction. The first group dislikes their large breasts because of the inconvenience and social embarrassment. The second group wants cosmetic breast reduction to achieve firm, well-positioned breasts, and are happy with C or D cup as long as the breasts look good.

Keep a **sense of proportion** when you're deciding what size you'd like your breasts to be. Your surgeon will have a good idea about what sizes are possible for your breasts.

THE OPERATION

While different surgeons have slightly different techniques for reducing the size of breasts, the basic operation is very much the same no matter who does it. It requires a general anesthetic and it'll probably take as long as four hours.

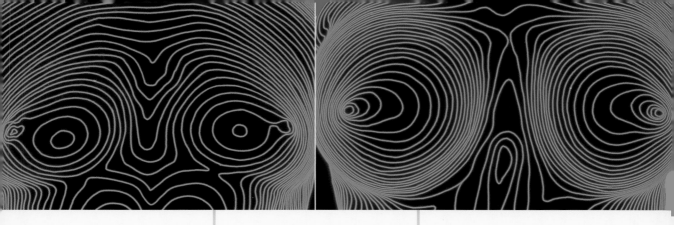

The nipples are important. Ask whether your surgeon's going to simply move your nipples up, or remove them and then graft them back in a different position. You can request that your nipple be preserved on a stalk of tissue – called a pedicle – so the tissue is taken from the sides and the underside of this stalk. This is essential if you want to breast-feed a future baby.

If you want to know exactly what's going to be removed in the operation, ask your surgeon to draw the shape on your breast with a pen.

The nipple can be lifted up and stitched into the breast at a higher level. The flaps of skin underneath are stitched together, resulting in reduction and some uplift. You'll be left with scars round the areola in a line from the nipple to the underside of the breast and in the skin fold where the breast joins the skin of the chest.

AFTEREFFECTS AND FOLLOW-UP

The results of the operation are usually extremely good. **Most women are thrilled**. This is a major operation so you can expect to have some discomfort for several weeks after. By the time you go home two or three days later, however, the pain should have subsided. Wear a bra day and night for support and to aid healing. The stitches should be removed within about two weeks, after which you could restart work. In a month you'll be **virtually back to normal**.

Women who are motivated to have breast reduction surgery because of their uncomfortable, pendulous breasts are nearly always more pleased with the results than those who are going for a purely cosmetic change.

Side effects are rare but include infection, a possibility with any operation. Your

surgeon can't predict whether you'll suffer loss of sensation because your response to surgery is entirely individual. If you gain weight, your breast size could increase again.

BREAST ENLARGEMENT

Breast enlargement can only be accomplished with the aid of implants, which are inserted in front of or behind the muscles of the chest wall – the pectorals – underneath the actual breast. Implants have received a lot of medical attention in recent years and their safety has been questioned by some experts.

Before undergoing breast enlargement, consider these vital factors:
• Breast augmentation can have complications, so read as much as you can about it. Ask your surgeon if he can put you in touch with someone who's had

Potential **WORRIES**

Breast cancer There's no proof of a link between silicone implants and cancer. It's important to realize that silicone is no longer injected directly into breast tissue and that data obtained from studies on cancer in rats can't simply be applied to human beings.

Autoimmune disease This association is speculative. There's no proof. Silicone gel has been known to leak out of the implant shell, and there have been sporadic reports suggesting that this causes connective tissue disorders like rheumatoid arthritis and systemic lupus erythematosus (SLE). A study performed by doctors at Harvard University over the past 14 years has found that connective tissue disorders occur equally in women who have not had implants and those who have.

Contracture The capsule of scar tissue that forms naturally around any implant can be quite thin and pliable, but it may contract and become as hard as wood. One research study puts the possibility of some contracture as high as seven out of ten at two to four years after surgery.

the operation so that you can go into it with your eyes open.
• Have a detailed discussion about the size you'd like your breasts to be. Be realistic. If your frame is small and you already have tiny breasts, think twice before going for a D cup. Your surgeon will probably advise against it anyway. The best prostheses now are shaped and are of standard width. You will be measured for the appropriate size and shape of these biodimensional prostheses.
• Make sure that your doctor checks for cysts in the breast that might require treatment in the future. It's difficult for a surgeon to interfere with the breast once an implant is in place.
• Discuss with your surgeon the possibility of contracture (see left) and ask where the scars will be.
• Ask whether the incisions will

interfere with breast-feeding or sensation in the nipple.
• Make sure that your surgeon tells you the size and the make of your implant in case it needs replacing at a future date.

THE OPERATION

Augmentation surgery will take a minimum of one and a half hours, the length of the operation being largely determined by where the implant is placed.

If it goes underneath the muscles of the chest wall, the operation will take less time than if it is placed underneath the breast tissue but on top of the muscle layer, because there's less bleeding in the former operation.

You might want to stay in the hospital for 24 hours to recover from the anesthetic, but then you can go home. You'll

Other **COMPLICATIONS**

Breast pain, loss of sensation in the breast, infection, and movement and leakage of an implant are all well-known complications. More uncommon is rupture of the implant, which can occur spontaneously or through physical force such as a blow. You'll need immediate surgery if this happens to remove all traces of silicone. Some authorities say half of all breast-augmentation patients will have some side effects by ten years after the operation; others estimate a one-in-three chance.

be asked to return to the hospital within about ten days to have any stitches removed.

IMPLANTS – SALINE OR SILICONE?

Silicone gel implants may feel the most natural, but in the US and Canada, only saline implants are used for general breast augmentation. In the US, silicone implants are available for reconstruction patients, such as women who have had breast cancer surgery, injury to the breast, or a birth defect that affects the breast. In Canada, silicone implants are approved on a case-by-case basis. The likelihood of contracture is about the same with both types of implant but obviously there's no risk of silicone leakage with saline-filled ones.

All implants used to be smooth, but nowadays a textured surface is preferred, since it seems to reduce the frequency of contracture.

NEW IMPLANT FILLINGS

Alternative implant-fill materials are currently being researched. It's hoped that these materials will be absorbed by the body if leakage occurs.

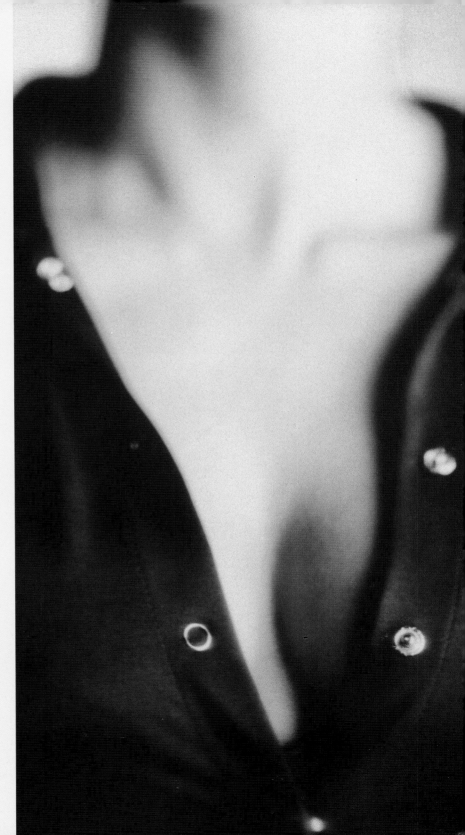

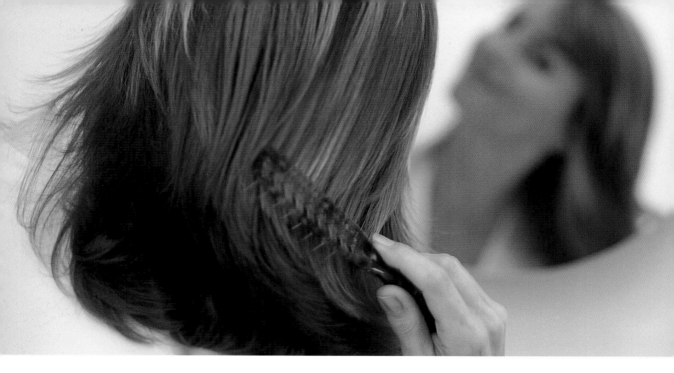

YOUR *crowning* GLORY

HAIR IS DEAD. YOU CAN USE MOISTURIZING CONDITIONERS AND SHAMPOOS THAT MAKE IT LOOK "HEALTHY" BUT NOTHING MORE. THE ONLY LIVE PART OF THE HAIR IS THE GROWING ROOT AND YOU CAN ONLY GET AT IT FROM INSIDE. A GOOD DIET WILL KEEP IT WELL NOURISHED.

Many women subject their hair to abuse from dyes and peroxide, hairdryers, sun, sea, and the elements. The injurious effects of these can be remedied, but only chemically, by moisturizing lotions and sprays. Tension on the hair caused by styles involving tight braiding, or by wearing curlers for prolonged periods, may also damage the hair, causing bald patches. To keep your hair looking good, get the best cut you can afford and have it trimmed regularly.

hair loss in women

The average person has about one hundred thousand scalp hairs and generally loses between 20 and 100 of them every day. Hair growth isn't continuous – a hair will only grow to a certain length before dropping out and being replaced by another.

For reasons unknown, certain parts of the scalp lose hair more readily than others, giving rise to the standard type of baldness that, though usually found in men, can be found in women – especially after menopause.

When hair follicles are permanently damaged, then growth ceases and may never start again. Only a trained dermatologist can tell you if your hair follicles are so badly damaged that hair loss is permanent.

TAKING CARE OF YOUR HAIR

◆ **Don't scrub** the scalp with your fingertips when you wash your hair, or you will loosen hairs from the soft wet hair follicles.

◆ **Don't tug** at wet hair as you comb it as this will remove or tear it. Use a wide-toothed brush or comb.

◆ **Don't brush** or comb your hair too frequently since this may irritate the scalp and stimulate oil glands to produce more oil, making your hair look lank and dull.

◆ **Don't use** antidandruff shampoos more than once every two weeks as they contain ingredients such as selenium that can irritate the scalp.

◆ **Use** the mildest shampoo you can find and only shampoo your hair once — shampoos are so efficient that shampooing twice is unnecessary. Mix two teaspoonfuls of shampoo in a glass of warm water and pour it over your already wet hair. Then massage the shampoo very gently into your hair. It's not necessary to scrub hard to work up a lather, just leave the shampoo on for about a minute and then rinse until the hair is clean. Always use a conditioner after hair washing to prevent tangling. After you've washed your hair, dab it dry with a towel rather than rubbing it vigorously.

what causes hair loss

Alopecia has many causes. Very rarely in sensitive people X-rays may lead to permanent baldness, even after a single dose. Chemical agents, like perms, may cause complete destruction of hair follicles, and baldness can occur with severe shingles, ringworm, and some scarring skin diseases. Certain drugs cause hair loss, the most common being cancer fighting ones, but hair always regrows when the treatment is complete.

Estrogen receptors in hair follicles maintain the health of each hair, which is why problems can occur at the time of menopause if estrogen levels are low. So it's possible that if you have a problem with hair loss it may be due to a hormone imbalance and **hormone replacement therapy might help**.

It's also possible that you have an underactive thyroid, as hair loss is one of the symptoms. A simple blood test can diagnose this. Iron deficiency anemia can cause hair loss and women who suffer with heavy periods are often deficient in iron. Rapid weight loss and stress are also thought to affect the hair follicles by constricting blood vessels that feed them and limiting their supply of oxygen.

Alopecia areata is a condition which causes bald patches of smooth skin to appear on the beard area or the scalp. It's an autoimmune condition — one part of the body's defense system attacks another. In this instance, hair follicles are attacked by white blood cells called lymphocytes in the mistaken belief that they represent foreign tissue (a little bit like the process that occurs in organ transplant rejection), but we don't know for sure why this happens.

It's thought that this type of hair loss can follow physical trauma, notably head injuries, and it's also believed that emotional stress alone may be a trigger. So, bereavement, loss, or anxiety of any kind might be the root cause, but hair loss could also be a side effect of something

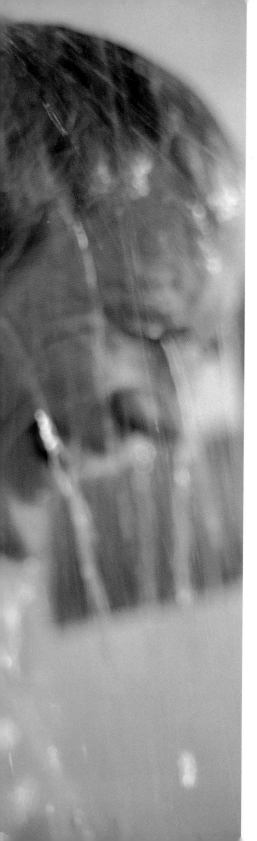

relatively minor of a physical nature such as uncorrected eyestrain. Spontaneous improvement can occur after a few months, but for others it can be a long-term problem. Specialized treatments like intradermal injections of steroids can help some people, but need to be prescribed by a dermatologist.

Alopecia areata is very unlikely to turn into a permanent problem and what should happen is that baby-fine hair will start to grow and will quickly turn into normal adult hair.

baldness in men

Most men feel that thinning hair is aging and it can cause loss or morale and great stress, so great that even the most questionable remedies are sought after. **Options are camouflage, drugs, or surgery**. Male baldness usually begins in the early twenties and is pretty well established by middle age.

DRUG TREATMENTS

There are both good medical and surgical treatments for baldness. The mainstays of medical treatment are drugs that were originally used for conditions completely different from thinning hair. For instance, during clinical trials with a new blood-pressure drug called minoxidil some patients noticed that they grew new scalp hair, so for once a drug's side effects could be put to good use.

Minoxidil is available on the market under the name of Rogaine and can be used as a lotion or cream for male pattern baldness. It must usually be rubbed into the scalp twice a day for at least three months before new hair growth is noticeable. Once hair has grown, the application must be continued indefinitely since the new hair tends to fall out if treatment is discontinued.

Don't raise your expectations too high. Fewer than one in ten report dense hair regrowth; nonetheless **Rogaine may stop or slow down balding** rather than replacing lost hair.

The only pill on the market to combat male pattern baldness is finasteride, a compound that's also used for treating men with benign enlargement of the prostate gland. Finasteride is marketed under the name Propecia. It's inappropriate as a treatment for women and may cause abnormalities in unborn babies. If a man wants to father a child, he may be told not to take the drug for a number of months prior to trying for a baby. The pill consists of 1 milligram of finasteride and stops most men from losing hair while two-thirds will have the beginnings of regrowth.

The drug works by inhibiting the enzyme that converts testosterone to dihydrotestosterone, the hormone that damages hair follicles and causes hair loss in men who are genetically predisposed to it. It takes six months before the effects are visible. Once the pill is stopped hair loss may start again.

SURGICAL TREATMENTS

A hair transplant is always worth considering though results can look somewhat "tufty" – a bit like doll's hair – if not done by a skilled and experienced practitioner. Hair from areas at the side and the back of the head that are spared from balding is used to fill up the spaces on the rest of the scalp where hair is thin.

For the best cosmetic results, hair transplants shouldn't be used in people who have advanced balding or where there's very little hair left. It's also important that the hair from the transplant area is of approximately the same color as the hair where it's going to be transplanted. The texture of the hair should also be similar. Tiny strips of tissue containing hairs are harvested from the donor site. Small incisions are made in the recipient site with a punch of a scalpel and then the grafts are carefully inserted and a turbanlike pressure dressing is applied.

Transplantation is a shock to hair follicles and the hair falls out immediately after transplantation. The initial results may be disappointing, but three months later the hair follicles have recovered and are growing new hairs. **Hair transplants generally result in the permanent replacement of hair –** though even when well established, it's not as luxurious as the hair you've lost.

Hair implant is a quasisurgical procedure – strips of hair are attached to the scalp by surgical threads implanted in the balding area. The implants are usually made of a synthetic material so a hairdryer mustn't ever be used. Quite a few hair follicles must be transplanted at the same session and the process needs to be repeated for bald areas to be covered.

CAMOUFLAGE

Hairpieces This is the safest and least painful way (in terms of health and money) to mask hair loss. Some hairpieces can be permanently attached to the head, either by being tied to existing hairs or by being sewn on to the scalp. The latter can cause infection and aren't often recommended for that reason. Another possible side effect is an allergic reaction to the adhesive used.

Hair weaving This is a nonsurgical procedure that adds replacement hair to existing hair in order to cover bald patches. The new hair is braided strand by strand on to the edges of the hair in situ. Hair weaving requires high maintenance and careful cleansing.

A colored spray that covers the head in an organic dust can disguise any bald patches.

COSMETIC *dentistry*

AS WE GET OLDER OUR TEETH TEND TO YELLOW WITH AGE AND GUMS MAY RECEDE. BOTH OF THESE AGING EFFECTS CAN BE MITIGATED BY GOOD HYGIENE AND REGULAR VISITS TO THE DENTIST.

The safest and by far the most efficient way to keep your teeth looking good is to visit a **dental hygienist**. When you're younger you should go every six months. **After the age of 50 you should go every three months** to remove plaque. If left, it causes inflammation in the margin of the gum and pockets form, leading to loosening of the teeth in the gums.

A good cosmetic dentist can alter the look of your teeth, your smile, the set of your mouth, and your facial expression. As we get older our teeth tend to be ground away, simply by use, by having especially strong masticating muscles, or perhaps by night grinding. Whatever the cause, our jawbones tend to fall closer together and this accentuates the aging folds on either side of the mouth. A cosmetic dentist can widen the distance between the jawbones by repositioning the teeth and stretching out the skin in your laughter line, making a **substantial difference** to your appearance.

caps, crowns, and bridges

Any badly positioned, ugly, or broken tooth can be given **a new look by capping or crowning** (the terms are synonymous). This is usually done by filing the tooth away to form a "peg" on to which the cap is cemented. This can still be done if your tooth is snapped off or has had to be removed right at the gum margin. Then, three or four posts are drilled into what is left of the tooth and the cap or crown can be fitted to them. Caps and crowns are made of a variety of materials. The most modern are made of strong porcelains or metals covered in porcelain, which come in a number of colors to match the rest of the teeth.

replacement teeth

If one or more teeth have to be extracted or are lost, they can be replaced by one of three different types of artificial teeth: a bridge, dentures, or a dental implant.

A **bridge** consists of one or more artificial teeth that are fixed permanently in the mouth, usually by being attached to the adjacent natural teeth.

REPOSITIONING TEETH

We think of cosmetic dentistry as involving complicated techniques with bridges, wires, and crowns, but many dentists use simple methods and materials to achieve results. For instance, it's possible to move the roots of the teeth within the jawbone by up to a millimeter if they're pulled or pushed in one direction for any length of time. Even such tiny adjustments make a difference.

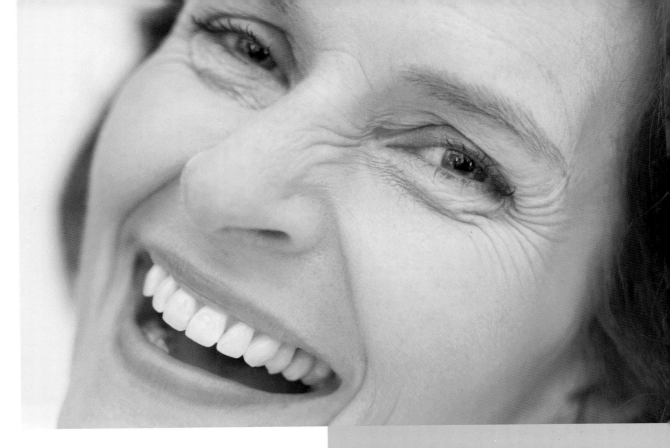

A **denture** is removable and may replace any number of teeth. Dentures have a metal or plastic base plate. They stay in place by resting on the gum ridges or they're held in place by clasps that fit on to the natural teeth. They can be removed for cleaning, either with a sterilizing solution or with a brush.

An **implant** is a permanent and effective method of replacing a single tooth. A hole is drilled in the jaw at the site of the missing tooth, and a screw is firmly fixed into the hole. A few weeks later when the site has healed, an artifical tooth is fitted to the top of the screw.

shortening or lengthening teeth

In some people with peridontal disease the gums recede, exposing the root surfaces of the teeth.

CHECK WITH YOUR DENTIST

Avoid using toothpastes that claim to whiten your teeth, unless your dentist recommends otherwise, because this whitening is nothing more than an optical illusion. The toothpaste contains a red pigment that turns your gums pink, making your teeth look whiter by comparison. Toothpaste that claims to give a white, polished smile makes the teeth shine by use of abrasives, including a very strong one know as "jeweler's rouge." These toothpastes are much too harsh on teeth and work by scratching the surface enamel. Prolonged use of such toothpastes damages and wears away teeth. It's far better to visit your dental hygienist, who will polish your teeth. This should make them several shades whiter, particularly if you are a smoker.

This can make the teeth very sensitive to hot and cold foods and make the crown of the tooth look very long – hence the saying "long in the tooth." With excellent oral hygiene, it may be possible to reposition the gum surgically to cover the exposed root surfaces and improve the appearance. Alternatively it may be possible to crown or shape the teeth. Some people have the reverse problem – the gums grow too far up the teeth so that they are, or appear to be, too short, or heavy grinding or clenching of teeth may wear the teeth away. Again, it may be possible to improve the appearance by crowning the teeth.

tooth whitening

This treatment uses a powerful gel containing hydrogen peroxide which is a potent, aging free radical. A liquid cream anesthetic is painted on the gums so the gel won't "burn" them. Then the gel itself is painted on followed by the insertion of a huge plastic mouth guard to hold the lips away from the solution. Once the teeth have been painted with the gel, a bright light on a stand is directed on to the teeth by the dentist and then left for 10 minutes after which the gel is removed and the whole procedure repeated twice more. The process is uncomfortable, but once over, you have new white teeth.

Tooth whitening is all the rage, but how safe is the process? Safe as can be, according to any dentist you care to ask, as long as it's performed in a dentist's office as a medical procedure. It's considered so safe that there is no recommended limit on the amount of hydrogen peroxide a dentist can use. And it's known that the higher the concentrations of hydrogen peroxide, the higher the risk to a patient of hypersensitivity.

In Britain, tooth whitening is classified as a cosmetic device, and in terms of products for cosmetics use the law says that 0.1 percent hydrogen peroxide is the maximum.

Dentists argue that even 3.5 percent, which could soon become the upper legal limit under a new European directive, is too mild to have any real effect. But if you put such a low concentration of hydrogen peroxide on teeth, it will have a negligible effect. Most dentists use 35 percent hydrogen peroxide and it doesn't remove enamel, damage teeth, or increase susceptibility to gum disease.

HOME TOOTH-WHITENING KITS

Home kits for tooth whitening are already fraught with danger if effective levels of peroxide are used. Safe home-kits are ineffective whiteners because they contain too low a concentration of peroxide.
◆ Whitening toothpastes don't whiten the teeth at all – they just remove surface stains, and they're costly.
◆ Over-the-counter whitening kits aren't a good option – some have high acidity or are highly abrasive, which can wear away the surface enamel.
◆ A home bleaching kit, supplied by dentists, consists of "trays" made to fit the teeth precisely. You apply a little peroxide gel (equivalent to 5–7.5 percent hydrogen peroxide) and leave the trays in your mouth overnight. Home bleaching takes up to two weeks to take effect.

RELAX *and* REJUVENATE

INSTANT REJUVENATION DOESN'T HAVE TO INVOLVE INTERVENTION. MANY OF THE MOST EFFECTIVE METHODS ARE WITHIN YOUR CONTROL – RELAXATION EXERCISES ARE JUST ONE OF THEM.

deep breathing

The depth and speed of breathing alters depending on your emotional state. If you're emotionally upset, your breath comes in short shallow pants from the top of the lungs. When you're relaxed, on the other hand, breathing is slower and deeper and uses more of the lungs. This is why **deep breathing lowers stress levels**. Try this instant tranquilizer. Take very slow, deeply inhaled breaths followed by long slow exhalations to a count of five – five in and then five out. Repeat two or three times.

yoga

There are different types of yoga, some of which emphasize exercises and others meditation. All types teach relaxation and breath control. Yoga postures exercise every part of the body and result in **increased suppleness, endurance, and strength**. Harmonization of breathing with yoga postures helps you achieve a state of relaxation and is very useful in relieving stress.

meditation

The goal of meditation is to **free the mind** from the usual everyday clutter. This promotes mental relaxation, which is then followed by physical relaxation. A relaxed mind is achieved by giving the brain a phrase, word, or mantra (a sound) to concentrate on, or an object such as a candle flame on which to focus very intently.

aromatherapy

Smells are interpreted by one of the most sophisticated parts of the brain which is the area concerned with emotions. Scents therefore tend to have a **powerful effect on mood and health**. Bad smells make us sick within a few seconds. I'm sure good smells confer a sense of well-being. Concentrated essences used by aromatherapists are a complex mixture of chemicals. Different essences have specific properties. Aromatherapy oil should never be taken internally, except for bergamot and rose and even then only in traces.

Interestingly, smell also seems to be quite strongly associated with **evoking memory**. Scents based on smells that older people might associate with earlier life have been used with some success to retrieve "lost" memories in people with Alzheimer's disease.

tense and relax

Once the body's major muscle groups are loosened the mind will also ease, resulting in a state of **deep relaxation**. Knowing if a muscle is very tensed is easy but it is less easy to be sure when it's really relaxed. In the tense-and-relax technique the main muscles are deliberately tensed as you breathe in and then consciously relaxed as you breathe out. Tense and relax muscle by muscle, working from your feet up to your face.

RELAXATION EXERCISE

Start by doing the exercise on your own in a quiet place, but you'll soon find you can do it anywhere, even with other people around you.

preparation

1 Sit on a chair with arms, shoulders, and head supported.

2 Clench your fists, hold the tension, and relax. Repeat until your hands feel relaxed.

3 With your mouth open, take a deep breath, hold it for five seconds, and let the air out. Repeat six times. You'll feel more calm and relaxed almost immediately.

legs

1 Stretch both your legs out, holding them in the air.

2 Point your toes away from yourself, holding the tension.

3 Pull your toes to point toward you and tense muscles.

4 Relax, letting your legs flop onto the floor.

5 Repeat until your legs feel loose and relaxed.

stomach

1 Contract your stomach muscles, take a deep breath, and hold the tension.

2 Relax, letting your breath out.

3 Repeat five times.

arms

1 Clench your fists, hold the tension, and relax.

2 Stretch your arms up (as if to touch the ceiling) and tense your muscles, reaching as high in the air as possible.

3 Relax, dropping your to your sides.

4 Repeat until your arms feel quite loose and relaxed.

shoulders

1 Shrug your shoulders so that they touch your ears. Then let them drop and relax. Repeat five times.

2 Push your shoulders forward and inward to meet each other, making a "hump" in your back (pushing arms forward).

3 Push your shoulders backward and inward, arching your back. Hold the tension and then relax, falling back into the chair.

4 Repeat five times.

neck

1 Move your head left and hold tension.

2 Turn your head to the right and hold.

3 Press your head forward with your chin on your chest and tense the back of your neck.

4 Relax, allowing your head to fall back onto the chair.

5 Repeat five times.

head and face

1 Raise your eyebrows, tense, then frown and tense. Repeat until your scalp and forehead are relaxed.

2 Close your eyes very tightly. Clench your eyes and hold the tension. Relax, letting your eyelids drop and close your eyes.

3 Clench your teeth, feel the tension, and then relax, letting your jaw drop slightly.

4 Clench your mouth into a whistling shape or "O," then tense your lips as if to make an "E" sound. Relax your mouth.

5 Concentrate on breathing deeply and regularly, letting your breath out slowly when exhaling.

6 Pick your favorite relaxing scene and fill your mind with it.

7 Let yourself sink, relaxed, into the chair. Remain like this for about ten minutes and let yourself enjoy it.

REMEMBER

◆ When you have finished relaxing, **slowly** open your eyes and stand up.

◆ **Never** jump up and rush around immediately.

◆ Use the relaxation technique on any part of your body that feels tense during the day.

◆ Deep breathing is useful anywhere to help you feel calm.

◆ Begin by doing each exercise in turn, working progressively through each part of your body. Later you will find that you can just sit down and relax in a moment, doing a few exercises.

DIRECTORY OF TREATMENTS AND TECHNIQUES

BEAUTY treatments

Treatment and claims made	What it does	Likely results	Who should avoid it
Face masks Said to cleanse and shrink the pores, remove dead cells from the surface of the skin, increase blood flow to the skin	A face mask, containing such ingredients as honey, egg yolk, peach, avocado, or glycerine, is applied to the skin. It is allowed to dry and then wiped away	A pleasant, relaxing few hours. Pores cannot be permanently shrunk and the feeling of tightness that follows the removal of a face mask wears off very quickly	Anyone with sensitive skin, eczema or dermatitis, or an infection of the skin, such as acne
Pressure spray toning Said to tone skin by increasing its water content	A fine spray of water under pressure is directed at the face, usually to remove a face mask	A psychological lift. Any water that enters the skin in this form will escape within about 20 minutes, simply because of evaporation	
Facial vacuum treatment Claims to improve the lymphatic drainage of the skin and the nutritional state of the tissue. Also helps to remove blackheads and oily secretions	Treatment with a facial vacuum may last 3–5 minutes for cleansing and 10–12 minutes for massage and drainage of the lymph nutritional state of vessels	A psychological benefit. It will cleanse and it may help to remove blackheads and oily secretions. It cannot improve the nutritional state of the skin, nor can it help lymphatic drainage. This is done most efficiently simply by the force of gravity because all the lymph vessels of the face, head, and neck drain downward	Anyone with any form of skin disease
Ozone therapy Said to dry, heal, and stimulate seborrheic skin, especially acne, and is beneficial to disturbed and blemished skin	Ozone, which is chemically related to pure oxygen but has one more atom of oxygen in the molecule, is applied to the skin, usually in the form of steam	Psychological benefit. At one time it was thought that ozone had all sorts of medical properties. These have never been clearly defined, let alone proven	Anyone with very sensitive skin or skin disease

ELECTRICAL treatments

Treatment and claims made	What it does	Likely results	Who should avoid it
Audiosonic vibration Said to increase the circulation of the blood in the locality being treated. Beauticians claim that it can increase "cellular activity" and so delay or arrest the development of wrinkles, crepy skin, and other symptoms of advancing age	The audiosonic vibrator may have a sponge or flat disk head which vibrates due to an electric motor	Psychological benefit only	
Vibrator treatments Said to stimulate circulation and have a relaxing effect	An electrical facial vibrator produces mechanical vibrations to simulate the effects of massage with the hands	You may feel relaxed after it and it may increase blood flow to the skin, but no more so than talking, chewing, eating, or laughing	
Diathermy Used for removing unwanted facial hair	A fine wire or metal point, which becomes red hot when an electrical current is passed through it, is applied to the hair root to kill it	Permanent removal of unwanted facial hair	Anyone with broken veins if the practitioner is not a medically qualified dermatologist
High frequency Said to dry, refine, and heal the skin and produce a germicidal effect on the surface to reduce the production of sebum	A high frequency current is applied to the skin	You may get permanent scarring of the skin if this is used in inexperienced hands	Anyone with skin disease

GALVANIC treatments

Treatment and claims made	What it does	Likely results	Who should avoid it
Iontophoresis Acidic substances are said to have an astringent effect. There is a variety of treatments packaged pseudoscientifically in ampules which beauticians apply for 3–12 minutes to moisturize or normalize the skin	Galvanic current (a very low strength electrical current) is used to introduce water soluble chemicals into the upper layers of the skin	Psychological benefit. Nothing can stay in the skin, not even an ion which is electrically pumped into the skin, because it is lost or shed in the skin cells within a few hours and in the case of water, a few minutes. The claim that frequent and regular prolonged courses of this treatment have a lasting effect on the skin is without foundation	Anyone with a skin disease
Disencrustation Said to remove blockages in the skin's surface oiliness and regulate secretions	There is special disencrustation fluid contained in ampules for use during iontophoresis. Many beauticians claim, however, that a simple solution of salt and water is as effective as the exotic ingredients contained in these ampules and indeed very often do use salt water with their client	Psychological benefit. The word "disencrustation" is a word entirely made up by beauticians: it has no scientific basis, nor can I find any true meaning for the word whatsoever. It is true pseudoscience	Anyone with very sensitive dry skin or any form of skin disease

REGENERATIVE CELL therapy

Treatment and claims made	What it does	Likely results	Who should avoid it
The most extravagant claims, ranging from curing diseases to putting off the effects of aging	Cells from the organs of animals are injected into people for the treatment of specific organ complaints. For instance, if you have a liver disease, then the liver cells from healthy animals are injected into your liver. Failures are claimed to be due to improper administration of treatment – not treatment itself	Psychological benefit at most. Despite exhaustive medical testing, has never been proven to have any medical effect	

SURGERY techniques

Operation	In or outpatient/ Length of stay	Postoperative effects	Stitches removed	Results/ Recovery time
Face-lift	Inpatient/ 1–2 nights	Red, swollen face, and numbness and tension in cheeks and neck	Some after 3–7 days, the rest after 2 weeks	Generally good results. Swelling goes down after 4 weeks
Brow lift Can now be done with an endoscope (viewing instrument)	one day	Shorter recovery time with endoscope method as only small incisions made	one week	Good – drooping eyebrows and frown lines smoothed so you look less tired
Blepharoplasty Reshapes eyelids and removes bags	Inpatient/ one night or a day's rest	Tender and bruised eyes	3–4 days	Very good results. Recovery takes 3 weeks
Soft-Form Polymer-like material inserted under skin to soften deep lines	Outpatient	Slight bruising and tenderness around stitches Sometimes slight swelling	Next day	Good, permanent results
Botox Injected into specific face muscles to smooth them	Outpatient	Slight bruising or swelling. If too much is used or surgeon is unskilled, brows or eyelids can droop or you can be left expressionless.	No stitches	Good results. Recovery takes one week. Boosters needed every 3–6 months.
Fat transfer Good for deeper wrinkles and smile lines	Outpatient	Risk of bruising where fat is removed and from injection of fat	None	Good results, lasts 10 years or more unless fat is absorbed by body
Breast Uplift, augmentation or reduction	Inpatient/ 1–2 nights	Bruising. Nipple sensitivity may be diminished	1–2 weeks	Good results. Recovery takes 1–2 months
Liposuction	Inpatient/one night or day	Temporary bruising and numbness	one week	Very good results. Recovery one week
Abdominoplasty Tummy tuck	Inpatient/ 3 nights	Temporary loss of sensation across wound	1–2 weeks	Very good results. Recovery takes 3 months

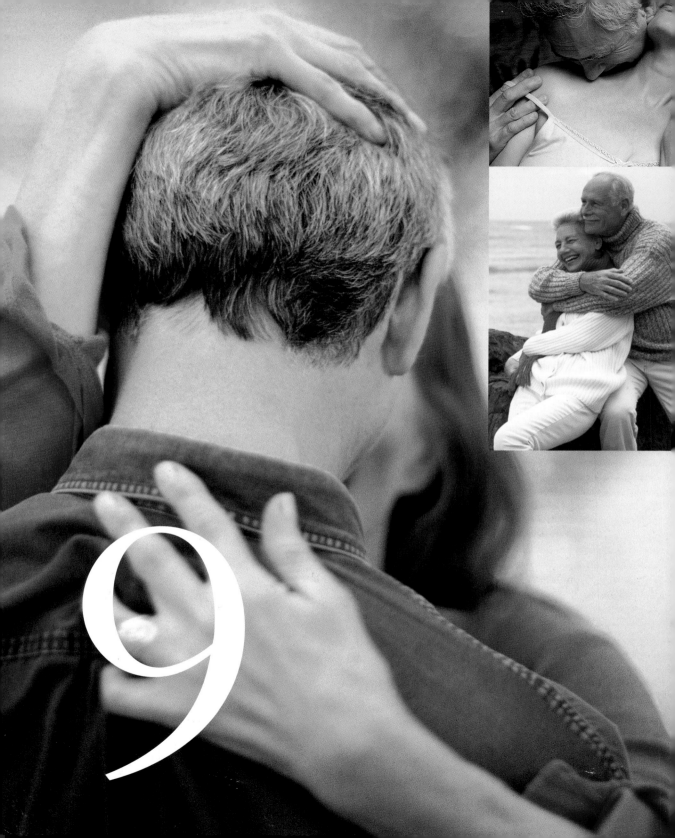

9

SEX

INTO THE SEVENTIES
AND BEYOND

As we get older we don't feel very different inside about anything, *particularly about loving*; we love just as strongly, just as passionately, and **just as tenderly** as we did when we were youngsters. Attraction, lust, passion are as *strong as ever*, though we may find new ways of expressing these feelings. Because the desires to love and be loved don't stop when we reach a certain age, we may look for **new ways** to express love. We may choose *companionship* without passion or expand the ways we express ourselves sexually. *We evolve sexually until we die* – it may be personal and private or it can be in **close intimacy** with a lifetime partner or a new one. It can be a very *thrilling* time.

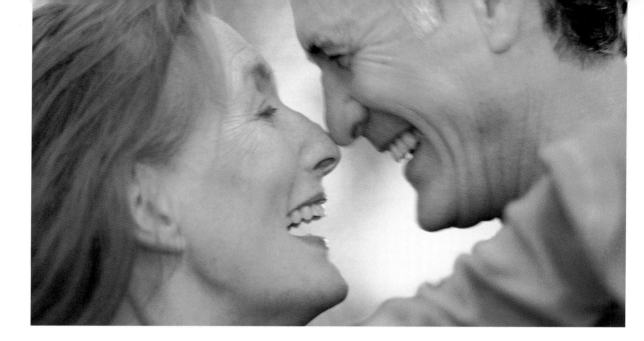

A *lifetime* OF LOVING

ONE OF THE BEST REASONS FOR MAINTAINING FITNESS AND HEALTH THROUGHOUT LIFE IS THAT FITNESS ALLOWS, AND MAY EVEN ENCOURAGE, THE ABILITY AND DESIRE TO CONTINUE SEXUAL ACTIVITY.

Being unfit certainly inhibits sex, and may even preclude it. Chronic illnesses affecting the lungs and heart, muscular strength, and joint mobility act as brakes on spontaneous sex. So it's worth planning well ahead of time to have **a fit, healthy, agile body as we get older** in order to be able to enjoy the particular benefit of **sex**.

I'm certain that fulfilment, happiness, maturity, and morality in a sexual partnership are largely the result of equilibrium, much more than quality and very much more than quantity. In other words, **it depends on two people being in balance**. To use oral sex as an example: a couple that is moved in any sense to use their mouths are in equilibrium; partners who both only like cunnilingus are in equilibrium; partners

who both only like fellatio are in equilibrium.

As we get older the meaning of sex and the frequency of sex have little to do with each other. A couple who has always shared strong physical affection is more likely to share caresses as they get older than a couple who has lost the habit of touching each other in middle age. **The frequency of sexual contact** is much less important. Between a devoted couple, sexual union is an affirmation of something that goes well beyond momentary pleasure. Years of giving and receiving love **strengthen the occasion**. For many couples, only one contact a month may be fulfilling enough, reflecting three, four, or five decades of intimacy. It also helps each partner to have a sense of being **desirable**, and to create the self-image of someone who is sexually alive. Anyone who has had an enduring relationship will miss the satisfaction and meaning of this kind of experience if it should end. Sensual awareness as we get older makes us **more vital, more attractive, and, yes, younger** in all sorts of relationships, not just sexual ones. Staying sexually alert helps us to avoid the drabness and grayness which a great many people wrongly associate with the older age group.

new ways of thinking about sex

Sex is a highly complex part of our lives, whatever our age, and it's influenced by our moods and emotions outside the bedroom. We go through times when sex is the last thing on our minds and our libido slumps. If we're depressed, tired, or ill, we'll have little inclination for it. But we don't have to dwindle into being sexless. There are always things you can do to **awaken your desire** for sex.

sensate focusing could be the key

If the suggestions in the circle below don't do the trick, "**sensate focusing**" might. This technique helps a couple focus on the sensations that arise when they gently explore and caress first their own and then each other's bodies. There's no intercourse or genital contact at first. The heat is taken out of the situation so there's no reason to feel anxious about your ability to enjoy sex. Relax and take your time.

The first stage involves only you, allowing you to explore your own body, massaging and stroking it to rediscover sensual feelings. Concentrate on yourself at this time and don't worry about sexual intercourse in the future.

The second stage involves your partner. Take it in turns to massage each other all over and talk about your feelings and what gives you pleasure. But you mustn't touch each other's genitals or the highly sensitive parts of your bodies. After a week or so when you feel comfortable it will be time to move on.

The third stage involves touching one another's sexually sensitive zones and the genitals. You should talk to each other all the time. During these sessions your partner may be eager for intercourse but it's essential to wait until you're both ready.

Not only may this exercise help to rekindle your sexual desire it may act as a template for **new and enjoyable sex** for the rest of your lives.

REAWAKEN SEXUAL DESIRE

◆ Make love somewhere other than in bed (on a chair, sofa, etc).
◆ Take a bath or shower together.
◆ Create an intimate atmosphere with music and candlelight.
◆ Give each other a massage with scented body oils.
◆ Make love at an unusual time.
◆ If you usually prefer some light, make love in the dark and vice versa.
◆ Last, but not least, allow enough time for lovemaking.

continuing sex and sexual relationships

I find it reassuring that the **majority of older people** still find sex thrilling and energy giving; neither their desires nor their capabilities vanish. Exactly as in relationships at a young age, attraction and love are followed by **sexual desire and sexual fulfilment**. The basic qualities in a relationship **strengthen** as we get older; they do not weaken.

In later life, most of us become somewhat more sophisticated at controlling intimate situations, and therefore feel **more at ease** in them and more capable of enjoying them. **All of us are the richer for loving and expressing love.** Sexuality – the capacity to respond to another person physically – is one part of that love, but there are many others.

friendships

The prevalent belief has been that it is simply impossible for a man and a woman to be just friends, a relationship of intimacy devoid of sexual connotations. Wherever a friendship between two people of the opposite sex is seen, society makes predictions about how the friendship is doomed to fail. The general view is that sooner or later, the relationship will get too intimate for comfort.

Relations between the genders have begun to rely more and more on **respect and friendship** and it is now understood that it is possible for a man and a woman to have a **friendship**, without the sexual implications.

Platonic friendships achieve a very real purpose. They help men to understand and perceive women as real people with real needs and problems, and not sex objects or playthings. Women also get a chance to see men as **caring people**, not creatures with nothing but sex and exploitation on their minds. A man who shares a healthy friendship with a woman is more likely to have **respect for women**.

Of course, there is always the possibility that platonic relationships will evolve into something more. But relationships that begin with friendships as their base are always far more stable. Both partners are more comfortable with

SEX ISN'T THE ONLY WAY TO LOVE

Most people have the potential to love in many ways and not all of them involve sex by any means.

◆ **Loving companionship** can be rich and rewarding in a deep, lasting way.

◆ Loving someone shouldn't just mean being "turned on" by them. There must also be a large element of **caring and sharing**, as well as **mutual respect** and trust, and tolerance.

◆ **A platonic relationship** can be defined as "a relationship where a person 'loves' the other but is not 'in love' with that person."

◆ As men and women interact more and more in various arenas, platonic relationships between the sexes tend to develop. Brought together by virtue of working together or sharing hobbies or interests, say at the local gym, social group, or even church, relationships tend to grow easily.

each other and there are no pretensions in the relationship.

It is relatively easy for a guy to be friends with a woman without a deep emotional attachment, but women tend to get attached very easily, especially if their emotional needs are being met. If it is a good solid friendship, then obviously the man will meet some of those needs and emotions will inevitably be involved.

a healthy sex drive

In both genders, the sexual urge declines with age but the general pattern differs in men and women. A **man's sex drive reaches a peak in the late teens** and thereafter gradually diminishes. A woman's sexual feeling reaches a maximum **much later in adult life** and is sustained on a plateau of responsiveness which, if it's going to decline, tends to do so only in her late sixties. There's much research supporting the existence of **a strong sexual urge in 70- and 80-year-old women**, just as there is in some men. There isn't usually an abrupt loss of sexual feeling coincidental with menopause, as many women fear.

About the time of menopause, a woman may become anxious about her loss of youthful attractiveness and the fact that any children she might have no longer need her maternal care. These insecurities may make her less ready to respond sexually. At the same time of life, a man has usually reached the most senior position he will attain in his work. If his early ambitions have not been fulfilled, and he feels threatened by younger men, his feelings may find expression in a lack of sexual interest or a feeling of sexual inadequacy. The "tired businessman" syndrome is

THE WHOLESOME TRUTH ABOUT OUR SEXUALITY

There's nothing but **good news about sexuality in our later years**. In fact, recent research has confirmed that sexual drive, sexual enjoyment, and sexual pleasure are greater in later life than they were when we were younger. This is why it's right to describe the *later years* as our prime time.

◆ Sex remains a **crucial part of life** during our older years and provides a sense of well-being and a positive feeling about ourselves.

◆ Sex makes older people feel beautiful, desirable, exhilarated, and mystical, and, for those who attach importance to the youth cult, **it makes them feel young**. Also, sex is relaxing and relieves tension. It may be one of life's exquisite moments, driving other problems out of our minds.

◆ Only a minority of people (less than 30 percent) feel there's a decline in sexual response and feelings. This is especially true of men who have problems with erection and so withdraw from sexual activities.

◆ Nearly two-thirds of older people feel that **sex is the same as it was when they were younger**; a third of older people say that sex is better than when they were younger.

◆ For those of us who find sex more gratifying when we are older, the key is having **the right partner**, loss of inhibitions, and a greater understanding of sex.

◆ For couples who get married for the first time or remarry in later life, **love, caring, and sharing and companionship** are emphasized, and so is sex. The majority consider that sex is very important in later life.

◆ About 80 percent of older people who are sexually active have sexual intercourse once a week or more; 30 percent have sexual relations three times a week; 20 percent report sexual relations twice a week.

◆ Sex brings **love, trust, approval, and warmth**; these are the same needs and desires for every age.

◆ A staggering 99 percent desire sexual relationships if they could have sex whenever they wanted to.

THE MATURE VIEW OF SEX

- ◆ The majority of us are satisfied with our sex lives the way they are.
- ◆ We consider **orgasm**, which may be stronger than earlier in life, to be **an essential part of our sexual experience**. Most women have had orgasms in their younger years, and are still having them.
- ◆ **Masturbation** is a perfectly acceptable outlet for our sexual needs.
- ◆ Many of us are very happy to live together without marriage. The majority of us, including widows, widowers, divorcees, and singles, **remain sexually active** in the last third of our lives.
- ◆ Many of us vary our sexual practices to achieve satisfaction.
- ◆ Many of us consider **oral sex** to be the most exciting sexual experience.
- ◆ We rarely show embarrassment or anxiety about sex if we're left to ourselves, and not bombarded with negative messages from the media and society.
- ◆ The majority of us like to be **naked** and enjoy nudity with our partners.
- ◆ When we think of an ideal lover, we choose someone close to our own age.
- ◆ Most of us see our sex lives remaining just the same as we grow older.

a reality to which many wives will attest. Both men and women may seek escape from this sense of decline by engaging in sexual adventures in a forlorn attempt to recapture the sexuality of youth. However, a satisfactory sexual relationship in an older couple is likely to be sustained if the couple enjoys a close understanding, companionship, and **mutual respect throughout their middle age**. This is entirely within the grasp of most couples, and it's worth planning and working for.

problems with sex

Problems with sex aren't the result of aging. In fact the same factors that lead to sexual problems in younger people – fatigue, emotional stress, drug abuse, alcoholism, disease, and eating too much – affect older people too, and these should be taken into account.

Most of us see our sex lives remaining just the same as we grow older and this isn't surprising.

Many people today live well into their eighties, which means that the years from 60 to 85 are more than a quarter of the total life span. Most of us, therefore, look forward to having more than one-third of our lives left after we pass our fiftieth birthday. We spend relatively few years at the beginning of our lives without sexual activity. **Why should we expect a curtailment of sexual activity toward the end?** We never lose the need to be touched, stroked, cuddled, and caressed. It's been known for years that **physical contact is a basic human need**, starting in the newborn infant, and, if anything it **becomes more powerful** in 60-, 70-, and 80-year-olds.

comfortable sex

All-consuming, passionate lovemaking is rare at any age, not just when we get older. If we set our sights on this romantic ideal and expect it to occur with any frequency, we'll almost certainly

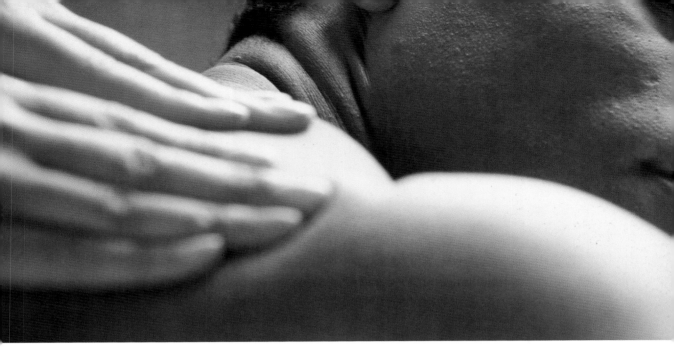

be disappointed. There are, however, many forms of enjoyable sex and **everyone can experience perfectly satisfying sex**, which can be quite different on different occasions, with the same partner. This is one of the thrills of a long-term relationship – discovering **new ways of enjoying sex** by being together over time and gradually making discoveries. For many women an **orgasm is not the be-all and end-all of enjoyable sex**, and as a man gets older he may not experience an orgasm every time he has sexual intercourse. Many men feel that they have to chase the elusive orgasm with every sexual union, but why, when there's so much satisfaction in **warm, less passionate sex**?

Several pitfalls await us if we continue to believe that sex must be exciting and that only exciting sex is good. This makes us tend to avoid having it unless we're sure that excitement will be an ingredient and, in this way, we narrow the spectrum of attainable experiences and deprive

ourselves of **peaceful, relaxing, joyful sex**. Another unfortunate result of this attitude is that sex becomes hard work and, as such, is boring and dull.

Hostility, resentment, contempt, and distaste can all ruin a good relationship, even a sound marriage, let alone sexual enjoyment. No good relationship requires an intense, permanent state of rapture or even a permanent emotional commitment. It does, however, require **goodwill, caring, thoughtfulness, a desire to comfort, and shared intimacy**. Problems are bound to arise when one partner has difficulty being warm and close with the other. There may be a steady pulling apart rather than a coming together if one person feels that the other is demanding more affection than he or she feels comfortable about giving. No couple can be close and intimate if there's no basic mutual respect and affection between the partners. In addition to this, no sex therapy can work.

SEX *and the* OLDER WOMAN

SCIENCE HAS RECENTLY SHOWN THAT UP UNTIL THE AGE OF 60, SEXUAL RESPONSES IN WOMEN DON'T CHANGE AT ALL, AND EVEN AFTER 60 THE CHANGES THAT DO TAKE PLACE ARE SLOW AND GRADUAL.

A man's sexual potency may decline more steeply, leaving too many women over the age of 60 desiring sex, but with partners who can't or won't fulfil their needs. Many older women find themselves without a regular sex outlet. Research has shown that for an older woman the only barrier to a more active sex life is the availability of a partner.

The fact is that even after her body has gone through menopause and is depleted of estrogen, a woman continues to manufacture male sex hormones, which are largely responsible for a desire for sex and the ability to respond and enjoy it. It's quite usual for a woman of 60 or 70 to find her **libido higher than ever** and her orgasms more thrilling.

The conclusion is that it's not age, but interest, opportunity, and availability that control the body's response. **"Use it or lose it,"** is a motto we'd be wise to remember. We should try to resist the emphasis that our culture places on menopausal changes which convert women's fears into self-fulfilling prophecies. There's absolutely no question that **powerful feelings of sexuality extend two decades and longer beyond menopause.**

women's attitudes to sex

Sexual repression died with the feminist movement. Today many women, particularly when older, have come to the conclusion that they have **just as much passion and sexuality as men** and, more importantly, that they have the right to make choices. Among older women there's a less willing acceptance of the old-fashioned male view of sex as being measured in performance only – how much, how often. **Many women are now seeking equality, quality, and variety.** And they're quite prepared to wake up their partners for sex when they feel in the mood.

how an older woman responds to sex

Most aspects of arousal remain identical to a younger age group. The arousal and erection of the nipple occurs in exactly the same way in older women as in younger ones, though engorgement of the areola (the pigmented area around the nipple) is not so intense as in younger women.

What's more important, however, is the fact that the **clitoris remains as responsive** as ever, at least until the middle seventies, and while there's a thinning and loss of elasticity in the vaginal walls with advancing age, plus a shortening of vaginal length and width, these changes have little effect on orgasm. People accept as fact that intercourse in an older woman must be painful because of a lessening in vaginal lubrication. **This is totally wrong – four out of five women report no such pain.**

orgasm and the older woman

Nearly 40 percent of women say that **orgasm is the most important part of sex**. This shouldn't be surprising. Much has been written suggesting that the female is superior to the male both in her capacity for, and her ability to sustain, orgasm. US doctor Dr. Jane Sherfey described the human female as "... sexually insatiable (even) in the presence of the highest degree of sexual satiation."

Sexologists Masters and Johnson were amazed by a woman's capacity for "... a rapid return to orgasm immediately following an orgasmic experience," and of "maintaining an orgasmic experience for a relatively long period of time." Though there are physiological changes, like vaginal lubrication – taking only 15 to 30 seconds in a younger woman, but perhaps one, two or even five minutes in an older woman – we're yet to have objective evidence that there's any real loss in sensation or feeling. The clitoris in both older and younger women remains the main organ of sexual stimulation, and the excitement generated by clitoral stimulation is **exactly the same in older women as it is in younger ones**. A woman of 80 has the same physical potential for orgasm as she did at 20.

In the older age group the proportion of women who haven't experienced orgasm is smaller than at any other age – less than two out of 100 women, and amazingly, not one of the women in the 80-or-over age group reported that they were nonorgasmic; 86 percent of women say that the frequency of their orgasms **is the same or better than when they were younger**.

helping a woman

Few women have any difficulty in reaching an orgasm through masturbation. You can make your lovemaking techniques **more successful** by modeling them on the way your woman masturbates. Feminist and sex researcher Shere Hite argues convincingly that an orgasm achieved through intercourse isn't necessarily a better orgasm than one achieved by other means. She also says that **women can have an orgasm whenever they want**. If intercourse doesn't work, you can help your partner reach a climax through manual or oral stimulation and this release is just as easy to accomplish for a woman as a man.

A man should be especially considerate to his partner during menopause years, especially if she fears menopause and aging. He should be open about her attractiveness and desirability with compliments and constructive suggestions. **Long, leisurely embraces, more attention to foreplay,** tender stroking, and kissing of the breasts and clitoris are rewarding at any time, but particularly for the older woman.

A woman of 80 has the same physical potential for orgasm as she did at 20

TIPS for successful lovemaking/MEN

◆ **Longer and stronger** foreplay, more tactile stimulation, including caressing, rubbing, and cuddling, and different sexual positions, help every woman enjoy sex.

◆ **Having frequent sex** is the best way to ensure a satisfying, continuing sex life. Many women, especially those who have regular intercourse – about once or twice a week – maintain a healthy vagina into advanced old age.

◆ **Use lubricating gels and jellies** – these can be a great help if vaginal dryness is a problem.

◆ **Masturbation** or using a vibrator increases lubrication and minimizes vaginal pain due to dryness. Few women have difficulty in reaching orgasm through masturbation so, if intercourse doesn't work, you can help your partner reach a climax through manual or oral stimulation.

◆ **Sensuous massage,** stroking her breasts and genitals, keeps a woman feeling attractive and desirable, and more liable to keep wanting to have sex.

◆ **Leisurely embraces** and a lot of attention to foreplay give an older woman the time she needs to lubricate and prepare for sex.

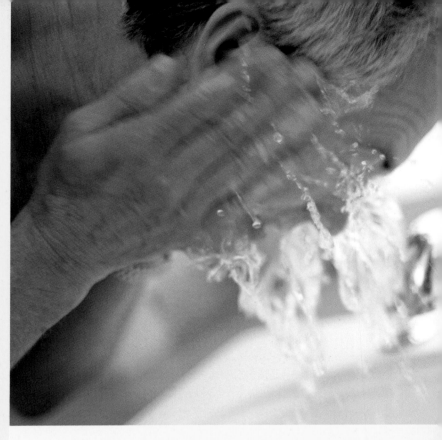

THE *older* MAN

SEXUAL POTENCY IS BY NO MEANS A PROBLEM FOR EVERY MARRIAGE, BUT IMPOTENCE CAN BE VERY DEMORALIZING WHEN IT HAPPENS. THE NEWS THAT A 60-YEAR-OLD MAN WILL NO LONGER BE ABLE TO SUSTAIN AN ERECTION CAN BE HORRIFYING FOR BOTH PARTNERS.

To most people it's tantamount to saying that their sex lives are over, but it shouldn't be. A sudden inability to achieve an erection may be due to past medical history or to fear alone. It may be that a man has had his prostate removed and is looking for an excuse to end his sex life. It may be that he's had a heart attack and is afraid of having another if he tries to have sex. This fear prevents him from having an erection. When this has happened several times, a man **quite wrongly** feels he's impotent. Older men need to know that any kind of therapy for impotence or premature ejaculation is as applicable to older men as it is to younger men, because most of these problems are **psychological in origin** and not physical. There's a lot of help available for older men and women and it's encouraging to know that the success rate is extremely high.

making adjustments

A few adjustments in expectations can make all the difference. It's unnecessary for a man to ejaculate every time. Get used to rest periods of several days before trying for another erection and orgasm. If older men hold back instead of feeling forced by macho instincts to have frequent sex, then the frequency of sexual relations is more under their control. It becomes easier for them to adapt their sexual relationship to suit their own personal needs as well as those of their partners. To feel comfortable with this changing pattern of sexual activity, it's important for men to be **open and honest** with their partners so that there's the mutual understanding to keep a loving relationship going.

One further point to remember is that the sensitivity of the penis to touch tends to decline with age so **more direct stimulation is needed**, usually with the hands and fingers and for longer. Masturbation can usually bring about an erection though it will take longer than when young. But many men can reach orgasm and ejaculation with a penis that's far from rigid, quite limp in fact, but sufficient to enter the vagina.

helping a man

You can help a great deal to make sure your man doesn't believe that his sex life is coming to an end. The most important thing is for you to **understand the new way your partner is functioning** and to see it as perfectly normal. Recognize his faltering patterns of erection and orgasm as normal, too. Both of you should discuss what's happening so that your expectations are realistic, and so that you can **adjust your sexual techniques** to whatever changes occur.

TIPS for successful lovemaking/WOMEN

◆ **Don't become afraid** or critical because your partner takes longer to get an erection. If you sense that he's apprehensive, reassure him that all is normal and if he takes longer it doesn't mean that he's unable. Your partner may be less aroused by seeing you naked or by thinking about sex; skillful manual and oral caresses can overcome this. Whatever you do, don't feel rejected. Don't think that because he can't attain an erection rapidly he's no longer attracted to you.

◆ **Don't worry** if he doesn't ejaculate but seems sexually satisfied. When your partner cannot attain a second erection within a short time, don't think this is the first sign of impotence.

◆ **Be a creator** and an initiator. Lead the way and introduce a changing pattern so that both of you create a new kind of sexual loving. A woman can find new ways of doing things which will fit her partner's new mood and will help to build his self-esteem rather than erode it.

◆ **Adapt foreplay** — more prolonged foreplay may be necessary for arousal — with you taking the lead.

◆ **Take a greater role** — try positions that let you control the pace and take pressure off your partner to perform.

SEXUAL *myths*

MISCONCEPTIONS ABOUT SEX ARE SUPPORTED BY THE POPULAR BELIEF THAT IT'S NOT QUITE THE THING FOR OLDER PEOPLE TO DO.

A common myth is that men in their fifties get a paunch, consider themselves less attractive, and suffer from impotence. A second is that women, once the fertile time of their lives is over, feel that their sex drive will dwindle into apathy. They fear that sexual excitement and pleasure will be things of the past.

Today, however, we recognize that with her child-bearing life behind her, a woman can look forward to **many years of a different kind of sexual loving**, more relaxed, more leisurely, and more exciting than ever before. A woman may even discover that **sex for pure enjoyment happens more often** than it did for procreation.

Unfortunately the good news about sex is kept secret. A recent newspaper survey revealed that many people in their seventies and older not only need to have, but actually do have, active sex lives. This news gets little publicity, remaining unknown to most people.

partners don't always have to be in sync

One of the most common and most frustrating difficulties a couple can face is that one partner wants sex much more than the other. No matter how well matched a couple are, there will always be times when their sex drives will be out of sync with each other. Like any other appetite our desires for sex waxes and wanes and various factors affect it. Our psychological and physical health has a marked effect on our sex drive and sometimes we have little inclination for it. For women in particular, the sex drive is a complex and somewhat delicate thing.

The brain is **our most powerful sex organ** and you might even call it the control center for our sexual desire and sex drive. There is a specialized sexual center within part of the brain called the hypothalamus, which responds to sexual stimulation of the receptors within the genital organs and is involved in the experience of orgasm. The largest "thinking" part of the brain, the cerebrum, enables us to have the sexual thoughts, perceive the sexual stimulation, and store the various sexual memories that between them go to make up the pattern of desire.

But differing sexual needs may show up for the first time in a mature relationship as a recent survey shows. Men between the ages of 57 and 64 have revealed they **value love and sex** more than at any time in their lives, but may find their needs are not met by their partners who, freed from family duties, are finding **new horizons** outside the home just at the moment when their men want to spend more time with them. Women are saying, sorry, I've got goals of my

the brain is our most

own, just as their men are saying, I want more intimacy. Women between 57 and 64 give sex a rating of 46 (out of 100) whereas men rate it 62.

lose your inhibitions

The oft-forgotten counterbalance to negativity is that more and more of us lose our inhibitions as we get older – at 60 there's no good reason to keep them. There can be a need to enjoy sexual pleasure which we've kept hidden, a sense that time is running out so we should follow our instincts. There's **freedom and energy** to be invested in pleasurable activities, including sex, and intimate situations are easier to control. There's more privacy, fewer interruptions, and many couples feel they have the time to savor the most beautiful moments in sex.

The newspaper survey mentioned previously also showed that the frequency of sex doesn't decline markedly from early adulthood. In the 1950s Kinsey stated that the average frequency of intercourse at 30 was 2.2 times a week and at 60 once every two weeks. The newspaper survey covered people aged 60 to 91 and the average frequency was 1.4 times a week. This figure matched the one that Kinsey reported in his 40-year-olds. Desire for sex was even higher.

These facts challenge the widely held belief that older people are beyond having sex. It may wane a little in frequency and vigor but not in **sweetness and satisfaction**. This is something we can all look forward to in our maturing years.

SO DOES OUR SEXUALITY DECLINE AT ALL?

Yes it does, in subtle and not so subtle ways and I list them only to alert you to what you might find happens to you so that you don't panic.

Men aged 50-89
◆ An erection takes longer and may not be as full or as firm as it was when you were younger.
◆ An erection subsides more rapidly after ejaculation.
◆ Ejaculation lasts for a shorter time and is not as forceful. The volume of semen is nearly always less than it is for younger men.
◆ It takes longer before you can have another erection and another orgasm.

Women aged 51-78
◆ A longer time is needed to respond to sexual stimulation.
◆ Lubrication is slower and generally takes longer than in younger women.
◆ The vagina is less capable of stretching than in younger women.
◆ After the age of 60 the clitoris shrinks but still remains responsive to stimulation.
◆ Orgasms are generally shorter and less intense than they were in younger years.

All these statements are **generalizations** – you can take each one and find valid research to show that it doesn't apply to the majority of people. This is what should be publicized. Then, instead of being terrified by the prospect of advancing years, we would look forward to them with joy and curiosity. If we did, growing older would be a great deal easier, we might even do it more gracefully.

powerful sex organ

SHIFTING *sexuality*

WE TEND TO THINK OF OUR SEXUALITY AS SOMETHING FIXED AND UNCHANGING, BUT THERE'S PLENTY OF EVIDENCE TO SUGGEST THAT THIS VIEW IS INACCURATE.

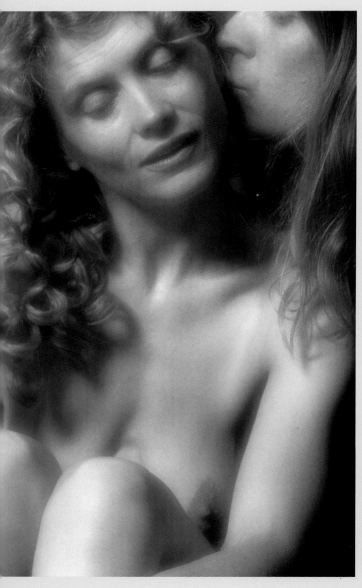

The popular image of society is that heterosexuals form one large group, homosexuals a much smaller minority, while a few bisexuals fall between both categories. Some behavior researchers believe that people don't fall into such rigid groups. **It's perhaps better to think of human sexuality as a linear arrangement.** At one end are a small group who could never be anything other than heterosexual, and at the opposite extreme are an equally small group who could never be anything but homosexual. The vast majority of us are somewhere in the middle, capable of **same sex relationships** – but only in certain circumstances. This could explain why homosexual relationships are more prevalent in certain situations – such as the confined environment of a prison – and at certain times in different cultures.

I think all this means is that we are all much more complicated than some people would want us to believe. It also explains why some people who have suppressed their true sexuality, even to the point of marrying and having children despite the inner conviction that they're homosexual, **take stock of their sexuality** when the children are in their late teens.

changing attitudes

By and large, men find the transition from a heterosexual lifestyle to a homosexual one easier than women because the gay network is more public and wider for men than it is for women. Plus it may take a women some time to realize that she's a lesbian, brought up as she has been with the traditional ideas that lesbianism is unnatural. Lesbianism is often the result of **a gradual change in attitude toward heterosexual relationships** and the standards of a heterosexual society, or a gradual realization that relationships with men are unsatisfactory, and therefore a lifestyle in which a heterosexual relationship is implicit will prove to be not only unpleasant but also impossible.

For that reason, many women (unlike men who often know they're homosexual from childhood) only come to realize that they are truly lesbians partway through their lives, when they are already married and have children. It's only with maturity, experience, and growing self-confidence that they're capable of revealing that both their marriage and lifestyle are unsatisfactory, and that they're no longer prepared to go on making concessions in so important an area of their lives.

Lesbianism does not solely imply a sexual preference for women – **it's much more a matter of lifestyle**. The majority of lesbians claim that sex occupies an important but small part of their lives. Much more important is contact with women, living with women, and planning a lifestyle that's built around **openness and freedom** in any sort of relationship between women.

There is, however, no reason whatsoever why you should give up your children. Even if your marriage ends in divorce, the judgement on custody may come out in your favor, but be prepared for the law courts to be one area of life where you will meet prejudice. Parenthood for lesbians is fraught with difficulties and if possible, lesbian mothers should seek out lesbian groups, all of whom are concerned to help and support lesbian mothers. The likelihood is that you will meet other lesbian mothers and so you will be able to introduce your children to other children with lesbian parents.

CELIBACY IS AN OPTION

It must be said that there's **nothing wrong in not wanting sex at all**. Sexual desire varies from none to a lot, and all variations are normal. There's absolutely nothing wrong with you if you don't want to have sex and don't have it. If you really don't want it, and are upset by having sex, be plainspoken and let it be known. Sex is supposed to be a pleasure and not a burden. If it's onerous and distasteful, **don't have sex and don't feel guilty about it**.

masturbation is normal

Both men and women feel the need to fill the gap in their sex lives left by the departure or death of a spouse. If they've opted to live alone and are not outgoing enough to seek new relationships they fall back on masturbation.

I receive thousands of letters from such people who feel ashamed of pleasuring themselves and even fear they may be doing themselves some harm – sexual myths still persist.

Just as sexual awareness starts in the teenage years with self-exploration, at the other end of life masturbation takes on the role of lone pleasuring and comforting. **Masturbation not only produces the most physically intensive orgasm** but it also brings both men and women to orgasm faster than any other type of sexual stimulation.

So it would be a pity for anyone to deprive themselves of this pleasure because they're caught up in misplaced guilt and fearfulness. There's **nothing abnormal or unhealthy about masturbation**, but that doesn't stop people feeling guilty about doing it.

Masturbation taboos have been drummed into our heads for many decades, and it's hard to shake them off. But masturbation means you can bring about a climax alone, whenever you feel like it and at your own pace – fast or slow, whatever your mood is at the time.

It's a normal part of life, and there's nothing in the least wrong about it.

What is important about masturbation is **why you're doing it**. If you're doing it as a way to release stress or for any number of healthy reasons, you can masturbate until the cows come home and not bother about it.

It's only when masturbation becomes compulsive and there's no room in your life for other pleasures such as friends that you'll need to think about what you're doing and consider reining yourself back.

SEX AND THE SINGLE PERSON

When a marriage fails or when a partner dies, men and women may decide to remain single but that doesn't mean they want to go without sex. I get thousands of letters from 50-somethings and 60-somethings who **are single but who miss a sexually-rich life** and wish to re-create one with or without long-term commitment. Indeed, some middle-aged singles would like to return to the free and easy singles life they enjoyed before marriage, and they do. This is easier for men than women, but in any case more divorced women than men opt to stay single.

Many women see nonmarriage as the simplest, if not the ultimate, way of achieving autonomy. After being enclosed in claustrophobic marriage **some women are attracted to living alone** so that they can be free and in control of their own lives. They reject marriage as a relationship that offers too few possibilities and choices to them.

Making the most of being single means being able to provide yourself with the kind of environment which will **enable you to grow**. This doesn't mean developing in isolation, but having a rich social life and a number of interests. Single women often find emotional fulfilment and sexual satisfaction hard to achieve, most often because of lack of opportunity. It's important therefore that you develop a degree of initiative and extroversion in order to develop relationships with people in groups. Joining a club or evening class, as well as becoming involved in community and volunteer work, are all useful ways of meeting new people.

WORRIES *about* ERECTION

FEW MEN ESCAPE ANXIETY ABOUT THEIR WANING SEXUALITY AS THEY AGE. BUT, FOR NEARLY ALL MEN, WORRYING ABOUT IMPOTENCE IS HARDER TO DEAL WITH THAN IMPOTENCE ITSELF.

I hope what I have to say will help alleviate some of that anxiety. Contrary to what men may expect, most women feel very sympathetic, so it's not fair to themselves or their partners to nurse hurt pride in secret. **Talking always helps to find a new way of approaching sex.** And it will help you (and your partner) if you know how an erection works and what might cause it to go wrong.

what happens in an erection

The stiffness of an erection depends on blood being pumped into specially designed spaces (the corpus cavernosum) in the penis in much the same way as we blow up a balloon with air. To keep the spaces full of blood, and an erection stiff, blood must be prevented from escaping from the spaces by valves snapping shut.

Both these events are controlled by nerves running down the sides of the penis which are in direct connection with the brain. Hence a man can see a sexual image and a split second later he'll feel his erection begin – the brain-penis connection.

Any interference with that connection, or damage to the penile nerves themselves, can result in too little blood getting into the penis to bring about erection (or only a limp erection). Alternatively, once in the penis, the blood necessary to maintain turgidity can simply seep away through leaky valves. It also has to be said

that, if the arteries bringing blood into the penis get clogged, there's insufficient blood to stretch the corpus cavernosum and expand the penis, so erection will be a pretty half-hearted affair. This could happen to any man who has hardening of the arteries.

WHY IMPOTENCE CAN HAPPEN

Despite the fact that one in ten men over the age of 21 suffers from impotence, very few understand why it happens. It can be a side effect of accidents, diseases, and most importantly, of prescription drugs. In addition, a quarter of all cases of impotence arise as a side effect of drugs given to treat other conditions (see page 244). This latter cause would fall into the category of medically induced, or "iatrogenic" impotence. Impotence can be a feature of medical conditions that are more common the older we get and include heart disease such as high blood pressure and angina, liver disease, thyroid disease, diabetes, chronic bronchitis, and emphysema.

Given this interaction of the brain, the nerves, and a healthy blood supply, it isn't difficult to see how the complicated mechanism of an erection can go wrong. And go wrong it will, if anything damages the health of the nerves and arteries of the penis.

AN APPROACH TO IMPOTENCE

The first step when tackling impotence is to make sure that you aren't overly tired. Something as simple as fatigue can often affect getting an erection.

◆ **Time of day.** Many men find that they're able to get an erection in the morning, but that it's quite impossible for them to do so at night. Also, it's good to remember that alcohol may increase sexual desire, but at the same time, it reduces the capacity to get an erection, so don't drink too much before sex.

◆ **Stop worrying.** You can reduce anxiety to a minimum by deciding not to have full sex but simply enjoy each other without trying to reach orgasm. In this way, the erection is nearly always strengthened.

◆ **Fear of failure.** It's easy for a man to fear he won't perform properly and become overly concerned about what his partner thinks of him. It will help if he's allowed to concentrate all his energies on his own sexual desires instead of worrying about what his partner may be feeling. He should just abandon himself to his own sexual feelings and think of nothing else at all.

◆ **A relaxing bath.** It may be helpful for you both to have a bath before having sex, or for your man to ask you to perfume yourself – smell can be an extremely potent sexual arouser. Some men will find that candlelight and playing soft music is helpful; others may prefer to make love in darkness and quiet. Use anything which is likely to increase sexual desire and get rid of anything likely to reduce it.

◆ **Give it time.** How long a man will take to respond varies by day, by occasion, by the hour, and you will have to be patient. It may be several weeks before your partner can achieve an adequate erection.

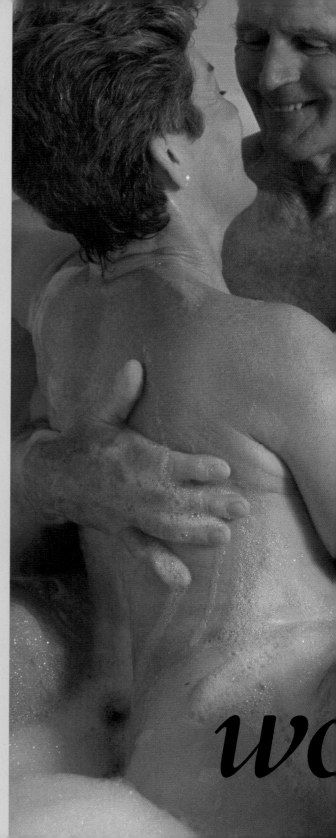

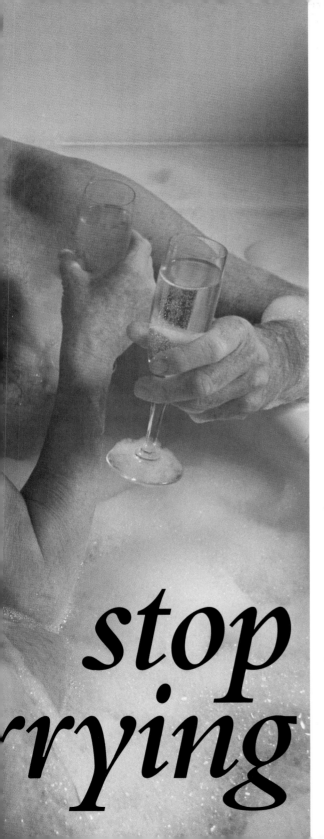

stop
rrying

impotence happens at every age

It's worth remembering that impotence is a common and distressing condition **affecting 10 to 30 percent of men on a regular basis** and involving all age groups. As men age, it's normal to find their ability to get and sustain an erection is more chancey than it was, but it's not a matter of life and death, and you can increase your chances with thought and preparation.

As you get older, you need a **longer time to get an erection**. Not only that, you need more direct and intense physical stimulation to get and maintain an erection. That's why many men find masturbation so satisfactory. Psychological stimulation (sexual thoughts, sexual fantasies), which was sufficient to get an erection when you were younger, becomes less and less effective. Even the ability to feel touch declines with age so an older man may require prolonged and firmer stimulation.

Studies here in the US reveal that men between 48 and 65 take on average five times as long to achieve an erection as men aged between 19 and 30. However, once an erection is achieved, an **older man has the advantage of being able to maintain it for much longer before orgasm.**

Due to the blunting of the ability to feel, an older man may have some difficulty in regaining an erection if he hasn't ejaculated. Contractions of the penis during climax aren't as strong as in younger times so the force of ejaculation is weaker. The seminal fluid is thinner and the quality is poorer.

Despite all of this, orgasm is still an intensely pleasurable experience. After ejaculation, the older man tends to lose his erection very quickly and it may be some time – hours or even days – before he's capable of getting another one.

Unfortunately age and medication act against some men, who may have to accept that they don't achieve orgasm every time they masturbate. However, there are many things you and your partner can do to have **years more of pleasurable sex**, though it probably means a change in approach and expectations. Sex shouldn't be any the less for that.

think about sex aids

Some relaxed couples have used **sex aids to spice up their sex lives** for years. Other, more reticent couples have never contemplated them. With loss of inhibitions older couples may feel the freedom to experiment a bit more and be more adventurous.

If you're a couple who feels curious I'd suggest you **follow your instincts** and talk about possibly using a vibrator which is especially effective for women, being many times more potent in stimulating the nerve endings of the clitoris than any part of a man. It's exciting for a man too, so you can experiment together and swap notes.

Then, don't turn your back totally on sexy videos and movies, magazines, even the internet to share your fantasies – **these can be a turn-on for all couples.**

DRUGS that may affect your sexual performance

Sleeping pills and tranquilizers	Phenothiazines (sedatives, antinausea pills) Benzodiazepines (tranquilizers and sleeping pills) Lithium (a drug used to treat manic depression)
Antidepressants	Tricyclic antidepressants e.g. amitriplyline, Monoamine oxidase inhibitors (MOAIs)
Almost all antihypertensives for high blood pressure and some heart drugs	Digoxin, diuretics, beta-blockers, ACE inhibitors
Endocrine drugs	Antiandrogens, estrogens (men)
Cholesterol-lowering drugs	Statins, fibrates
Drugs used to treat an enlarged prostate gland	Any of them
Others	Cimetidine (antiulcer drug) Pherytoin (antiepileptic drug) Carbamazapine (antithyroid drug)
Recreational drugs	Alcohol, nicotine, marijuana, amphetamines, barbiturates

SEX POSITIONS FOR OLDER LOVERS

Take **a fresh look** at the positions you're using for intercourse. **Traditionally,** the missionary position has been the most popular with couples. This is the position where the man lies on top of his partner supporting his weight on his arms. It can be tiring for the older man and uncomfortable for the woman, especially if her partner is heavier than she is. Lying side by side, with the man behind, is probably a more suitable position since it's less tiring and also provides the opportunity for maximum manual stimulation.

Experience more than compensates for any lack of energy that we might feel as we get older. Understanding our partner's body as we do makes us confident and considerate enough to concentrate on pleasing our partner.

Foreplay Remember that lovemaking is not just about penetration; skilled and loving caresses can be just as fulfilling as intercourse itself. Since the clitoris may also require a little more stimulation we will enjoy and benefit from long, loving embraces during foreplay.

Woman on top Here the emphasis for both partners is on comfort. The woman lowers herself on to her partner's penis. She can then face him and gently rock to and fro.

Spoons With the man curled up behind his partner and hands free to fondle her breasts, sex can be intimate and untaxing. The woman has her hands free to masturbate or use a vibrator.

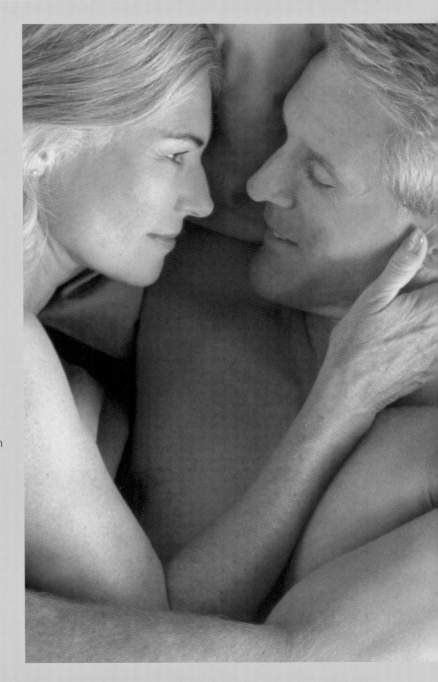

CHRONIC MEDICAL CONDITIONS

If you and your partner want to have sex, few medical conditions should stop you. You just need to be open to adjustment and willing to embrace new approaches.

heart disease doesn't necessarily mean you'll have to eliminate sexual activity altogether unless it's very severe. In fact, in many cases of heart disease **sexual activity can be beneficial**, since sexual activity can be the equivalent of performing moderate exercise with an increased heart rate, slightly increased blood pressure, and improved oxygen consumption. A study has shown that less than one percent of all coronary deaths occurred during, or after, intercourse. Most doctors believe that the **therapeutic benefits outweigh the risks**. Total abstinence can bring a great deal of psychological stress which will worsen any heart condition. All in all, the news on heart disease and sex is extremely good. Doctors now realize that a normal sex life can actually *benefit* many men who suffer from heart attacks, but it's important that they don't get overly tired. It's possible that the pattern of sexual relationships has to change to mornings, when both partners are feeling rested. A new sexual position can also help people with heart conditions. Lying next to each other on your sides, face-to-face, is more restful than the missionary position. You can find positions that avoid muscle cramps and tension, with the affected partner doing the least work.

high blood pressure Many people with high blood pressure believe that sexual activity is dangerous for them. This isn't necessarily so, although quite a number of patients who take drugs for high blood pressure say that they suffer loss of potency and some drugs for high blood pressure do cause impotency. If you're prescribed treatment for high blood pressure, make sure you're getting one of the drugs that won't affect your sexual potency.

diabetes Impotence is fairly common among diabetics. Men find that they have difficulty in attaining erections and ejaculation and women may have difficulty with vaginal lubrication. Research has revealed lower testosterone levels in diabetic men and it has been suggested that male impotence may result from malfunction of the nerves which supply the penis as part of diabetic neuropathy. Premature ejaculation may be a symptom too.

arthritis can affect your sex life by causing discomfort during intercourse. Painful, stiff joints may make the face-to-face position difficult but the adoption of a new position – such as with the woman on top (if it's the man who's arthritic) can often bring success. Taking analgesics before having sex can help. Even if the problems involved in making love are so severe that you decide to forego full intercourse, **don't give up other sexual activities** if you or your partner desire them. Physical closeness through touching and caresses can provide **a great deal of comfort and reassurance**. If you're used to sleeping with someone, it's better to get in an extra single bed for the occasional troublesome period, than to switch to twin beds permanently.

VIAGRA

THERE'S BEEN A LOT OF HYPE
ABOUT THIS DRUG BUT THE
REALITY IS QUITE SOBERING. MANY
MEN THINK VIAGRA INCREASES SEXUAL
DESIRE – IT DOESN'T. WHAT IT DOES IS
INCREASE SEXUAL RESPONSE IN THOSE
WHO HAVE THE CAPACITY TO RESPOND.

For Viagra to work the penis needs adequately healthy nerves and arteries (see page 241). A man of 80, for example, is bound to have some hardening of the arteries, which won't have spared the arteries to the penis. So, while Viagra may be worth a try if you have a condition such as diabetes, in trials only half the diabetic men tested had an improvement in their erections.

If your pelvic nerves or pelvic arteries have been damaged by an accident or by surgery, Viagra might not perform miracles for you either. The success rate is only 40–50 percent.

IS VIAGRA SAFE?

As a rule of thumb you have to be **fit enough to walk up a flight of 20 stairs** without getting breathless to qualify for Viagra. The manufacturers say **it shouldn't be taken with heart drugs which include nitrates**. There are also side effects. The US Food and Drug Administration reported the most common were headache, flushes, upset stomach, stuffy nose, urinary tract infection, changes in vision, and diarrhea.

is Viagra available to all men by prescription?

In the US and Canada, Viagra is available by prescription only and is used in men with erectile dysfunction, including those with prostate cancer, kidney failure, spina bifida, Parkinson's disease, and those who have had polio. It has also been found to be helpful in men who have undergone radical pelvic surgery or had their prostate removed and those suffering from spinal cord injury, diabetes, and multiple sclerosis. Other men distressed by their impotence may also consider consulting their doctor. Viagra is not used in men with certain medical conditions nor in those taking medication that contains nitrates, found in many prescription drugs, so it is vital to discuss your medical history with your doctor before taking Viagra.

would Viagra work for women?

Clinical trials are underway and it looks as though drugs like **Viagra should work for some women** – it depends whether you have a **big G-spot**. How do you know if you have? Well – there's still debate about whether the G-spot even exists, so an Italian team decided to look for biochemical markers of sexual pleasure in the area where the G-spot is supposed to be. They decided on PDE5, an enzyme that gets rid of the nitric oxide in the penis (and clitoris, incidentally) that triggers erections. Viagra works by blocking PDE5, leaving enough nitric oxide to cause an erection. So would it work on the clitoris – the penis simply being an enlarged clitoris?

We've known for ages that there's nitric oxide activity in the clitoris and now PDE5 has been found in the vagina. The enzyme is clustered close to where the G-spot might be. Also buried in the flesh of the alleged G-spot are the **Skene's glands**, the female equivalent of the prostate.

In men, the prostate produces the watery component of semen. Skene's glands also produce a watery substance that may explain female "ejaculation." The tissue surrounding these glands swells with blood during sexual arousal, including the part of the clitoris that reaches up inside the vagina – which accounts for the type of female orgasm that seems to ascend from the clitoris upward, deep into the vagina.

However, some women are underprivileged – not all of us have Skene's glands and for those who don't, a vaginal orgasm is anatomically impossible. Viagra and similar PDE5 inhibitor drugs such as tadalafil and vardenafil should have the greatest effect on women who have large Skene's glands and a lot of PDE5. Trials of Viagra in women have so far had mixed results probably because female sexual anatomy varies so much.

So how do you tell if you've got a G-spot? Sadly, because Skene's glands are so well hidden, no visual examination can reveal if a woman has them or not. Only personal experience reveals if you're one of the chosen few.

But even for those with no G-spot at all, **Viagra-type drugs might still have some effect** as PDE5 is found in the clitoris, too, and most women are more than happy with a clitoral orgasm. Other drugs that stimulate arousal via the brain could soon become available. However, the female orgasm is so wondrously complex that drugs alone are unlikely to work for everyone.

ENJOYABLE sex

Sex in the second half of our lives can be more relaxed, varied and diverse than at earlier times. **Social mores** no longer bother us, **inhibitions don't curtail experimentation,** curiosity, or adventurousness and we know our bodies and our sexual predilections better than ever. Seen this way **sex becomes an expanding universe,** not a restricted one. And we're more prepared to laugh at ourselves, at our own frailty, and at our falsely high expectations. **Laughter** can help couples through many sexual embarrassments and lead the way to more enjoyable sex.

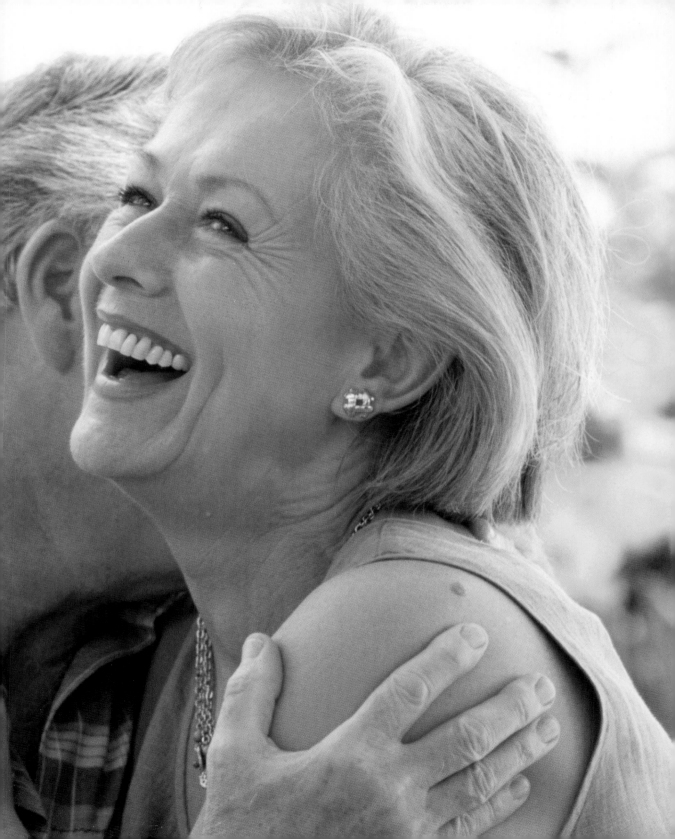

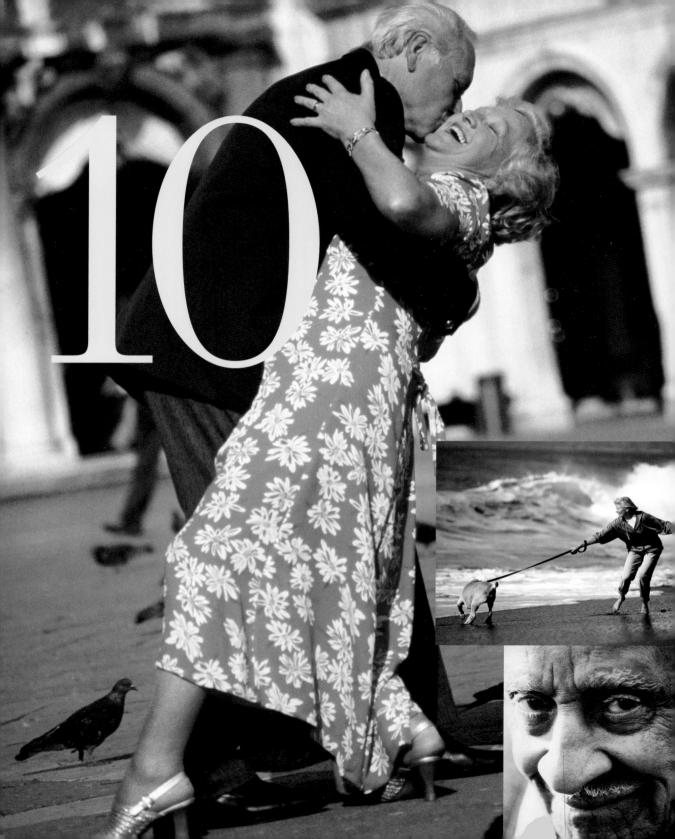

10

THE BEST YEARS
ARE THE
LATER YEARS

All through my life each decade has been **better** than the last and now with *grandchildren*, my own business, and a **garden** to tend in France, this is still the case. My body and mind are in the *best condition* I can remember. My body responds when I call on it to perform **strenuously** and my **brain** works as fast and as clearly as it did when I was 27.

Add to that *experience* and a smattering of wisdom collected along the way and I find myself still taking life at full speed. If asked what the **magic ingredients** of my life are I'd have to say that by good luck or good management, much of the *age-defying lifestyle* that I've described in this book finds expression in my own life.

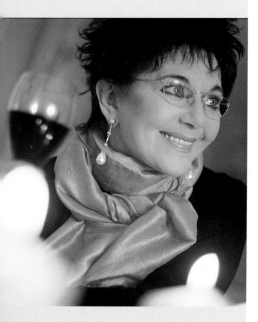

Here's what works **FOR ME**

◆ My brain is stretched by several jobs and by working with a team of young people.
◆ I give myself lots of time-outs.
◆ My husband is supportive and encouraging.
◆ My family and extended family are in touch all the time.
◆ I have a close circle of loving girlfriends.
◆ I eat healthily 90 percent of the time (12 or 13 fresh fruits and vegetables a day, lots of fish, and few fatty foods).
◆ I don't smoke.
◆ I exercise every day.
Also, because I'm in better shape than I've ever been, I find I have more hours in the day to live life to the fullest. I no longer tire out in the early evening as I used to when I didn't get regular exercise.

BE*optimistic*

YES, I'M HAPPY WITH THE HAND LIFE HAS DEALT ME, AND THAT, AS YOU'LL SEE IF YOU READ ON, IS AN IMPORTANT PREREQUISITE OF LIVING A LONG LIFE.

The fantastic news is that you can have the time of your life when you reach your sixties and seventies and this chapter will help you to avoid the pitfalls. Work, mortgage, and worries about bringing up children will all be in the past and you'll have in abundance the one thing that younger people want but can't buy – **time to enjoy yourself**. Time is such a gift that it's worth making an effort planning what you want to do with your newfound freedom.

This optimistic view of our later years stems from a study in Britain, based on nearly 10,000 people aged between 15 and 90 and performed over four consecutive years. Professor Ian Stewart Hamilton, a professor of psychology at University College, Worcester and an expert in gerontology – the scientific study of aging – has conducted many surveys into attitudes about older people. **He says the standard cliché that people in their later years are devoid of any fun is utterly false.**

More and more septuagenarians who are enjoying life retire late, sometimes not until they are over 70. And having lived full working lives **they continue to live full social lives**. At 70 of course there's the danger of losing your partner, possibly from a marriage spanning 40 years or more, and anyone would become depressed after the death of a partner with whom one has spent a long and loving life. But a surprising number of older people pull themselves out of depression, **join the social mainstream**, get out and about, meet new friends, and have fun.

satisfaction with life

Research shows that the overall satisfaction with life of people between the ages of 15 and 90 resembles a U-shaped curve. As you'd expect, teenage optimism puts them at the top of the chart but that *joie de vivre* swiftly plummets by 18, flattens out in the twenties, dips in the thirties and forties, then begins to rise again during the midfifties. By 70 people's contentment reaches its peak. Although the happiness graph begins to dip again, **people up to the age of 90 still register a higher score of overall satisfaction with life than people half their age**.

What we're all doing during our forties and fifties is juggling with several demanding roles. After that the benefits come. There's time for traveling, time for sightseeing, for taking bicycling vacations, for spending weeks on a tennis or golfing vacation, for the trip to Machu Picchu you've always longed for. People who've lived a bit appreciate what life has to offer and are grateful for what surrounds them. **Seventy-year-olds are by and large embarrassingly enthusiastic about life**.

Other than satisfaction with health, which shows a steady decline from the teenage years, contentment with most other aspects of life improves with age – satisfaction with spouse, partner, house, and income all register a greater sense of well-being among 70-year-olds.

This may be because older people know how to enjoy their leisure time. People of 35 are least likely to be happy with the amount they have, whereas those over 70 are the most satisfied.

age is no barrier to anything

These days age isn't a barrier to doing almost anything, as long as you have your health and enough money to pay for your pastimes. At 75 you're spurred on by the thought that time's running out and **you have to hurry and get on with things** before it's too late. So if a spouse dies, it's time to do a lot of traveling, not sit at home and mope. And even though trekking in the Himalayas would test you to the limit, you could still try walking in the jungle or a safari in Africa.

One of the greatest reasons for life satisfaction as we get older is that **we're happier because we've lived and learned a lot**. You can do the things you want how you want: you can choose to be where you want, with whom you want. And of course, after retirement, couples have a lot more time to do things together.

OPTIMISM

If I were to choose one factor above all others to increase longevity it would be optimism. Optimism can give you real resilience as you get older – it's a great healer. Research has shown that people with optimistic attitudes have fewer illnesses and recover more quickly from illness. Optimists are more likely to feel that they can take charge of their health and not just passively slide into old age. They tend to take better care of themselves too. They sleep better, don't drink or smoke too much, exercise regularly, and are freer from depression. They live longer and age more gently. It's worth cultivating optimism, believe me.

PESSIMISM

Pessimism, on the other hand, weakens the immune system. Pessimists have high levels of T-suppressor cells which can interfere with immunity. People with the most negative and hopeless attitudes are at a greater risk of developing heart disease. Some researchers say that pessimism begins to have a negative effect on health around 35 to 50. Believing that your health problems are the result of aging is a dangerous supposition. You're much better off believing illness has a treatable cause because then you'll seek treatment rather than accepting infirmity as inevitable. It's important to distinguish pessimism from true depression, which is eminently treatable.

UNDERSTANDING *stress*

STRESS IN OUR LIVES IS UNAVOIDABLE BUT WE CAN ALL LEARN TO MANAGE IT. IN FACT, BY THE AGE OF 60, MANY OF US ARE EXPERTS AT COPING WITH STRESS AND CAN EVEN TURN IT INTO A POSITIVE FORCE.

So stress can age you, but it doesn't have to. There's good stress and bad stress, and we can learn to turn bad stress into good stress. By that I mean we can manage stress so that it **increases** our productivity rather than **lessening** it. Plus we all differ markedly in how we react to stress. Many people thrive on challenges; others react with fear, anxiety, and worry. So the stress you feel depends on how you personally respond to stress. **If you react positively there's little problem and you'll probably live longer.** But people who don't

What **STRESS** does to your body

Response to stress	Why it occurs	Effects if stress is long-term
Adrenaline, noradrenaline released into bloodstream	Physical and mental faculties focused	High blood pressure, frustration, worry, impatience, anxiety, insomnia
Liver releases energy stored as glycogen	Energy is provided	Inability to relax, hyperactivity, irritability, fatigue, buildup of cholesterol in blood
Rapid breathing and pulse rate	Oxygen supply in bloodstream increased	Breathlessness and high blood pressure, hyperventilation, dizziness, fainting
Muscular tension	Readiness for action. "Fight or flight"	Dizziness, faintness, heart palpitations, headaches, hypertension, muscles continually tensed and aching
Digestion inhibited	Energy diverted to muscles	"Butterflies" in stomach, nausea, loss of appetite, vomiting, indigestion, constipation, peptic ulcers
Profound sweating	Clammy hands, body cools as it prepares for action	Nervous rashes, eczema, sweating
Need to empty bladder and evacuate bowels	Body weight reduced in preparation for "fight or flight"	Frequent urination, defecation, diarrhea
Emotional tension	Preparation for effort	Crying, nervous laughter, aggression, angry outbursts, depression, panic attacks, hyperventilating, dizziness, fainting

handle stress well live shorter lives. So **dealing calmly with stress** is a trick it's worth learning in order to ensure a longer and happier life.

One useful device to master if you can is to think of stress as **energy generated by change**. As such you can see that life without stress of any kind would be a nonevent. On the other hand, too much stress, particularly if it never lets up, can cause serious health problems.

stress relievers

We all develop our favorite antidotes to stress that experience has told us work for us. By the age of 60 we should have quite a menu to choose from – the following are a few ideas.

smiling to relieve stress

When we smile it acts as a trigger to the mind and body to release chemicals that induce pleasant emotions. **A smile feels like love** and that's regardless of your mood before you smile. The same thing happens when someone smiles at you and you can store this **good feeling** in your memory. You can call up this memory of good feelings whenever you want to. A smile can be seen as a **source of energy** to make you feel good.

• Recall in your mind the **sensation of smiling** and visualize an image that makes you feel like smiling.
• Hold the image in your mind and breathe slowly and calmly. Smile back at the image. The change in your facial muscles may be very slight but you'll feel a **peaceful** sensation overtake you.
• Become fully aware of that sensation and embrace it – all you need do is smile to yourself inwardly to feel it.

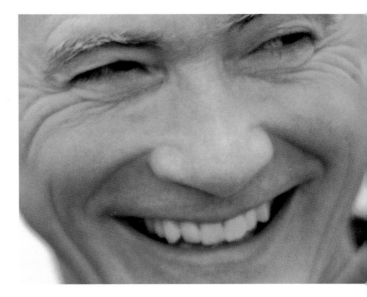

• Practice smiling into the various parts of your body, smile into your heart, lungs, stomach, liver, and especially the parts of your body you don't like very much.
• Cultivate the **loving feeling** that arises from a smile.
• **Share your smile** with as many people as you can, especially children and people you don't like very much.

meditation

Meditation sounds intimidating but it isn't. It's simply a means of quieting the mind and you can do that how you want. With a quiet mind comes a **sense of peace** and an **absence of stressful feelings**. When we meditate we empty our minds of all thoughts and problems and focus on nothingness. This allows us to be in the present moment and nowhere else, rather than being separated from it by our thoughts, feelings, plans, and expectations.

Nearly everyone who starts to meditate finds concentrating on focused breathing can be very helpful and it's a good way to start. It's the simplest and most direct method of developing your concentration skills and it will help you prepare for your meditation by relaxing your mind and body.

Here's a simple meditation exercise:
• Sit comfortably with your spine straight.
• Focus your attention on your abdomen as you inhale and exhale in a natural way.
• Take a few deep breaths without straining.
• Let the flow of your breath settle into its own natural rhythm while keeping focused and aware during the whole process.

• Allow your attention to focus on the changing rhythms of your inhalations and exhalations. When your attention begins to wander, gently but firmly bring it back to your breathing.
• Count your breaths: on exhalation count one, on the next exhalation count two, and so on for a count of ten, then start over again.

If you practice focused breathing you'll find that your **concentration skills and attention will improve** and your mind will become **clearer and calmer**. You can do this anywhere and anytime, though it's important to find a time and a place that are comfortable for you. Twenty minutes a day of meditation seems to work well for most people, but anywhere from 10 to 40 minutes, once or twice a day, is usually enough.

focused breathing helps to

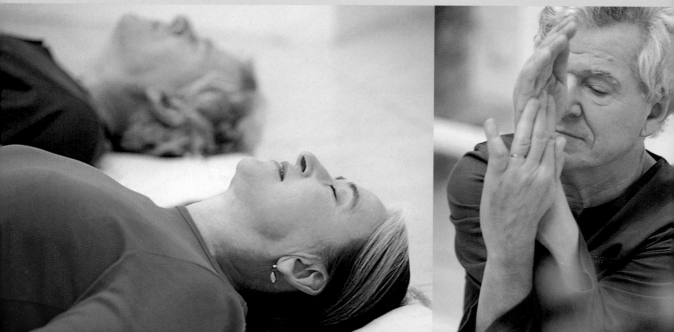

relaxed abdominal breathing exercise to try

The following simple abdominal breathing exercise is extremely effective in **calming the mind, releasing tension, and energizing the body.** You do it lying down to begin, but once you can breathe easily in this position you can go on to practice the exercise in a sitting or standing position, wherever you feel most comfortable.

• Lie on your back in a comfortable position on a bed, couch, or well-padded floor.

• Loosen any tight clothing, especially around the abdomen and waist.

• Place your feet slightly apart, rest your hand comfortably on your abdomen near your navel, place the other hand on your chest, and close your eyes.

• Inhale through your nose and exhale through your mouth.

• Quietly concentrate on your breathing for a few minutes and become aware of which hand is rising and falling with each breath.

• Slowly exhale most of the air in your lungs.

• Inhale while counting slowly to four, about one second per count. As you inhale slightly extend your abdomen, causing it to rise up about an inch, and feel the movement with your hand.

• As you breathe in, imagine warmed air flowing in and imagine this warmth flowing to all parts of your body.

clear and calm the mind

MEDITATION TIPS

◆ Talk to friends, do a little research and reading, then choose the form of meditation that you intuitively feel most comfortable with.

◆ Try to set aside a specific time of day to meditate – **it's not essential that you meditate at the same time every day** but at the beginning it makes it easier to get into the habit.

◆ **Aim for 20 minutes** but if you find that too difficult, start with five or ten minutes then gradually work yourself up to 20 minutes by adding an extra minute or two every couple of days.

◆ Just find a quiet comfortable spot wherever you are – even your car will do.

◆ Before sitting down to meditate, **take a few minutes to stretch** or do one of the relaxation experiences already described (see page 216).

◆ Allow your thoughts, feelings, and sensations to drift in and out of your mind without fixating upon them or trying to chase them away.

◆ **Avoid overanalyzing the meditation**, forcing the process, placing too much emphasis on the perfect technique, or trying to turn off your thoughts.

◆ It's fine to meditate on your own without professional guidance, but it's a good idea to find a teacher when you begin.

BE KIND *to your* MIND

JUST AS WE BECOME LESS PHYSICALLY RESILIENT AS WE GROW OLDER, SO WE ALSO BECOME LESS MENTALLY RESILIENT AND MORE PRONE TO FEELINGS OF ANXIETY.

There are anxiety centers in the brain that are tripped more easily in some people than in others, so everyone has their own threshold of adventurousness before they begin to feel anxious. As we age, these anxiety centers in the brain become more sensitive and we gradually lose our ability to distinguish between the negative kind of anxiety that comes from stress and the more positive types of anxiety that are an integral and exciting part of experiencing something new. We find ourselves becoming more fearful and begin to avoid situations that make us feel anxious, including relatively safe activities such as walking, hiking, swimming, or foreign travel. In my own case it's simple things like wearing high-heeled shoes (I now feel insecure in them), and skiing (I haven't got the nerve for steep black runs any more, even though my technique is better that it's ever been).

WORDS TO USE, WORDS TO AVOID

Don't use	Do use
I can't	I won't
I should	I could
I hope	I know
If only	Next time
It's not my fault	I'm responsible
It's a problem	It's an opportunity
What will I do?	I can handle it
Life's a struggle	Life's an adventure
Sorry	

So we start viewing all feelings of anxiety in the same negative way. It's the lumping of positive and negative feelings together that makes people want to feel safe and comfortable all the time. And it's why, as we get older, we may become content to sit back and be observers instead of being participants.

Playing it safe, however, can be the same as trying to escape from living. The one responsibility we have to ourselves from which there's no escaping is to be responsive. **Keep your mind open and responsive to what life offers you.**

WAYS TO KEEP OPEN AND RESPONSIVE

- ◆ Retain your curiosity.
- ◆ Match your skills to the challenge.
- ◆ Be prepared to learn a new skill.
- ◆ Take small, simple steps.
- ◆ Don't push yourself into dangerous situations.
- ◆ Make sure you have a buddy.
- ◆ Keep your sense of humor.

resisting social isolation

Very few of us keep up the pace and diversity of our social lives which were the norm when we were younger. Most of us begin to withdraw from the social whirl through choice and because our obligations are fewer. We're at the peak of our engagement with society during our middle years because this is the time that many people depend on us and we're in great demand.

From adulthood to retirement age we go through a transition that involves **a natural withdrawal** from the activities and obligations that had previously linked us and our circle closely together.

Withdrawal from the social mainstream is dramatically punctuated when we decide to retire. We no longer meet with colleagues or work friends and have less to do with the social side of our jobs. Ties of friendship are weakened. Relatives and children are likely to be widely scattered. It's a sensible attempt on our part to **distribute our reduced energies and resources over fewer but more personal occupations**. Effort is conserved and we escape from demands which we cannot or don't wish to meet.

We all disengage differently, some of us willingly, others stubbornly. Although some of us fight all the way, some disengagement is bound to come. Ideally, disengagement is graded to suit our declining biological and psychological capacity on the one hand and the needs of family and friends on the other. The degree to which we can engage has as much to do with personality as it has with aging.

However, the net effect might be a shrinkage in the range of our activities and a lessening in the amount of contact we have with other

self affirmations

You can teach yourself to think well of yourself. Being negative about yourself usually stems from experiences that have marked you and stuck with you from childhood, and they can be difficult to erase. Positive affirmations in the form of positive "self talk" can help get rid of a negative self image and help you rebuild self-confidence and self-esteem. Of course you can design your own affirmations to suit yourself, but here are some to start with. Read them and say them over to yourself, out loud if you want. The sound of your own voice saying positive things about yourself can be very potent.

• I'm a good person.
• I believe in my potential to succeed.
• I can make my life better and better.
• I love and accept myself for who I am.
• I wasn't put on Earth just to please others.
• I'm getting stronger, healthier, and more energetic.
• I deserve to be happy.

people. Gradually, our lives could become separated from the lives of others. We could see other people less often, become less emotionally involved, and more absorbed in our own problems and circumstances.

This would be a damaging and unnecessary form of disengagement. It's healthier and more enjoyable to see the narrowing of horizons as being **a form of specialization**, of focusing on these things in life that give us the most pleasure, and a greater emphasis on pleasing ourselves.

Finding yourself **ALONE**

When my marriage ended, I found myself single and on my own for three years. Without my girlfriends, who rallied around me and with whom I stayed in constant touch, I'd have been without a lifeline to the outside world.

My instinct was to retreat into my personal world, but my girlfriends kept me looking outward. I also realized **I had to literally force myself to stay in the mainstream** – to stay a participant rather than an observer of life.

So I sought a handful of "walkers," men friends, who'd accompany me on an evening out – a son, a colleague, an old friend, or a new friend met at a professional meeting or a dinner party. I became adept at opening lines like: "Do you like opera? Oh, I have a couple of tickets."

It was important to me not only that I was **seen** to be engaged with life, but also to **feel** that I was.

loneliness

Loneliness isn't the same as being alone. A person will always have times when they choose to be alone. Loneliness, rather, is the feeling of being alone and feeling sad about it. **And, of course, all of us feel lonely some of the time**. It's only when we seem trapped in our loneliness that it becomes a real problem.

Loneliness is a passive state. That is, it persists by our passively letting it continue and doing nothing to change it. We hope it will go away, eventually, and we do nothing but let it envelop us. Strangely, there are times when we might even embrace the feeling of loneliness. Yet, embracing loneliness and sinking down into the feelings associated with it usually leads to a sense of depression and helplessness, which, in turn,

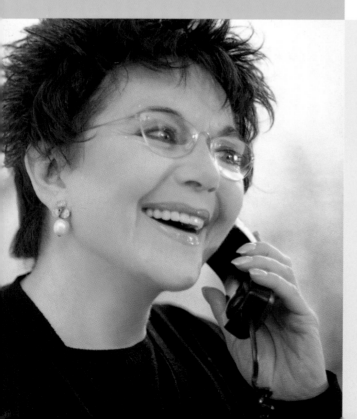

start socializing

Starting some sort of activity or joining a club can accomplish several things. It can **take our minds off feeling lonely** as we get involved in the enjoyable activity and can actually **change our mood directly** in this way. It can give us opportunities to meet people with similar interests and practice our people-meeting skills. It can provide some structure in our lives so that we have **things to look forward to**. And it can remind us of how good we might have felt in the past doing similar things.

These effects may come very quickly or more slowly. We might really need to push ourselves to go to meetings, talk to people, and make friends or attend several activities before we begin to

can lead to an even more passive state and more depression.

To stop feeling lonely, **we first must accept that we are feeling lonely**. Sometimes admitting that to ourselves is difficult. We then have to express those feelings of loneliness in some way. We might find ourselves keeping a journal, writing an imaginary letter to a friend or relative, drawing or painting a picture, making up a song, or doing anything else that lets us begin to express the feelings we have inside us – including **talking with other people**!

Expressing our feelings might lead us to discover that we feel a number of things which might be connected to our feelings of loneliness, including sadness, anger, and frustration. We might be able to see where these feelings are coming from – what they're connected to in our lives. As we begin to see the connections we'll be more able to begin to make changes.

The big change, of course, is to **stop being passive and to become more active**. If we're missing someone, such as parents, family, or friends, we can telephone, write, e-mail, or visit them. **Talking to an understanding friend can often help change our moods as well**. If we don't have an understanding friend, talking with a therapist or clergyman might be a place to start.

Maybe in the past you've been looking in all the wrong places to make new friends. Activity clubs and organizations are the best places to meet friends – people who share your interests and enthusiasms. There are literally tens of thousands of clubs out there.

feel comfortable with what we are doing and begin to see progress.

It's best not to join a club or organization or to develop a new interest just because we think it will make us a better or more interesting person. A better strategy might be to get involved in something because **we know we've enjoyed it in the past** or because we think it might be fun. That way we're more likely to find ourselves **enjoying** what we're doing and being with people who genuinely enjoy the same things. We may also find out that some people **like us for the way we already are**. A bonus is that we might also begin to realize that we could choose to engage in some of those activities or interests entirely on our own without feeling lonely.

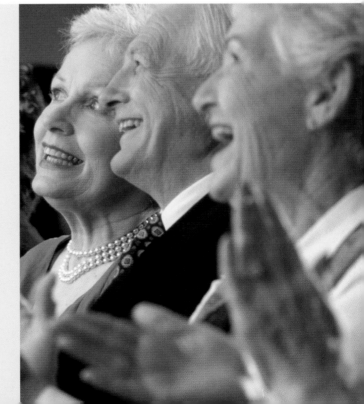

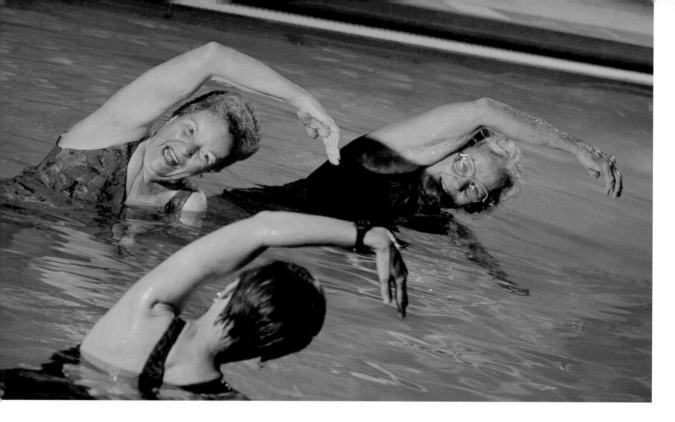

don't isolate yourself

Building relationships takes time. Many people will participate in an activity club for one meeting, decide that people are not friendly, and not go back. They then come to the conclusion that most people are not very friendly and give up making an effort to make friends. In reality, most people feel uncomfortable meeting new people and it takes a few meetings for people to open up. Have you ever noticed when you go to a party that most people hang out only with the people they already know, rarely risking meeting someone new?

Here are some reasons why clubs are such great places for meeting people.

• Unlike a party where the primary purpose is to socialize, at a club you are there to participate in an activity that you enjoy.

• Although the primary purpose is not to socialize, casual conversations will occur and you will meet people and make friends.

• Activities are already arranged so you don't have to feel uncomfortable calling people to organize the activity.

• You can meet far more people than if you only met people through normal friendship-making channels, which include work, neighbors, and friends of the family.

making friends

You'll find that after about three visits to a club or organization where you see the same people, both you and they will begin feeling much more comfortable and open toward speaking with each other. **The secret is being persistent.** Before you make new friends, you have to decide who you want to be your friends. Most people like to have friends who like to do the same kind of things they do. That doesn't mean you have to be exactly like each other, just that you enjoy many of the same things.

The quickest way to make a friend is to smile. When you smile, other people will think you are friendly and easy to talk to. One easy way to start a conversation with someone is to **say something nice** about them. Think about how great you feel when someone says something nice to you. Doesn't it make you want to keep talking to that person?

Many shy people are fearful that when meeting someone new they won't know what to say and will be embarrassed. When first meeting someone, it's important to get them talking about themselves without asking complicated questions. In other words **small talk is the key for opening someone up.** It's the only way to get to know what they're like AND it's the only way they'll know that you are interested in them.

You can give to friends and take from them and any real friendship needs a good measure of both. **Friends really need to be able to trust each other.** You can't expect friends to stick around forever if you keep letting them down. Even if you're busy with other things in your life, **try to keep in touch** with the friends you value and let them know what you're doing. Make sure that they know you care about them.

don't let fear of rejection stop you

If you really value other people and how they feel about you, it's natural that you would feel some fear of rejection. Whenever there's the possibility for actual rejection, most people feel some fear. Fear of rejection is increased by the importance of the other person to you, by your perceived inexperience or lack of skills in dealing with the situation, and by other factors.

However, some people suffer more intense levels of rejection for longer periods in their life than other people. Deeper issues such as those listed below may be increasing your fear of rejection.

• Underlying your fear of rejection might be a fear of being or living alone. You might fear ending up all alone in the world with no one who really cares.

• The thought of being all alone in the world is not in itself something to panic about. While

GET TALKING

The key is asking simple questions to get people talking about themselves. Here are some ideas.

◆ Hi, my name's James. What's yours?
◆ Do you live around here?
◆ Did you grow up around here?
◆ How did you hear about this event?
◆ Do you work around here?

Make sure you have something to add to the conversation too. When someone asks you a question, do you have an answer for them? If you don't know who your favorite singer is, or what your hobbies are, think about it. There's nothing that will stop a conversation quicker than a shrug for an answer.

some people panic at the thought – others delight in it. If you believe that you can take care of your own needs well and be happy even if you are alone, **then being alone is nothing to fear.** If you believe that you need others to take care of you and "make" you happy, then you are too dependent on others and their absence is something to "panic" about.
• Examine the degree to which you can create your own happiness – even when alone.
• Examine how too much dependence on other people for happiness can undermine your feelings of confidence with others and lead to fear of rejection.

The more you want to be wanted by another person, the more anxiety it will cause. Many people develop a fantasy or script about what love should be like. For example, many people expect to marry their "first love," or the person who they've called their "soul mate." Letting yourself plan and fantasize about the future with a person increases attachment and anxiety about the expectations or plans not coming true. Any little event that makes the plan seem likely makes you feel elated; any event that makes it seem unlikely makes you feel devastated. You can get on an emotional roller coaster, dependent upon these little signs of success or failure in the relationship. You may then drive the person away by being too emotional or needy.

To prevent this emotional roller coaster, don't develop expectations prematurely. Don't fantasize and plan for the future too soon. Always accept that it may not work out and have alternative plans that you know you can be happy with.

The less confident you are that you can create a happy relationship or get close to the person you like, the more likely you are to pick someone with whom you will not be satisfied. Or you may wait for others to approach you. People who may use or dominate you may be the very type of more outgoing person who will seek you out. Then you may later wonder why you keep getting into relationships with people who don't treat you well. **Learn to be active in the process of meeting others and getting involved in a relationship.** Keep the initiation of mutual activities closer to a 50-50 level, and don't just go along for the ride when you are seeing red flags.

REJECTION IS THE OTHER SIDE OF BEING LOVED

Sharing life events increases attachment. Just being together in a variety of circumstances seems to build some degree of closeness. Sharing important life events, sharing of one's innermost feelings and thoughts, and physical intimacy are powerful forces that can lead to very strong attachment and you must allow yourself to be vulnerable and risk rejection. If you're lonely, your reticence about coming forward may be making you miserable. Taking the open approach really can't be any worse, can it? Approach new experiences as opportunities to learn rather than occasions to win or lose. Doing so opens you up to new possibilities and can increase your sense of self-acceptance. Not doing so turns every possibility into an opportunity for failure and inhibits personal growth.

SOME THOUGHTS ON **REMARRIAGE**

Two people who have shared intimate years of joy and sorrow can buffer each other from the contingencies of the outside world.

a new loving relationship With a loving partner we can find the reassurance that we're still individuals and that our emotional needs haven't been forgotten. In each other's arms we can be ourselves, rather than the image of an old person which society forces us to be. This sense of **togetherness against the world**, the joy of small, shared intimacies, and quiet conversation that insulates us from the rest of the world is **life-affirming and precious**.

men and women see remarriage differently. As it happens, widowers are much more likely to get married than either bachelors or divorced men, especially if they were happily married before. Once they have gotten over the initial shock of losing their wives, widowers begin to miss domesticity after the years of companionship and loving. Women, on the other hand, may be deterred from marrying men over 40 because they think that they're marrying a potentially disabled person, especially if their future husband has diabetes, a heart condition, or high blood pressure. However, even a healthy man, if he's over 50, is risky too. Women over the age of 50 are also something of a health risk, but none of these facts necessarily spell pessimism.

it's difficult to overestimate the importance of a long-standing loving relationship as we go through life. Sex on its own isn't to be slighted, but **love brings much more than physical pleasure**. Each partner is sure of their identity as a person and feels that they can offer something valuable and worthwhile. **A body which is no longer young can still be a means of giving and receiving pleasure**. Older lovers like and understand their bodies. People of 50 and over who enjoy an active sex life have more confidence in themselves than those who decided to go into their old age celibate. You have to decide whether the companionship of a few years of remarriage is worth the risk of living with chronic illness later. Only you can decide this for yourself. There's a lot to be said for having someone to share life with.

you know how much or how little you really want to get married. Examine the kind of person you are. Be entirely honest with yourself and examine your feelings about this particular man or woman. Then make your decision. There's one golden rule which should be applied during your older years, if not at all other times – **there's no point in marrying anyone unless you would trust them with everything of yours, and unless you're attracted to them**. You're going to spend an awful lot of time with your new partner. If you're over 50 your new partner may be ready to retire. He or she may already be semiretired or fully retired. This means that you will be thrown together much more frequently than a younger couple. But then that may be one of the pleasures you seek – the companionship to do everything together, no holds barred.

release from work
can be like
a new lease
on life

PLANNING*retirement*

WE SPEND THE REST OF OUR LIVES IN RETIREMENT SO IT'S
WORTH PLANNING FOR AND THINKING SERIOUSLY ABOUT. AT A
YOUNGER AGE WE'D NEVER CONTEMPLATE THE NEXT 25 YEARS WITHOUT
A GAME PLAN AND SOME GOALS. DON'T NEGLECT THEM NOW.

Retirement means different things to different people, depending upon their gender, how well off they are, and their psychological makeup. In general, however, we give up a job and this changes our lives in terms of our daily timetable, social contacts, and our standard of living. If unplanned, retirement can be rapid and sudden, moving from a financially secure state to a financially uncertain and relatively dependent state. This raises all kinds of social, ethical, psychological, and financial issues and it shouldn't.

If we're proactive, **there's no need to be forced into a sudden, enforced dislocation of our working lives**, which will almost inevitably result in feelings of rejection and physical or mental ill-health.

With thought and planning, the release from exacting work can be like a new lease on life with more **enjoyable leisure time, closer family ties, and better physical health**.

With retirement come 40 or more hours in the week that we can spend in new and unfamiliar ways, hours previously spent in connection with work. **Many retired people say they miss nothing.** Some say they miss work itself and, of course, money. To a lesser extent, others miss the feeling of being useful. You'll find your attitudes change fairly rapidly during retirement and it isn't age, but the passage of time, that explains the differences between us.

imagining retirement is often worse than the reality

It's often the prospect of retirement, rather than retirement itself, which leads to a morbid state of mind. Studies have shown that, given reasonable physical health and financial resources, the average retired man or woman soon adapts to the changed circumstances and shows an improvement in physical health and outlook.

THOUGHTS ON RETIREMENT

Retirement, from the point of view of prolonging your life, is a mixed blessing. Men over the age of 65 who continue to work a few hours generally seem less lonely and better adjusted than retired men, but not *because* they're working. Physical health and personality underlie both morale and working capacity in later life. Over many decades there has been **a gradual but absolute improvement in the health and welfare of retired people** and in their standard of living. Morale is highest when financial status approaches that of other working adults. Reduction in income and living standards after retirement is the greatest concern for most of us. Coupled with natural regrets of leaving friends and familiar activities, that concern may escalate into a temporary depression or anxiety.

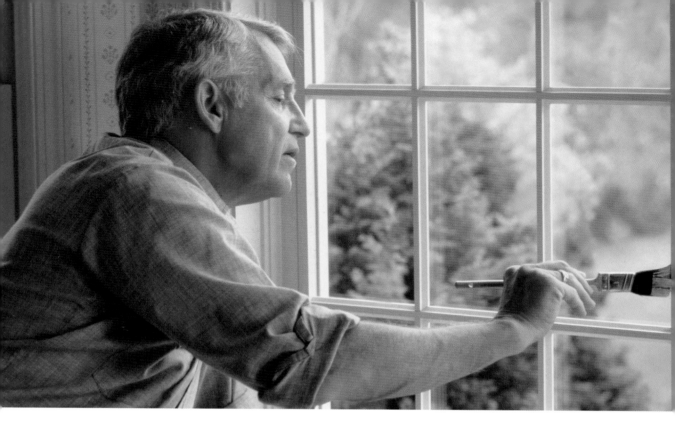

It isn't so much old age and retirement as the transition to old age and retirement that can create difficulties of adjustment. Retirement is rapidly becoming a normal and expected phase of our lives to be looked forward to, prepared for, and enjoyed over a long time.

planning retirement

Preparation for retirement is now a widely recognized need. Many companies, volunteer organizations, and centers for adult education cater to it. The financial and leisure demands of retirement can be met only by long-term planning. Many people don't face the changes soon enough and reach retirement inadequately prepared. Preparation means putting money aside, buying and disposing of personal property and assets, attending to health needs, getting

IMPORTANT AREAS TO PROVIDE FOR

◆ Income and assets to provide for our **material well-being** when we retire.
◆ Some continuation of working activities or social relationships to promote a sense of **belonging** and participation.
◆ **Attention to health** to make for more activity and security.
◆ Gainful use of **leisure time** to provide a kind of dividend in feelings of achievement, usefulness, and happiness.

MEN AND RETIREMENT

Disengagement from working life will work best for you if you have maintained some **professional continuity** throughout your life and have a vocation rather than a job. As a professional man you can pursue some aspects of your work and maintain your professional contacts right up to the end of your life. Moreover, you have the time, money, and opportunity to prepare for your retirement and to cultivate interests and activities which carry over into later years. This continuity of activity, relationships, and attitudes helps you adjust smoothly from your busy adult working life to a **more leisurely but satisfying retirement**.

Most men, however, spend a large part of their adult years in fairly routine jobs which earn them a living and a retirement pension, but which do little to provide opportunities beyond their jobs. Some men find that retirement presents problems of adjustment, since it often occurs abruptly at the age of 65, with neither the continuity, which is important for good adjustment, nor the time, money, or opportunity to prepare for a satisfactory retirement.

Better provision for retirement and courses in preparing for retirement will help you to use and enjoy your later years. A shorter work week, longer vacations, and a gradual retirement from paid work in years to come will all give you ample opportunities to cultivate interests and activities throughout your working life. These will carry you over into retirement. **Increased opportunity for personal outlets** might do much to improve your emotional stability and could lessen the social stigma sometimes attached to retirement.

information and advice about leisure time interests, and generally changing the balance between disengagement and activity.

women and retirement

If you're a working woman you're usually **more closely bound to family life** than a man is. Because of of your continued activities in the home and established social patterns, you have to deal with with fewer demands for readjustment than men. So by and large **you find disengagement from professional life easier** than men do because, unless you're single, you aren't faced with the problem of suddenly having to adjust to an abrupt retirement. A man often depends on his job and his earning capacity for status, prestige, and authority in the home and the transition from

work to retirement may be difficult. You, by the very fact of your family network and ties, retain **prestige, status, and friends through kinship links**.

However, the departure of children from the home changes the environment of the middle-aged mother and a partner's retirement calls for a further readjustment. Additionally, more married women eventually become widows, which requires them to readjust yet again.

Disengagement proceeds differently for most women as compared with men and some of the stages – loss of children, disability, and bereavement – may occur relatively early. In addition to the differences in temperament and attitudes which are a result of gender, a man's absorption in his job and outside interests provide him with powerful supports and these

TIPS ON RETIREMENT FOR MEN AND WOMEN

Preparation is the key to successful retirement. Here are some ideas of ways to help yourself make the most of your retirement years:

you'll reap untold rewards, not to mention peace of mind if you plan retirement, even pre-retirement, several years in advance of it actually happening, certainly in terms of housing, financial arrangements, and health care as well as cultivating hobbies, interests, and activities that can be continued into retirement.

get the best advice you can to make your money work for you during your retirement years; get the best counsel on investments and insurance, mortgages, and wills. An accountant or a bank manager will be happy to give you advice. Try to make a budget even if you've never made one before.

as a practice run, it's a good idea to start living on your retirement income about six months before you or your partner retires. If you start to ease into retirement this way, before you are under the strain of the other changes that go along with retirement, any financial adjustments may be easier to manage. You will also have saved up the money that you didn't use in the previous six months, which will give you a nest egg and a sense of security. You may get a pleasant surprise and find out that managing on your retirement income isn't nearly as difficult as you thought it would be.

if one partner retires and the other goes on working, you may find that your days get out of sync. Instead of both being up early in the morning, both getting home in the early evening, and both wanting to go to bed at the same time, one may be exhausted when the other is raring to go. Sit down and talk about it. Examine the problem and find a solution that will work for both of you. Make a particular point of doing things together on weekends when your clocks become synchronized again.

if you find yourself at home with a lot of time on your hands, feeling lost, lonely, unwanted, and left out, then it's probably a sign that you haven't made the emotional transition to retirement. Your partner can help by figuring out with you how best to spend your leisure time together. Discuss a rotation for the chores. Make a list of all your friends and relatives who are free during certain parts of the week whom you haven't seen for several years, and match up your interests with those people. What can be done with whom? A partner should be prepared to change his or her routine.

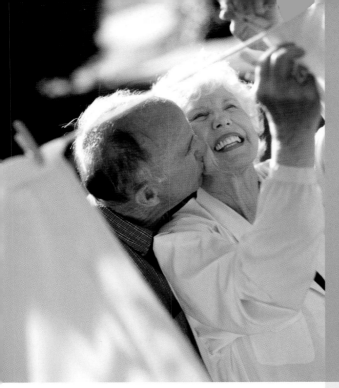

Getting used to spending
24 HOURS TOGETHER

For men

◆ If you retire but your partner is still working, it's time for an **egalitarian form of domestic arrangement**. It's only fair that you should do some of the domestic chores while your partner is out at work.

◆ If you do start to take a pride in the home, you shouldn't become rigid and fussy. Men can be particularly prone to do this if they don't have interests outside of the home, and that is the best solution – to find important jobs to do that take you out of the house.

can weaken his emotional involvement with his family. He may not react to family events with the same intensity as a woman. If your children have grown up or you have lost your husband, you may often find other women in similar circumstances who will form a support network, but retired men or widowers are less likely to have a large pool of friends and they may feel isolated unless they can turn to their families.

planning your newfound time

You can make the most of retirement by **letting it make things easier for you**. For one thing, you can place yourselves at the top of your priority list. You can choose to be by yourselves; you don't have to adjust your schedules to meet others' needs; you don't need to answer to anyone but yourselves; you can give priorities to spending your time, money, and resources in ways that you prefer; you can decide exactly

For women

◆ It's tough on both of you if you try to be a perfectionist when your husband retires. **Try not to put too much stock in keeping your house spick and span** with everything in its place. And try not to complain about newspapers or books on tables, unwashed dishes, and a messy kitchen. Adjustments have to be made. If you're working and can't relax, you may have to consider early retirement yourself.

◆ If you've retired while your partner is still working, **start new projects and take up old interests**. Remember old passions and renew them. If you have got a lot of spare time then spend some of the day pampering yourself. Sleep late, read in the afternoon, put your feet up whenever you feel like it.

◆ If your partner is retired and you're still working, **don't resent their freedom**, though you may have to get up early while they are still sleeping.

where and how to live. These are solely your decisions from now on.

Success or failure in the second half of life, measured in terms of happiness, is determined more by how you're going to use or abuse your leisure time than by any other factor. The trick is to learn how to **enjoy leisure activities** without feeling guilty. Some people have to learn not to work so that they can enjoy leisure. Just like work, **leisure has to be planned** and you have to stick to the plan to enjoy it. Now that you have so much time, leisure isn't a second-rate activity – it's very important. It pays to adapt to it in exactly the same way as you adapt to a new job. You have to be positive and enthusiastic about it and give it all you've got, **devoting all your energy to enjoying yourself.**

Appointments for leisure activities should go into the datebook and be honored in the same way as our professional appointments in the past.

Just because you have more leisure time, don't fall into the trap of feeling that all your time has to be spent together as a couple. It doesn't. More leisure time can mean more time for **private activities** as well as those you do as a couple.

Although retirement may demand a good deal of flexibility and adaptation, it can lead to a **time of great happiness and contentment** once negotiated. The critical period for adjustment is shortly before retirement. During this time people tend to become increasingly agitated about the consequences and potential problems. **Being old is manageable** – it's becoming old that's frightening.

BEING A *grandparent*

ONE OF THE JOYS THAT MANY OF US HAVE IN STORE AS WE GROW OLDER IS THAT OF BECOMING A GRANDPARENT.

Once past the childbearing age, many women begin to look forward to their **second chance for mothering,** and find that few experiences exceed those of being with, teaching, and learning from their grandchildren. To my mind, grandparents are an extremely important part of the family, be it nuclear or extended. I personally see a family as a fundamentally stable gathering, encompassing strong and lasting relationships among an extended group of people in which a child can grow up feeling **secure and loved,** to which he or she must contribute, and in

which his or her voice is always heard. I also consider it important that a child becomes able to relate to people of all ages, and therefore should be close to older relatives and friends.

being valued as a grandparent

When grandparents are fully integrated into the family and it operates as a **cooperative three-generation unit,** it's a win–win situation. Everybody's life is enriched and the pressures that can sometimes exist within the parent–child relationship are eased. Of course not all families

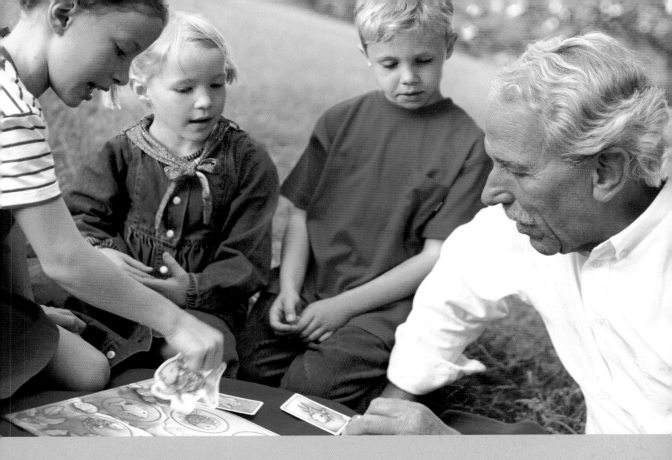

live within a distance of grandparents that enables them to be in contact on a daily, weekly, or even monthly basis. But then visits of a few days or a week or more take on a vacation air. As soon as children can spend a few days on their own with their grandparents it's a good idea to make such visits a regular feature. They give immense pleasure to grandparents, **children feel really special** because their presence is so valued, and parents get breathing space and some welcome time on their own.

why relations with grandparents are so important

Let's be clear about it: children won't be actively hurt if you don't play an active part in their lives, though they will certainly have missed out on one of childhood's great pleasures. Having somewhere where she's always welcome and appreciated, having someone who is always interested in her affairs, who takes delight in caring for her, all do wonders for a child's self-esteem and for her sense of security. People who never knew their grandparents or lost them when they were very young often feel great regret when they see how wonderful the relationship can be. In some areas there are adopt-a-grandparent programs because families without grandparents feel such a need for their input to the family. It's an excellent idea, not only for the difference it can make to family life but also because it widens a child's horizons and gives her the opportunity to see people's lives that are different from her own.

WHY GRANDPARENTS ARE GREAT

My own mother, when she held her first grandchild for the first time said, "This is a baby that I'm just going to enjoy." And maybe the key lies there.

◆ Parenthood is a huge responsibility. It entails worry as well as contentment. For a grandparent the ultimate responsibility lies elsewhere.

◆ Children sense this feeling of ease in their grandparents and respond to it joyfully.

◆ No matter now hard we try with our own children, we don't always come up to our own expectations. A grandparent has the chance to do it again, but perhaps even better this time around.

◆ Normally, by the time we become grandparents, a lot of our rough edges have been worn down. We know what really counts and the happiness of a child comes high on the list.

◆ Grandparents can find enormous satisfaction in knowing that they are useful to their children and grandchildren. If someone in the family is sick, who better to lend a hand than grandparents?

◆ Our genes probably have a part to play too. Grandchildren are the living proof that we have accomplished one of our basic biological tasks, successful reproduction.

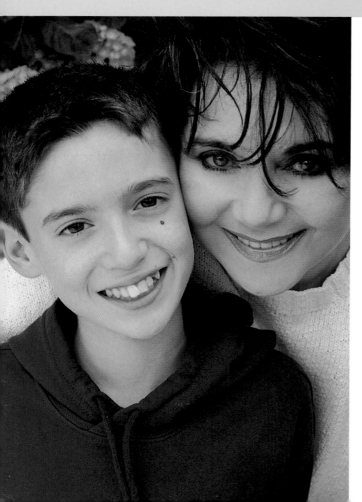

getting the most out of being a grandparent

The best grandparents can interpret warning signs, anticipate problems, and head them off. They pacify by distraction, not by insistence, and so handle young children comfortably. Unlike those parents who rule by force, **grandparents will more often than not persuade with patience**. It's said that grandparents spoil their grandchildren. This must be a misuse of the word "spoil." If spoiling a child means giving explanations instead of dismissals, suggesting alternatives instead of negatives, and helping instead of ignoring, then grandparents do spoil children. **The presence of grandparents in the house can often be a boon to the family** and, given that they don't cause friction with the parents, they're often welcomed.

Grandparents can renew earlier joys with their grandchildren. A grandmother can teach her young granddaughter the art of sewing, bird-watching, or gardening. A grandfather can once again enjoy tranquility while he's teaching his grandson to fish, and discover a new sense of purpose and usefulness if he can take the young baby for a walk and chat with his friends on the way. Grandparents should live **along with their grandchildren** but it's important that they don't live through their grandchildren rather than **through their own direct experience**. If they do, they may suffer an emotional setback if misfortune strikes the younger generation.

the special role of grandparents

In the past grandparents were the authorities on what was right and wrong. Grandparents no longer have that role. In fact, as a grandparent you may find yourself casting around as to what you can do to help. **The best thing you can do is to show your children and your grandchildren how to deal with change.**

You have lived through the most drastic changes the world has ever known. You have lived longer than any of your family so you have had to deal with a rapidly changing society more than anyone who is close to you. Your granddaughter may be very depressed because she can't get a job. Only you, with a historical perspective on unemployment, and knowing how much it demoralizes people, can help your granddaughter to develop a healthy critical distance between the refusal she gets at job interviews and her feelings about herself. **You can share with her what you remember about unemployment in your time**.

You can allow your grandchildren to see you as a real person for the first time, drawing a parallel between their development and yours.

How your grandchildren BENEFIT from you

◆ Your unconditional acceptance of your grandchildren counts for a lot.

◆ It generally falls to the parent to insist that homework is done and household tasks completed, to arrange trips to the dentist and unwanted haircuts, to attend parents' evenings at school, and perhaps hear unwelcome news. **By comparison, relations with grandma and grandpa have few constraints.**

◆ You have **more time** to spend playing board games, helping with puzzles, shopping for favorite snack-time treats or letting the children help make them, and for a lot of talk.

◆ Your grandchildren also find **psychological comfort with you**. With the best will in the world, children and parents sometime clash and it's good for a child to be able to confide his grumbles to you because he'll get sympathy but also reason and advice on how to smooth things over.

◆ Children who have a close relationship with their grandparents also have a much more rounded view of society at large. **From an early age they learn that life can be shared in different ways with different age groups.** As they grow older, they begin to feel protective toward their grandparents and this can give them an understanding that nurturing and help is especially necessary for those at both ends of our life span.

◆ **As their grandparents age,** children and young people begin to appreciate that every time of life has its satisfactions and its difficulties. Really old age has perhaps more than its share. If your child continues to take a real interest in his grandparents' lives, and he should, he will in some measure be able to repay a little of what they gave him in time, patience, wounds healed, games played, stories told, hurt feelings soothed, interminable interest in his doings, and everything else that goes into the love of a grandparent for a grandchild.

In a conversation on politics, for instance, you can stop being a wrinkled, white-haired old person and describe how you felt about the world in your youth. You can recount some of your experiences, possible moments of glory. **There isn't a grandchild in the world who won't be riveted and learn much from that kind of story.**

You can show your family that you aren't a doddering, useless grandparent. **You can be independent and act so.** You can be mobile and agile so that you can join younger members for a walk, or take a stroll around the golf course while they play a few rounds. You can also listen. Parents don't have a lot of time for that. But you can listen without giving advice, you can tell your family what experience you have had in your life and what it has led you to believe.

You will also find that you have a lot more in common with teenage grandchildren than you had ever thought. At opposite ends of life you are both searching for changing identities and both asking the same questions: "Who am I?" "What do I really want to do?" "How should I do it?" **Adolescents often have more in common with grandparents than they do with their own parents.** Parents often are too busy or too ambitious forging ahead in life to be self-examining and introspective. The relationship with younger grandchildren, even babies, is also very special.

a unique kind of loving

Grandparents can give a unique kind of loving and caring which can only come from them. Young children usually adore them, and also enjoy knowing that they have a very special place in their grandparents' lives. You shouldn't be surprised if it turns out that you and your partner are different as grandparents. After all, you might have been different as parents. One of you might have been the disciplinarian and the other more permissive. Or it might be that one was strict with a daughter, but lets a granddaughter get away with murder.

In a family this ability to change roles is a very good thing. It means you and your partner **have different strengths and make different contributions to your family** than you have made in the past. This results in rich relationships which are special.

Of course the later years aren't all sweetness and light; they bring their own challenges, and stress in one form or another is ever-present. An increasing number of families now spans four generations so you might be lucky enough to enjoy the double dose of happiness of being a grandparent with your own parent(s) still alive.

Young children usually *adore* grandparents and enjoy knowing that they have a very *special place* in their grandparents' lives

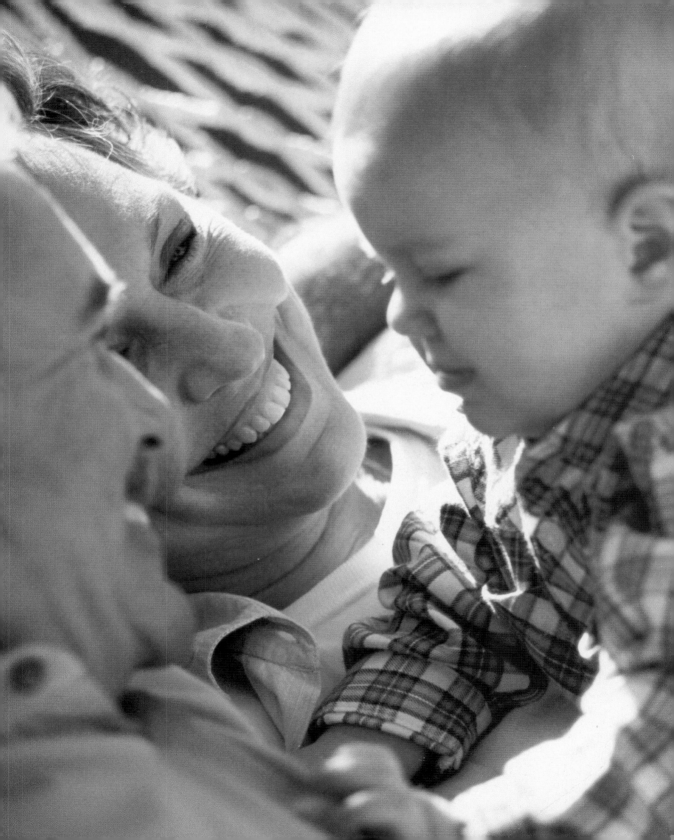

LIVING*wills*

THE LIVING WILL, ALSO KNOWN AS AN ADVANCE DIRECTIVE, ALLOWS YOU TO DECIDE WHICH TREATMENTS YOU DON'T WANT IF YOU BECOME SERIOUSLY ILL AND CAN'T INDICATE HOW YOU WANT TO BE TREATED. A LIVING WILL HELPS GUARANTEE THAT YOUR WISHES WILL BE RESPECTED.

The living will, also known as an advance directive, gives you the option to veto treatments you do not want in the event that you become seriously ill and lose the capacity to communicate your wishes.

Through a living will, you can make sure you're not given life-prolonging treatment if, for example, you are suffering from a medical condition from which there is no hope of recovery.

It's your chance to take **control over your treatment** and make sure that you're not kept alive in a situation you might find intolerable, such as being kept alive indefinitely on a life-support machine.

why have a living will?

With the best of planning you never know what's around the corner or what lies in the future for you. By the time you find out, it may be too late to make any decisions for yourself because you're not physically or mentally able to do so. This leaves your friends and family caring for you with difficult decisions to make about your treatment, hampered by not knowing what you would have wanted. You may have a serious or terminal illness, brain damage due to stroke or injury, dementia, Alzheimer's disease, or advanced nervous system disease such as motor neuron disease. You could have severe or lasting brain damage due to an accident. You could be left on a life-support machine or in a deep coma, being fed through a tube or intravenously, with all your bodily functions being under the control of a machine to keep you alive. Treatments may offer you little or no chance of recovery and they may have side effects that you would consider worse than the illness itself, or leave you in a condition you would find unbearable. You may feel strongly that you don't want to go through this treatment to make you live longer.

Is a living will **LEGALLY** binding?

Although there's no US law that governs the use of living wills, in common law refusing treatment before you need it will have a legal effect as long as it meets the following conditions:

1 You're mentally able, aren't suffering any mental distress and are over 18 when you make the request.
2 You were fully informed about the nature and consequence of the living will at the time you made it.
3 You're clear that the living will should apply to all situations or circumstances which arise later.
4 You weren't pressured or influenced by anyone else when you made the decision.
5 The living will hasn't been changed, either verbally or in writing, since it was drawn up.
6 You're now mentally incapable of making any decision because you are unconscious or otherwise unfit.

That's what a living will is for – to ask doctors not to subject you to any medical intervention or treatment aimed at prolonging or sustaining your life beyond a certain point.

A living will is a legal document. In the US, you can get a living will form from a hospital, the US Living Will Registry, the Internet, or create your own with the help of a lawyer. In Canada you can contact The Provincial Health Ethics Network for advice. Doctors and organizations like AARP and The Provincial Health Ethics Network recommend that people develop such legal documents.

updating your living will

If you have a living will, **it's sensible to read it through and reconsider and reconfirm it every few years**. Updating a living will isn't a requirement of US law. Nonetheless, it makes good sense to review it, reassuring medical staff that it's current and you haven't changed your mind.

Every three to five years, simply resign and redate every copy of your living will. It's also a good idea to check that your doctor still has your living will on file.

advantages of the living will

The living will makes sure you won't have treatment you don't want, even if you can't tell the doctors your decision at the time.
• The living will ensures that your family and friends are not left with difficult decisions because they are not sure what you would have wanted.
• **Knowing what you want** will help doctors to make the right decision in difficult situations.
• The living will gives you the chance to **discuss your views** calmly with both the medical team treating you and your close family and friends long before a decision has to be taken.
• When a medical team is faced with a difficult choice about what treatment or care to give you when you aren't able to make a decision, a living will helps the team understand what you would have wanted if you'd been conscious.

However, the living will still has to be interpreted to make sure that the situation it describes applies to the patient.

MAKING *your* WILL

MAKING A WILL ISN'T A NEGATIVE MOVE, IT'S MERELY GOOD PLANNING, AND HAVING MADE ONE WE CAN FEEL A SENSE OF JOY AND SATISFACTION THAT WE'VE DONE OUR BEST FOR LOVED ONES.

Forget any morbid thoughts you may have about making a will – think instead of how it will help those nearest and dearest to you.

Even if you think that you don't have much to leave, not making a will could make life much more difficult for your family after your death. Wills can be a sensitive subject so making your wishes clear prevents giving additional stress to relatives left behind.

Even with a very simple will it's best to see a lawyer, so make that your step. This way you avoid any misunderstandings that might arise after your death. You can, however, make your own will from a preprinted form available from most stationery stores. If you're going to do a will yourself here are a few tips.
• Make sure that at the beginning you say this will revokes all others (even if you have never made a will before), otherwise your heirs may wonder if you've left different instructions in another will.
• Decide who will be executors, the people named in the will to deal with your affairs.
• Choose whom you want to be the main beneficiary or beneficiaries of your estate (a beneficiary is someone who benefits from a will and your estate includes all your money, property, and possessions); and then name them to receive the remainder of your estate
• Name anyone you want to receive specific sums or goods. If they die before you, the gift will revert to your estate, unless you specify it should go to someone else.
• Be precise – put the full name and relationship of any beneficiary and full details about any possessions or money you wish them to have.
• Make provisions in case any beneficiary dies before you.

What about **ESTATE TAX?**

There's no federal inheritance tax when everything is left between husband and wife in the US. Beyond that relationship, the assets of your estate will be federally taxed. US tax laws, however, are in flux. Sweeping changes were made to estate tax laws in 2001. The revisions are on federal estate and gift taxes. Oddly, the law repeals the current Federal estate tax in the year 2010 and then brings it right back one year later to the way it was! In the meantime, though, some of these estate tax changes will be phased in over time. For example, the estate tax exclusion amount ($675.00 in 2001) rises, over time, to $3.5 million in 2009, and the top (federal) estate bracket will fall from 55% in 2001 to 35% by 2010.

WHO SHOULD WITNESS MY WILL?

Your signature to the will must be witnessed by two independent people, present at the same time. Your husband or wife should not witness it. Witnesses and their husbands or wives must not benefit from the will so it's important to select people who are not named in the will.

HOW DO I FIND A LAWYER?

The American and Canadian Bar Associations list lawyers by state or province. However, it is up to you to check the disciplinary record of any lawyer you may wish to hire. For low cost legal information, contact a nonprofit group such as AARP. The cost of making a will varies according to its complexity. Ask at the outset what the cost is likely to be. Some lawyers are prepared to visit you in your own home, care facility, or hospital.

CHOOSING AN EXECUTOR?

You should choose an executor to carry out your wishes, as stated in the will. Normally, people choose their spouse or

What will happen **IF I DON'T** make a will

No matter what size your estate is, it is important to make a will. A will allows you control over how your estate and how its assets are allocated after your death. If you do not make a will, your intentions for the division of your estate may not be honored. Without a will, there will be delays in the distribution of your assets and state law will dictate how your assets are divided. State laws in the US usually distribute assets to your natural or adopted relatives, leaving nothing to charities or friends. If you have no relatives, the estate goes to the state. Though some property can be passed through joint ownership, it is still important to establish a will.

one of their children. It's a good idea to choose two executors in case one dies before you. Make sure that the person you choose can deal both with day-to-day matters to do with your home and with handling the business or administering the estate. Make sure you ask their permission before naming them. They can be beneficiaries under the estate and can claim from the estate for expenses in performing the task, e.g. postage.

CAN I REVISE MY WILL?

If you marry or remarry, your will becomes invalid unless it was made with your marriage in mind and it refers to your proposed marriage. If not, it

should be revised. Divorce does not automatically make a will invalid. Codicils (supplements to a will) can be added to an existing will for minor changes. These must be correctly witnessed, but the witnesses don't have to be the same as for the original will. If anything substantial needs to be changed you should make a new will revoking the former one. NEVER make alterations on the original document. Any change must be by codicil or a new will.

WHERE SHOULD I KEEP MY WILL?

Your will should be kept at home with your other important papers, with a lawyer, or at your bank.

BEREAVEMENT

THE GRIEF OF BEREAVEMENT ISN'T ALWAYS EASY TO DESCRIBE. THERE MAY BE AMBIVALENCE AT THE TIME. FOR EXAMPLE, SORROW AND DISAPPOINTMENT MAY BE MIXED WITH ANGER, GUILT, AND ANXIETY.

Bereavement's a stress which can precipitate mental illness, psychosomatic illness, or sometimes even suicide. The reorganization of daily life that's called for following the death of a spouse is an added source of stress in regard to both emotional deprivation and living arrangements. It is so stressful, it brings the possiblility of death itself to the bereaved person.

The importance of GRIEF

Most people think of grief as a natural response to bereavement. Nearly all of us see grief as therapeutic, and we're often told "Get it off your chest and have a good cry."

Grief's a more complicated process than that. It's dynamic and we live through its vicissitudes. We go through several steps, each of which is hard work. It isn't a passive process of *letting out* pent-up feelings. It's an active process of *pushing out* pent-up feelings. It's an active process of adjustment. It's a positive "letting go" of something or someone who's been very precious to you for a long time.

Grief's important in that it's a half-way stage between the experience of losing something and coming to terms with the loss.

ANTICIPATION It's uncommon for bereavement to strike out of the blue. But even when death comes at the end of a long illness there's still the reality and shock of loss. When death and bereavement are sudden the shock is greater still.

LOSS This encompasses a feeling of emptiness. There is a space where that person used to be, even if the person was hated.

NUMBNESS This is a protective mechanism. It's a primitive shutting down of all our emotions — a kind of mechanical shut-down which stops us from feeling any more hurt.

ANGER Here we get indignant, rebellious, and resentful that something we cherished so much has been taken away. We may feel self-pity. We may wonder what we have done to deserve this grief. We may feel that we have been unfairly singled out.

DENIAL Here we deny to ourselves that we aren't going to find our loved one. We may believe that he or she is just around the corner.

ACCEPTANCE This occurs when our anger eventually burns itself out.

LETTING GO At last, with acceptance, we know that our loved one has gone.

REGROWTH This stage takes a long while to complete. Ultimately, if we have gone through all the different stages, regrowth takes place and we gradually return to normal.

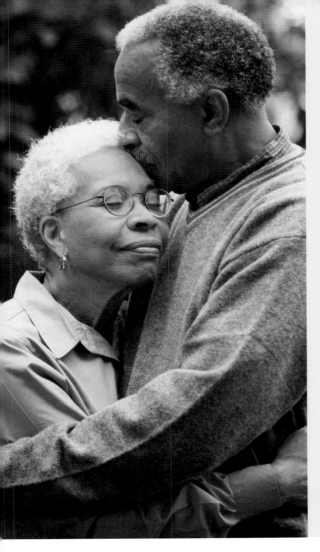

the chaos of grief

There's no right way to grieve. The point about grief isn't how it's done but that it should be done somehow. Things may go wrong. Grief may be denied totally, or it can begin and then be inhibited. It may be turned inward instead of outward to relationships with other people.

If grief is delayed or inhibited, superficial relief is only gained for a short time.

If grief is denied altogether, the person may slip from grief, which is normal and healing, into a depressive illness, which is distressing and abnormal. When grief is turned inward into the body, it may cause physical illness. Widowers often complain of heart trouble which may literally go on to result in death from a broken heart. Widows consult their doctors with gastric upsets and rheumatic conditions.

It's very easy to confuse grief with depression. A bereaved person feels sad and lost. Appetite goes away, and sleep is interrupted. There may be reproach for not having cared more or done more for the lost one.

dealing with bereavement

It's important to realize that **the feelings you're experiencing are normal**, so don't spend a lot of emotional energy on self-recrimination.

Try to find an understanding person to talk to. You can work out quite a lot of your anger, guilt, shame, and grief on someone who'll just listen, correct you when you overreact, and sympathize with what you're going through. At this moment when you're in the depth of despair, an objective viewpoint which doesn't see life as entirely white or entirely black is one of the best helps you can have.

Grieve in your own time. Don't pay any attention to people who encourage you to snap out of it or get back to normal. You'll know when your grieving is done, because you'll feel it's worked its way out of your system and you'll feel like starting afresh, so if you really want to have a good cry or if you want to have a conversation with your dead partner, go ahead.

Once the grieving is over, it is important that you start to think about regaining your identity, or even possibly building a new one. Resist the temptation to live in the past and to continue living through your dead partner. You should try to become **your own person** and to assert your **own identity**. Start shaping your life as it suits you by doing things that you are really interested in rather than continuing a past way of life.

Don't make any big decisions quickly, rather let yourself grow into them gradually. Some decisions may be quite hard to take at first. If left for several months or a year, a problem which seemed insoluble will have a very ready solution. Trust your own judgement and go on your own gut feeling which has always served you well throughout your life. Don't choose this moment to start doubting yourself without reason.

keep control

Don't neglect your finances. This isn't the time to let them to get out of control and find yourself in debt. So keep an eye on your money, budget your expenses, and keep tabs on all your sources of income.

Though it seems unlikely while you're grieving, life does go on and you will live again and be happy again. Meanwhile, take good care of yourself. Treat yourself, give yourself a vacation, see family and friends. Whatever you do, try to stay mobile, and don't retire to your bed or sofa.

DRUGS of a lifetime

Statins
HRT
Selegiline (for Alzheimer's)
Retinoic acid (for the skin)
Aspirin

FOODS of a lifetime

Fatty fish
Fresh food
All fruits and vegetables
Eat vegetables rather than meat
Oatmeal every morning
Carrots, tomatoes, and a few nuts and seeds every day
Dark-colored fruit and vegetables – dark red or black fruit and dark green leaves

SUPPLEMENTS of a lifetime

Vitamin E
Cod liver oil
Selenium
Gingko biloba (but only this form: EG6761)
Folic acid

HABITS of a lifetime

Don't smoke
No salt
No sugar
Eat vegetables rather than meat
A glass of young red wine every day
Drink tea
Eat slowly
Putter around all the time
Keep learning
Avoid undue stress
Keep in touch with friends

INDEX

ACKNOWLEDGEMENTS

Miriam Stoppard would like to thank:

For their support and interest I'd like to thank Corinne Roberts, Lynne Brown, Rosamund Saunders, Peter Jones, and Michelle Crane. I should add that for their diligence, patience, and intelligence I'm indebted to Jinny Johnson, Kathryn Gammon, and Daniel Park.

Dorling Kindersley would like to thank the following for their help in the making of this book:

Specially commissioned photography: Slater King, Justin Leighton, and Guy Drayton
MODELS: Annie Godwin, Lawrence Jackson, Farah Diggins, Trevor Diggins; John Fisher, Tom Tsuchihashi, and members of the Mortlake Anglian and Alpha Boat Club; Lynne O'Neill, Michael O'Neill, Isabella Baker, Ted Kinsey; Sheila Tait, Peter Taylor; Angela Cameron, Kimberley Thomas; Rena Nicholaou, Maya Slater, Nicholas Slater; Elaine Banham, Greg Sherriff.
MAKEUP: Anne Marie Simak; Toko.
PROPS, LOCATIONS, AND PROFESSIONAL ADVICE: Gossypium (www.gossypium.co.uk) organic, fair-trade yogawear; Toast (www.toastbypost.co.uk) futon-style yoga mats; Agoy (www.agoy.co.uk) yoga mats ; Bodum Shop, Neal Street, London; The Filofax Centre, Conduit Street, London; Totally Fitness (www.totallyfitness.com) exercise bike; YHA/Karrimor Adventure Shop, Southampton Street, London; Natural Living (www.Starlight-tables.com); Mortlake Anglian and Alpha Boat Club and Blackheath Tennis Club for providing locations; Rena Nicholau for yoga instruction.

Editorial acknowledgements: KFA National Trainers for their assistance in developing the exercises shown in this book. Contact: KFA (Keep Fit Association), Astra House, Suite 1.05, Arklow Road, London SE14 6EB Telephone: 0208 692 9566. Email: kfa@keepfit.org.uk. Website: http://www.keepfit.org.uk; Dr. Laurence Errington for compiling the index; Constance Novis for proofreading.
References: Carper, Jean *Stop Aging Now: the ultimate plan for staying young and reversing the aging process.* HarperCollins, 1995
Le Fanu, James *How to Live to 90.* Constable and Robinson, 2000
Perricone, Nicholas *The Wrinkle Cure* Vermillion, 2001.
Charts on pages 185–89 are based on information from the following publication:
Ernst E. (ed) *The Desktop Guide to Complementary and Alternative Medicine: an evidence-based approach.* London: Mosby (Harcourt Publishers Ltd), 2001.

The publisher would like to thank the following for their kind permission to reproduce their photographs:

(Abbreviations key: t=top, b=bottom, r=right, l=left, c=center)

1: Getty Images/Imagebank/Anne-Marie Weber; 3: Masterfile UK/Kevin Dodge; 10: Science Photo Library/Chris Knapton (l); 12: alamy.com/David Young-Wolff (tr); 14: Getty Images/Stone/Kellie Walsh; 17: Masterfile UK/Kevin Dodge; 20: Getty Images/Image Bank/Rob van Petten; 26: Powerstock/Superstock (cl); 29: Getty Images/Image Bank/David Epperson; 38: alamy.com/Linda Burgess (c), Getty Images/Taxi/Nick Dolding (cr); 43: Getty Images/Stone /Joe McBride; 44: Corbis/Michael Keller; 45: Getty Images/Stone/ Gerard Loucel (tr); 50: Zefa/Benelux; 65: Getty Images/ Image Bank/Rita Maas (bl); 74: Getty Images/Image Bank/Ghislain and Marie David de Lossy (c), Image Bank/Yellow Dog Production (tr), Getty Images/ Photodisc Collection (tc); 77: Corbis/Ronnie Kaufman; 79: Getty Images/Stone/Alan Thornton; 85: Getty Images/Image Bank/Mike Brinson (tr); 95: Science Photo Library/Dr. P. Marazzi; 104: Getty Images/Taxi/Jerome Tisne; 107: Corbis/George Shelley; 108: Science Photo Library/TEK Image; 113: Getty Images/Allsport Concepts/Ancil Nance; 125: Powerstock/Superstock; 127: Getty Images/Stone/Tom Stock; 143: Getty Images/Taxi/Deborah Jaffe; 144: Getty Images/Taxi/ Deborah Jaffe (t); 149: Science Photo Library/TEK Image; 151: Getty Images/The Image Bank/Britt Erlanson; 160: Getty Images/ Photographer's Choice/Robin MacDougall; 168: Corbis/ Jose Luis Pelaez, Inc (cr); Zefa/Benelux (c); 170: Science Photo Library/Alan Sirulnikoff; 179: Science Photo Library/Gusto; 181: Corbis/Claudia Kunin; 182: Getty Images/The Image Bank/Yellow Dog Productions; 190: Getty Images/Stone/ Lisa Peardon; 207: Science Photo Library/ Dr. Robin Williams (tl), (tr); 209: Photonica/ Christopher Thomas; 215: Getty Images/Stone/Ian O'Leary; 224: ImageState/Pictor/StockImage (cr); 231: Getty Images/Stone/Bruce Ayres; 238: ImageState/Pictor/AGE Fotostock; 242: ImageState/Pictor/ AGE Fotostock; 245: Corbis/Larry Williams; 250: Getty Images/Stone/ Bruce Ayres (br), Getty Images/ Stone/Christopher Bissell (cr), Getty Images/Stone/Steven Rothfeld (c); 261: Corbis/Chuck Savage; 262: Getty Images/Stone/Zigy Kaluzny; 266: Getty Images/Taxi/ Andre Lichtenberg; 268: Corbis/ Robert Wagoner; 271: Getty Images/ Taxi/ Antony Nagelmann; 273: Zefa/ Creasource; 277: Masterfile UK/Kevin Dodge; 279: Getty Images/Stone/David Hanover; 283: Getty Images/Stone/Donna Day.

All other images © Dorling Kindersley. For further information see: www.dkimages.com